Rhinosinusitis

Erica R. Thaler · David W. Kennedy

Editors

Rhinosinusitis

A Guide for Diagnosis and Management

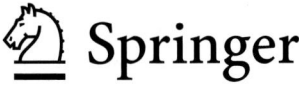 Springer

Editors

Erica R. Thaler, MD
Associate Professor
Department of Otorhinolaryngology-Head
   and Neck Surgery
University of Pennsylvania
Philadelphia, PA, USA
Erica.Thaler@uphs.upenn.edu

David W. Kennedy, MD
Professor
Department of Otorhinolaryngology-Head
   and Neck Surgery
University of Pennsylvania
Philadelphia, PA, USA
David.Kennedy@uphs.upenn.edu

ǀ

ISBN: 978-0-387-73061-5   e-ISBN: 978-0-387-73062-2
DOI: 10.1007/978-0-387-73062-2

Library of Congress Control Number: 2008935646

Printed on acid-free paper

springer.com

Thank you to all the contributors to this book for their hard work and gracious donation of time; and thank you to my family, who provide the perfect antidote to such an undertaking.

Erica

Preface

Sinusitis and rhinitis are ubiquitous medical problems, comprising a set of conditions most commonly today described together under the term rhinosinusitis, that occupy a significant portion of time in many outpatient care providers' offices, be it pediatrician, family practitioner, internist, primary care provider, or otolaryngologist. Indeed, rhinosinusitis is one of the most common of all health care complaints, reported to be present chronically in fully 14% of the American population. Chronic rhinosinusitis has also been shown to have a much greater impact on overall quality of life than previously recognized and is indeed a potentially debilitating disorder. Because rhinosinusitis is managed by such a wide variety of practitioners, there is a lack of cohesiveness in patient care and much contradictory literature about the best approach to patient management. Additionally, the chronic form of rhinosinusitis can be an enormously difficult problem to manage, with under-treatment and over-treatment of patients both equally possible to lead to poor outcomes.

This book aims to provide a unifying guide to the diagnosis and management of this complex health care problem. It covers the entire width and breadth of rhinosinusitis, from etiology and pathophysiology, to diagnosis, to medical and surgical management, both pediatric and adult. In recognition of the ever increasing role of alternative medicine in our health care management, there is a special chapter devoted to this topic. Systemic contributions to the disease process are discussed, and there is a chapter on what is frequently referred to as the unified airway, the special relationship between rhinosinusitis and pulmonary pathology, particularly asthma.

We hope this book provides practitioners with a useful tool in the care of patients with rhinosinusitis. The assembled authors represent true experts in the condition, with a wealth of clinical and basic science experience to bring to bear on their writings.

Erica R. Thaler, M.D.
David W. Kennedy, M.D.

Contents

Contributors

Megan Abbott, MSN, CRNP
Department of Otorhinolaryngology, University of Pennsylvania,
Philadelphia, PA, USA

Walleed Abuzaid, BSc (Hons), MBBS (Dist)
Department of Otorhinolaryngology – Head and Neck Surgery, University
of Pennsylvania, Philadelphia, PA, USA

Marcelo B. Antunes, MD
Department of Otorhinolaryngology – Head and Neck Surgery, University
of Pennsylvania, Philadelphia, PA, USA

Benjamin S. Bleier, MD
Department of Otorhinolaryngology – Head and Neck Surgery, University
of Pennsylvania, Philadelphia, PA, USA

Rakesh K. Chandra, MD
Assistant Professor, Department of Otolaryngology – Head and Neck Surgery,
Northwestern University Feinberg School of Medicine, Chicago, IL, USA

Alexander G. Chiu, MD
Assistant Professor, Department of Otorhinolaryngology, University of
Pennsylvania, Philadelphia, PA, USA

Noam A. Cohen, MD, PhD
Assistant Professor, Department of Otorhinolaryngology – Head and Neck Surgery,
University of Pennsylvania, Philadelphia, PA, USA

Lisa Elden, MS, MD
Assistant Professor, Department of Otorhinolaryngology, Head and Neck Surgery,
University of Pennsylvania School of Medicine, The Children's Hospital of
Philadelphia, Philadelphia, PA, USA

Jean Anderson Eloy, MD
Rhinology and Skull Base Surgery Fellow, Department of Otolaryngology, Head
and Neck Surgery, University of Miami – Jackson Memorial Hospital, Miami,
FL, USA

Satish Govindaraj, MD
Department of Otolaryngology, Head and Neck Surgery, Mount Sinai School
of Medicine, New York, NY, USA

Joel Guss, MD
Department of Otorhinolaryngology, Head and Neck Surgery, University
of Pennsylvania, Philadelphia, PA, USA

Richard J. Harvey, BSc (med) MBBS FRACS
Department of Otolaryngology, Medical University of South Carolina, Charleston,
SC, USA

Christina F. Herrera, MSN, CRNP
Department of Otorhinolaryngology, Hospital of the University of Pennsylvania,
Philadelphia, PA, USA

Rohit K. Katial, MD
Associate Professor of Medicine, Department of Medicine, Division of Allergy
and Immunology, National Jewish Medical and Research Center, Denver, CO, USA

David W. Kennedy, MD
Professor, Department of Otorhinolaryngology – Head and Neck Surgery,
University of Pennsylvania Medical Center, Philadelphia, PA, USA

Todd T. Kingdom, MD
Department of Otolaryngology, University of Colorado Health Sciences Center,
Aurora, CO, USA

Karen A. Kölln, MD
Chief, Rhinology, Allergy and Sinus Surgery, Department of Otorhinolaryngology –
Head and Neck Surgery, University of North Carolina at Chapel Hill, Chapel Hill,
NC, USA

John H. Krouse, MD, PhD
Professor and Vice Chair, Director of Rhinology and Allergy, Department
of Otolaryngology, Wayne State University, Detroit, MI, USA

Laurie A. Loevner, MD
Professor, Departments of Radiology and Otorhinolaryngology – Head and Neck
Surgery, University of Pennsylvania, Philadelphia, PA, USA

Roxanne S. Leung, MD
Allergy and Immunology Fellow, Department of Medicine, Division of Allergy
and Immunology, National Jewish Medical and Research Center, Denver, CO, USA

Richard R. Orlandi, MD
Associate Professor, Division of Otolaryngology – Head and Neck Surgery,
University of Utah School of Medicine, Salt Lake City, UT, USA

James N. Palmer, MD
Department of Otorhinolaryngology – Head and Neck Surgery, University of
Pennsylvania Health System, Philadelphia, PA, USA

Christine Reger, MSN, CRNP
Department of Otorhinolaryngology, University of Pennsylvania, Philadelphia,
PA, USA

Rodney J. Schlosser, MD
Department of Otolaryngology, Medical University of South Carolina, Charleston,
SC, USA

Brent A. Senior, MD
Department of Otorhinolaryngology – Head and Neck Surgery, University of North
Carolina at Chapel Hill, Chapel Hill, NC, USA

Edwin Tamashiro, MD
Affiliated Otorhinolaryngologist, Faculty of Medicine of Ribeirão Preto,
Department of Ophthalmology, Otorhinolaryngology, Head and Neck Surgery,
University of São Paulo, São Paulo, Brazil

Erica R. Thaler, MD
Department of Otorhinolaryngology – Head and Neck Surgery, University of
Pennsylvania, Philadelphia, PA, USA

Lawrence W. C. Tom, MD
Associate Professor, Department of Otorhinolaryngology, Head and Neck Surgery,
University of Pennsylvania School of Medicine, The Children's Hospital
of Philadelphia, Philadelphia, PA, USA

Kevin C. Welch, MD
Department of Otorhinolaryngology – Head and Neck Surgery, University of
Pennsylvania Health System, Philadelphia, PA, 19104, USA

Chapter 1
Etiology and Impact of Rhinosinusitis

Walleed Abuzaid and Erica R. Thaler

Definition of Rhinosinusitis

Rhinosinusitis is a broad diagnostic label that encompasses a spectrum of disorders involving concurrent inflammation of the mucosa of the nose and paranasal sinuses [1,2]. The wide range of clinical signs and symptoms associated with rhinosinusitis has complicated the establishment of a working clinical definition. Furthermore, patients with rhinosinusitis may present to a variety of practitioners including internists, family care physicians, pediatricians, allergists, pulmonologists, and otolaryngologists. A standardized definition of rhinosinusitis has been sought to facilitate communication among physicians and to promote uniform reporting of the disease. Such a definition facilitates further elucidation of the pathophysiology of sinusitis, the development of a clinical staging system, and the introduction of new treatments based on robust clinical data [3].

Past attempts at defining rhinosinusitis have been largely symptom based. Approximately 87% of visits for the diagnosis and management of rhinosinusitis are in the primary care setting where nasal endoscopy and computed tomography (CT) imaging are not routinely used for diagnosis. Consequently, a variety of national and international consensus meetings have developed symptom-based definitions for the initial diagnosis of rhinosinusitis [3–5]. For example, in 1997, the Task Force for Rhinosinusitis of the American Academy of Otolaryngology identified a range of major and minor factors (Table 1.1), as well as the duration of symptoms, to diagnose and classify rhinosinusitis (Table 1.2) [3]. Nasal endoscopy and imaging modalities such as CT were not considered necessary to confirm the diagnosis. This scheme and other similar symptom-based diagnostic systems conform to standard practice in the primary care setting [5].

Recent studies have demonstrated that symptom-based definitions for rhinosinusitis are imperfect in predicting whether a patient truly has disease. Approximately 73% of chronic rhinosinusitis patients diagnosed using a symptom-based

E.R. Thaler
Department of Otorhinolaryngology – Head and Neck Surgery, University of Pennsylvania, Philadelphia, PA, USA
e-mail: Erica.Thaler@uphs.upenn.edu

E.R. Thaler, D.W. Kennedy (eds.), *Rhinosinusitis*, DOI: 10.1007/978-0-387-73062-2_1,
© Springer Science+Business Media, LLC 2008

Table 1.1 Factors associated with adult rhinosinusitis as identified by the Task Force on Rhinosinusitis

MAJOR FACTORS	Facial pain/pressure (only suggestive of rhinosinusitis in presence of another major symptom) Facial congestion/fullness Nasal obstruction/blockage Nasal discharge/purulence/discolored postnasal drainage Hyposmia/anosmia Purulence in nasal cavity on examination Fever (suggestive of acute rhinosinusitis only in presence of another major symptom)
MINOR FACTORS	Headache Fever (all nonacute) Halitosis Fatigue Dental pain Cough Ear pain/pressure/fullness

Source: Reprinted from Lanza DC, Kennedy DW. Adult rhinosinusitis defined. Otolaryngol Head Neck Surg 1997;117:S1–S7 by kind permission of Elsevier [3].

scheme had no supporting objective endoscopic or CT findings to confirm the diagnosis [6]. There is a significant lack of correlation between symptom score and disease presence as diagnosed on CT, with several of the aforementioned "major" factors not elicited in patients with a positive CT [7,8]. Overall, more than half the patients who meet the criteria for the diagnosis of rhinosinusitis will not have evidence of disease on CT scans [7]. Symptom-based diagnostic instruments have good sensitivity but extremely poor specificity for detecting a positive CT scan [9,10]. This limitation has called into question the reliability of the diagnostic criteria used in symptom-based definitions of rhinosinusitis.

There is increasing recognition that, at present, the accurate diagnosis of rhinosinusitis is reliant on a combination of symptoms and objective investigations. The recent European Position Paper on Rhinosinusitis recommends that a diagnosis of rhinosinusitis should be based on the following[1]:

• Two or more symptoms, one of which should be either nasal blockage/ obstruction/congestion or nasal discharge:

  ○ ± Facial pain/pressure
  ○ ± Reduction or loss of smell

• Additionally, there should be objective signs of disease on nasal endoscopy and/or paranasal CT scan.

  ○ Endoscopic signs of polyps; and/or mucopurulent discharge primarily from the middle meatus; and/or edema/mucosal obstruction primarily in the middle meatus
  ○ CT evidence of mucosal changes within the ostiomeatal complex and/or sinuses

Table 1.2 Classification of adult rhinosinusitis as outlined by the Task Force on Rhinosinusitis

Classification	Duration	Strong history	Include in differential	Special notes
Acute	≤4 weeks	≥2 major factors; 1 major and 2 minor factors; or nasal purulence on examination	1 major factor; or ≥2 minor factors	Fever or facial pain is not suggestive in the absence of other nasal signs/symptoms. Consider acute bacterial rhinosinusitis if symptoms worsen after 5 days, if symptoms persist >10 days, or in presence of symptoms out of proportion to those typically associated with viral infection
Subacute	4–12 weeks	Same as chronic	Same as chronic	Complete resolution after effective medical therapy
Recurrent acute	≥4 episodes/year with each episode lasting ≥7 to 10 days and absence of intervening signs/symptoms of chronic rhinosinusitis	Same as acute	–	–
Chronic	≥12 weeks	≥2 major factors; 1 major and 2 minor factors; or nasal purulence on examination	1 major factor; or ≥2 minor factors	Facial pain is not suggestive in the absence of other nasal signs/symptoms
Acute exacerbations of chronic	Sudden worsening of chronic rhinosinusitis with return to baseline after treatment			

Source: Reprinted from Lanza DC, Kennedy DW. Adult rhinosinusitis defined. Otolaryngol Head Neck Surg 1997;117:S1–S7 by kind permission of Elsevier [3].

Epidemiology of Rhinosinusitis

The true incidence and prevalence of rhinosinusitis is unknown as many cases do not present to a medical practitioner [11]. Estimates of the prevalence of acute rhinosinusitis are largely based on CT evidence demonstrating that 90% of patients with colds have concurrent viral or bacterial rhinosinusitis [12]. Each year, children and adults average between six and eight and two to three upper respiratory tract infections, respectively. Therefore, more than 1 billion cases of acute rhinosinusitis occur annually [2]. The difficulty in establishing a standardized definition of rhinosinusitis and resulting diagnostic challenge has made it difficult to estimate the prevalence of chronic rhinosinusitis. Nonetheless, recent data indicate that rhinosinusitis, in all its forms, is one of the most prevalent health care problems in the United States [2]. Among a representative sample of 100,000 U.S. adults who participated in the 2005 National Health Survey, 13.4% of respondents indicated a diagnosis of rhinosinusitis in the preceding year [13]. Based on census data, this percentage translates to approximately 32 million Americans medically diagnosed with rhinosinusitis annually [14].

Etiology of Rhinosinusitis

Multiple factors have been implicated in the development of rhinosinusitis (Table 1.3).

Environmental Factors

Microbial Pathogens in Rhinosinusitis

Acute bacterial rhinosinusitis complicates approximately 0.5% of adult and 5% pediatric cases of viral upper respiratory tract infections [15–17]. The mucosal lining and immune defenses of the nose and paranasal sinuses can be damaged by viral infection (common cold) predisposing to bacterial superinfection, the most important cause of acute rhinosinusitis [1]. The species most commonly implicated

Table 1.3 Potential etiologic factors in the pathogenesis of rhinosinusitis

ENVIRONMENTAL FACTORS	Infectious microbial pathogens
	Allergy/atopy/asthma
	Air pollution
ANATOMIC FACTORS	Concha bullosa
	Septal deviation
	Mucociliary impairment
SYSTEMIC DISEASE	Genetic disorders
	Immunodeficiency states
	Endocrine disorders
	Laryngopharyngeal reflux

(a)   (b)

Microbial pathogens in adult acute bacterial rhinosinusitis   **Microbial pathogens in pediatric acute bacterial rhinosinusitis**

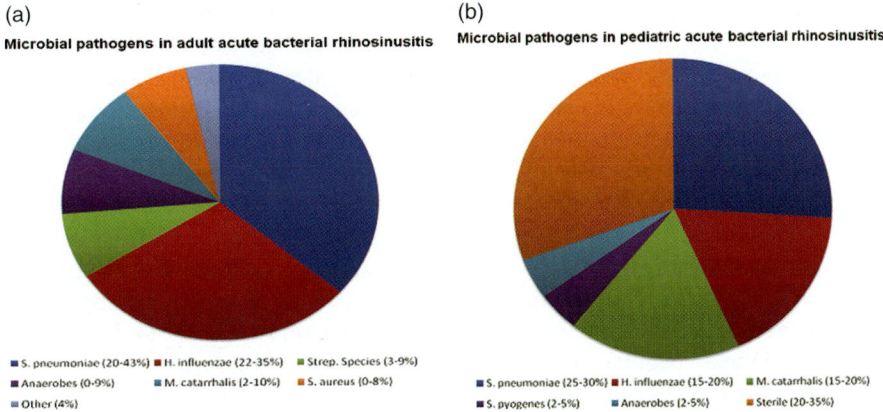

S. pneumoniae (20-43%)   H. influenzae (22-35%)   Strep. Species (3-9%)
Anaerobes (0-9%)   M. catarrhalis (2-10%)   S. aureus (0-8%)
Other (4%)

S. pneumoniae (25-30%)   H. influenzae (15-20%)   M. catarrhalis (15-20%)
S. pyogenes (2-5%)   Anaerobes (2-5%)   Sterile (20-35%)

Fig. 1.1 Sinus culture isolates in (**a**) adult and (**b**) pediatric acute bacterial rhinosinusitis. *S. pneumoniae, Streptococcus pneumoniae; H. influenzae, Haemophilus influenzae; Strep. species, Streptococcus species; M. catarrhalis, Moraxella catarrhalis; S. aureus, Staphylococcus aureus; S. pyogenes, Streptococcus pyogenes.* (Reprinted from Anon JB, Jacobs MR, Poole MD, et al. Antimicrobial treatment guidelines for acute bacterial rhinosinusitis. Otolaryngol Head Neck Surg 2004;130:1–45 by kind permission of Elsevier [23].)

in acute rhinosinusitis are *Streptococcus pneumoniae, Haemophilus influenzae,* and *Moraxella catarrhalis* [18–22] (Fig. 1.1a,b). This is not surprising because these pathogens reside in the nasopharynx and are, therefore, ideally situated to produce secondary overgrowth following viral infection. Generally, the bacteria that induce acute rhinosinusitis in children are the same as those found in acute otitis media [22]. A smaller proportion of cases are attributed to other *Streptococcus* species, *Staphylococcus aureus,* and anaerobic species [18,20,23] (Fig. 1.1a,b). Aerobic gram-negative rods, particularly *Pseudomonas aeruginosa,* are common in acute rhinosinusitis of nosocomial origin, immunocompromised individuals, and those with cystic fibrosis. Fungal sinusitis is most common in the immunocompromised and diabetic populations [22].

Antibiotics are often prescribed empirically for acute rhinosinusitis, although the cause is often viral. Consequently, the resistance of respiratory pathogens to antibiotics has been increasing yearly [1,23–25]. The penicillin resistance rate in *S. pneumoniae* has increased dramatically from 4% in the 1980s to 37% in 1997. The prevalence of β-lactamase producing penicillin-resistant *H. influenzae* and *M. catarrhalis* has increased over the past several decades to around 40% and 98%, respectively, in the United States [26]. High levels of resistance to first-line antibiotics including penicillin, erythromycin, co-trimoxazole, and older fluoroquinolones have been demonstrated in sinus cultures from patients with acute rhinosinusitis [26]. The widespread antimicrobial resistance among pathogens that cause rhinosinusitis allows for the persistence of infection and the development of chronic rhinosinusitis.

It has been postulated that chronic rhinosinusitis evolves from acute rhinosinusitis, but this has never been definitively proven [1]. The role of bacteria in the development of chronic rhinosinusitis is controversial. Investigators have isolated both aerobic and anaerobic species from the diseased side and the contralateral, nondiseased side of patients with chronic rhinosinusitis, suggesting that colonization does not directly translate to disease [27]. Several studies have consistently isolated a variety of microbial pathogens from the sinuses of chronic rhinosinusitis patients. The majority of these isolates (86%) are aerobic, although anaerobes are isolated in a minority (8%) of patients. There are several distinct differences in the microbiology of chronic rhinosinusitis when compared to acute disease. The most commonly isolated organisms in chronic rhinosinusitis are *Staphylococcus aureus* (36%) and coagulase-negative *Staphylococcus* (20%). *Streptococcus pneumoniae* (9%) is found far less commonly than in acute bacterial rhinosinusitis [28]. Similarly, *Haemophilus influenzae and Moraxella catarrhalis* do not appear to be major pathogens in chronic rhinosinusitis [2]. Aerobic organisms may be gradually replaced by anaerobes as disease duration lengthens. This is potentially mediated by antimicrobial agents that select for resistant microbes, as well as changes in the local sinonasal environment including reduced oxygen tension and pH. Polymicrobial colonization is also a common feature of chronic rhinosinusitis [1].

Fungi have also been isolated from the sinus cavities of rhinosinusitis patients, but no evidence has been demonstrated for causality. Although fungal proliferation and invasion by species such as *Mucor, Alternaria, Candida, Curvularia, Bipolaris, Sporothrix schenckii,* and *Pseudallescheria boydii* can occur in immunocompromised patients, the inflammatory response cascade triggered by fungi is likely to be a more important factor in the etiology of chronic rhinosinusitis [2]. Consequently, desensitization to fungal antigens has proven to be useful in symptom control among certain patients with rhinosinusitis [2]. However, the use of antifungal agents has inconsistent efficacy in patients with chronic rhinosinusitis [1].

Allergy

The suggested association between atopy and rhinosinusitis is based upon the concept that the mucosa of the nasal airway is in a continuum with that of the paranasal sinuses. Mucosal swelling and edema in the region of the ostiomeatal complex may facilitate obstruction of the sinus ostia, reducing ventilation and permitting negative pressure to develop in the sinus cavities. Oxygen tension within the sinuses is reduced, disrupting ciliary function and thereby impairing mucus drainage; this increases the risk of secondary infection [1,29]. Repeated exposure to allergens further reduces the response threshold of the mucosa to other allergens, pollutants, and irritants, increasing edema and effectively "priming" the mucosa for secondary bacterial infection [29].

There is some evidence for a relationship between allergies and rhinosinusitis. Around 50% to 84% of patients with chronic or recurrent rhinosinusitis had at least one positive skin prick test [30,31]. Sixty percent of the allergic cohort demonstrated significant allergic sensitivity, with 52% positive for multiple allergen sensitivities, particularly house dust mites [31]. However, the prevalence of allergies in many of these studies may be optimistic because cases were often recruited from allergy or otolaryngology clinics, creating a selection bias [1]. Interestingly, although multiple studies report a higher incidence of positive CT findings in rhinosinusitis patients with the highest degree of sensitivity, other studies indicate that the severity of the allergy does not necessarily correlate with disease severity as assessed on CT scan [31–33]. This suggests that, although allergies may predispose to rhinosinusitis, the eventual development of symptoms is a multifactorial process [31]. Indeed, epidemiologic studies investigating chronic rhinosinusitis reveal no increase in the incidence of disease during pollen season in pollen-sensitized patients, refuting a causative link between allergy and chronic rhinosinusitis [34].

In studies of acute rhinosinusitis, 25% of patients had evidence of allergy after skin testing, nasal smears, and allergy questionnaire versus an allergy prevalence of 16.5% among control cases. Despite this difference, allergic patients did not suffer more acute rhinosinusitis episodes than their nonallergic counterparts, nor did they have significantly different bacteriological or radiologic findings [30].

Overall, the role of allergy in rhinosinusitis remains unclear, which will likely continue to be uncertain until a well-designed prospective study investigating the relationship between allergy and infective rhinosinusitis is conducted. Nevertheless, from a practical standpoint, it is evident that failure to adequately control allergic symptoms reduces the likelihood of successful pharmacologic and surgical intervention [1].

Asthma

Initial evidence for a link between lower and upper respiratory tract disease comes from the observation that asthma and rhinosinusitis coexist in patients at a higher frequency than either condition alone in the general population [35]. The prevalence of asthma in patients with allergic rhinitis is approximately 17% to 38%, considerably higher than the 5% to 8% prevalence of asthma in the general population. The inverse association also holds true, with 60% to 80% of patients with asthma suffering from rhinosinusitis compared to only 10% to 20% of the general population [35,36]. Chronic rhinosinusitis is associated with a 20% prevalence of asthma, approximately fourfold higher than in the general population [37]. One-fifth of patients with chronic rhinosinusitis have coexisting polyposis and, in this subset, the prevalence of asthma is 50% [38]. Furthermore, patients with severe asthma were observed to have more significant sinus disease on CT scan than those with mild asthma [39]. However, these results must be viewed critically since sinus abnormalities detected on imaging in sensitized patients may be a consequence of the underlying allergic state rather than sinus disease [1]. In addition, the true incidence of atopy in the rhinosinusitis population may be lower than estimated in many of these studies. For example, one study indicated that 39% of patients with chronic rhinosinusitis had asthma as well as eosinophilia and elevated IgE, but only 25% of patients had true markers of atopy [40]. Although there does appear to be significant evidence that asthma and rhinosinusitis are associated, the nature of this relationship and the implications for management have yet to be elucidated.

Pollution

Multiple studies have explored the association between outdoor air pollution and chronic rhinosinusitis. An epidemiologic study from Brazil demonstrated that chronic exposure to urban air pollution was associated with a higher prevalence of rhinosinusitis and upper respiratory tract infections than was diagnosed in children from a rural, pollution-free environment. This effect was correlated with an observed increase in ultrastructural damage to the cilia of the airway epithelium in rats exposed to similar levels of urban pollution [41]. In contrast, a report from Korea found that there was no significant difference in the prevalence of chronic rhinosinusitis between rural and urban areas [42]. Recently, an investigation into the association between air pollution and chronic rhinosinusitis that was conducted in Germany revealed that the spatial distribution of chronic rhinosinusitis correlated with areas in which air pollution exceeded a relatively low threshold [43]. Cigarette smoking has also been associated with a higher prevalence of rhinosinusitis, although further studies have failed to confirm this finding [1]. Environmental factors undoubtedly play a role in the pathophysiology of rhinosinusitis, but confirmatory in vitro histopathological evidence remains scarce.

Anatomic Factors

Mucociliary Impairment

Intact ciliary function is a key defense mechanism against infection of the paranasal sinus and nasal mucosa. Mucociliary flow is compromised by viral rhinosinusitis, which produces increasing ciliary damage during the first week of infection. Regeneration of ciliary function does occur, but initially consists of short and immature cilia that are not as efficient in maintaining mucociliary flow. Consequently, the risk of bacterial superinfection is increased, which, in turn, results in further loss of cilia and compounds the ongoing infection [1,44,45]. As a result, a secondary ciliary dyskinesia develops as a result of chronic rhinosinusitis, permitting persistence of infection. The importance of mucociliary clearance is highlighted in primary ciliary dyskinesia, Kartagener's syndrome, in patients who frequently present with recurrent and chronic rhinosinusitis. Similarly, patients with cystic fibrosis produce viscous mucous secretions that directly impair ciliary function, predisposing to chronic rhinosinusitis [1].

Anatomic Variations

Anatomic variations of the lateral nasal wall and nasal septum have long been implicated in the etiology of chronic rhinosinusitis. These assertions are based on the concept that certain anatomic features can disturb nasal physiology by impairing mucous flow and, hence, predisposing to infection [1,46]. For example, nasal deviation can potentially force the middle turbinate laterally, narrowing the middle meatus and compromising airflow and mucous outflow from the paranasal sinuses. This problem could be compounded by a concha bullosa, which further narrows the middle meatus [46]. Obstruction of the associated ostiomeatal complex can lead to ethmoidal and maxillary sinus disease [47].

Considering the relative preponderance of anatomic variation in nasal structures (64.9%–86%), the relationship between anatomy and rhinosinusitis could be highly relevant [48]. Concha bullosa is detected in 13.2% to 50% of healthy individuals and in 33.8% to 72.6% of cases with symptoms of rhinosinusitis [46]. Although there have been reports linking this anatomic variant to rhinosinusitis, there is also evidence that there is no significant difference in the incidence of concha bullosa between healthy and diseased individuals [49]. Another study demonstrated that rhinosinusitis often occurred on the opposite side to the concha bullosa, further arguing against a causal role for this anatomic variant in the disease process [46]. Septal deviation of greater than 3 mm from the midline has been correlated with chronic rhinosinusitis in some studies [50,51]. This finding has also been refuted in the literature [42,52]. The lack of a significant correlation between any anatomic variant as detected on CT and rhinosinusitis has been demonstrated repeatedly [1,48,53]. In the absence of a study that definitively demonstrates obstruction of the ostiomeatal complex by an anatomic variant, a causal role for paranasal anatomy in rhinosinusitis cannot be assumed.

Systemic Disorders and Rhinosinusitis

Immunodeficiency

Immunocompromised states have been associated with an increased risk of rhinosinusitis and, as a result, immunological testing is a critical component of the diagnostic workup of chronic or recurrent rhinosinusitis [1]. Low levels of immunoglobulin (Ig) G, A, and M have been found in 17.9%, 16.7%, and 5.1%, respectively, of patients with refractory rhinosinusitis. Approximately 10% of these cases are a result of common variable immunodeficiency, and a selective IgA deficiency was diagnosed in 6% of cases. Forty percent of the study cohort was anergic, and subsequent assessment of T-lymphocyte function revealed that 54.8% of cases showed an abnormal proliferation response to recall antigens [54]. Ataxia telangiectasia and X-linked agammaglobulinemia have also been associated with rhinosinusitis [1].

With the increasing incidence of acquired immunodeficiency syndrome (AIDS), several investigators have studied the relationship between human immunodeficiency virus (HIV) infection and the risk of rhinosinusitis. The development of suppressed humoral and cellular immunity, impaired mucociliary clearance, and increased levels of IgE in AIDS patients could theoretically increase the risk of rhinosinusitis [1]. Interestingly, rhinosinusitis has not been consistently associated with HIV infection, although low CD4 cell counts do appear to predispose to sinus disease [55]. The increased risk of infection and colonization of the sinuses with opportunistic microbes such as *Aspergillus* species and *Pseudomonas aeruginosa* in patients with AIDS may also account for sinonasal symptoms in these individuals [1].

Bone marrow transplantation involves a period of acquired immune deficiency and, in allogeneic transplants, involves significant immunosuppression to facilitate graft success. In one study, all patients receiving an allogeneic bone marrow transplant demonstrated symptoms and signs of rhinosinusitis, and 70.5% were diagnosed with chronic rhinosinusitis despite receiving prophylactic antimicrobial therapy [56]. Common causative organisms include *Pseudomonas aeruginosa*, *Serratia marascens*, and various fungi [1].

Genetic Disorders

As discussed previously, mucociliary impairment is a component of cystic fibrosis and primary ciliary dyskinesia. Cystic fibrosis is an autosomal recessive condition. Due to the high prevalence of the common F508 mutation in the Caucasian population, this diagnosis must always be considered in children presenting with rhinosinusitis and/or nasal polyps. Chronic rhinosinusitis and nasal polyps are found in 25% to 40% of cystic fibrosis patients above the age of 5 years [1].

Laryngopharyngeal Reflux

The role of laryngopharyngeal reflux in the pathophysiology of rhinosinusitis is an area of recent interest. Patients with reflux who undergo pH monitoring often demonstrate intermittent acid reflux as high as the nasopharynx [57]. Children are particularly susceptible, with gastric pepsin often detected in the effusions of secretory otitis media [58,59]. Control of reflux has been associated with an improvement in chronic sinus symptoms in both children and adults [60,61]. In addition to the ciliary impairment resulting from exposure to low pH, the role of sinus exposure to *Helicobacter pylori* during episodes of laryngopharyngeal reflux has also been investigated. A recent study has not demonstrated an etiologic role for this organism in rhinosinusitis [62]. Continued research in this area is needed because proof of causality between laryngopharyngeal reflux and rhinosinusitis could potentially impact the management of a significant number of patients.

Endocrine State

The hormonal changes that occur in pregnancy have been associated with increased nasal congestion in approximately 20% of women during the course of their pregnancy. The precise mechanism behind this observation has yet to be elucidated, but potentially includes the effects of estrogen, progesterone, and human placental growth hormone on the nasal mucosa and underlying vasculature [1]. Nasal congestion may not necessarily predispose to rhinosinusitis. In a prospective study, 61% of pregnant women had nasal congestion during the first trimester, but only 3% were diagnosed with rhinosinusitis. The incidence of rhinosinusitis was comparable in the pregnant cohort relative to controls [63].

Economic Impact of Rhinosinusitis

The economic implications of rhinosinusitis are significant because of high direct medical costs, including the expense of office visits, diagnostic tests, medication, surgical procedures, hospitalization, and the complications of treatment [2]. In 1996, the total direct costs of rhinosinusitis in the United States were estimated to exceed $5.8 billion annually [64]. In that same year, direct medical costs for physician visits that resulted in a diagnosis of rhinosinusitis were conservatively estimated at $3.39 billion, representing an increase of more than $1.1 billion from the 1992 estimate [64,65].

This level of expenditure funds the 18 million or more physician office visits annually within the United States for rhinosinusitis [66]. In 2000, there were approximately 11.6 million physician office visits resulting in a diagnosis of chronic rhinosinusitis and a further 1.2 million visits to hospital outpatient clinics, emergency departments, and walk-in clinics. Additionally, more than half a million ambulatory and inpatient procedures are performed annually for rhinosinusitis [11]. Surgical costs for chronic rhinosinusitis average $6,490 per patient [67]. Analysis of direct medical costs at a single health maintenance organization revealed that patients with a diagnosis of chronic rhinosinusitis made 43% more outpatient and 25% more urgent care visits than the general population. The cost of treating a patient with chronic rhinosinusitis was estimated at $2,609 per patient annually if costs of imaging, hospitalization, and prescriptions are included. The cost of chronic rhinosinusitis care in isolation was estimated at $206 per patient per year, translating to an overall cost of more than $6 billion for chronic rhinosinusitis [68].

Furthermore, there has been a rapid increase in the rate of antibiotic prescriptions for rhinosinusitis. By 2002, rhinosinusitis was responsible for 9% of all antibiotic prescriptions in children and 21% of prescriptions for adults in the United States, making it the fifth most common diagnosis for which antibiotics were prescribed. Approximately, $400 to $600 million is spent annually on antibiotic prescriptions for the treatment of acute rhinosinusitis alone [23]. A significant proportion of this expense results from overtreatment of uncomplicated rhinosinusitis. For example, several reports indicate that primary care physicians prescribe antibiotics for 85% to 98% of patients with suspected rhinosinusitis without necessarily establishing the presence of a bacterial etiology [69–71]. Once a diagnosis of chronic rhinosinusitis is established, expenditure increases even further. Indeed, the annual cost of pharmacologic management for chronic rhinosinusitis has been estimated at $1,220 per patient per year [67]. The transition to newer, and more expensive, antibacterial and antifungal agents, the longer duration of treatment, and the increasing use of systemic antibiotics will further escalate costs in the future [2,23].

The adoption of a standardized definition of rhinosinusitis to ensure appropriate diagnosis and management of this condition by both primary health and specialist medical practitioners will assist in alleviating the economic burden of rhinosinusitis.

Quality-of-Life Impact of Rhinosinusitis

The lifetime prevalence of chronic rhinosinusitis is approximately 15% [1]. Our imperfect ability to diagnose and manage rhinosinusitis and the recalcitrance of illness means that patients may carry the diagnosis with attendant morbidity for many years [72]. Studies have investigated the subjective impact of symptoms on patient well-being, decreased work productivity, decreased enjoyment, and compromised socialization [73]. Several validated quality-of-life assessments are in use clinically including the Sino-nasal Outcome Test (SNOT-20) and Chronic Sinusitis Survey (CSS) [73,74].

Rhinosinusitis has been ranked in the top 10 most costly health conditions to employers in the United States as 85% of patients with chronic rhinosinusitis are of working age (18 to 65 years old). Employers pay $60.17 per employee per annum for rhinosinusitis, and nearly half of this cost was secondary to absenteeism and disability [1,75]. The impact of rhinosinusitis symptomatology on patients is significant. A recent study indicated that nasal obstruction and facial congestion were the most common symptoms, affecting 95% and 85% of chronic rhinosinusitis patients, respectively. These symptoms were also rated as the most debilitating among these patients. Headache and fatigue were the most common and severe minor symptoms [72]. The decreased quality of life resulting from these symptoms, among others, leads to absenteeism and ""presenteeism" or decreased productivity at work. Approximately 12.5 million work days are missed annually secondary to rhinosinusitis. An impressive 58.7 million days are marked by depressed productivity secondary to restricted activity [64]. Compromised quality of life undoubtedly contributes significantly to the staggering economic burden of rhinosinusitis.

In summary, rhinosinusitis is a pervasive medical condition, affecting many among us with adverse impact on quality of life. It is imperative for physicians caring for these patients to understand the many and varied aspects of the disease in its presentation, diagnosis, and treatment.

References

1. Fokkens W, Lund V, Mullol J. European position paper on rhinosinusitis and nasal polyps 2007. Rhinology 2007:1–136.
2. Benninger MS, Ferguson BJ, Hadley JA, et al. Adult chronic rhinosinusitis: definitions, diagnosis, epidemiology, and pathophysiology. Otolaryngol Head Neck Surg 2003;129:S1–S32.
3. Lanza DC, Kennedy DW. Adult rhinosinusitis defined. Otolaryngol Head Neck Surg 1997;117:S1–S7.
4. Kaliner MA, Osguthorpe JD, Fireman P, et al. Sinusitis: bench to bedside. Current findings, future directions. Otolaryngol Head Neck Surg 1997;116:S1–S20.

5. Fokkens W, Lund V, Bachert C, et al. EAACI position paper on rhinosinusitis and nasal polyps executive summary. Allergy 2005;60:583–601.
6. Tahamiler R, Canakcioglu S, Ogreden S, et al. The accuracy of symptom-based definition of chronic rhinosinusitis. Allergy 2007;62:1029–1032.
7. Stankiewicz JA, Chow JM. A diagnostic dilemma for chronic rhinosinusitis: definition accuracy and validity. Am J Rhinol 2002;16:199–202.
8. Stewart MG, Johnson RF. Chronic sinusitis: symptoms versus CT scan findings. Curr Opin Otolaryngol Head Neck Surg 2004;12:27–29.
9. Orlandi RR, Terrell JE. Analysis of the adult chronic rhinosinusitis working definition. Am J Rhinol 2002;16:7–10.
10. Hwang PH, Irwin SB, Griest SE, et al. Radiologic correlates of symptom-based diagnostic criteria for chronic rhinosinusitis. Otolaryngol Head Neck Surg 2003;128:489–496.
11. Anand VK. Epidemiology and economic impact of rhinosinusitis. Ann Otol Rhinol Laryngol 2004;193:3–5.
12. Gwaltney JM Jr, Phillips CD, Miller RD, et al. Computed tomographic study of the common cold. N Engl J Med 1994;330:25–30.
13. Pleis JR, Lethbridge-Cejku M. Summary health statistics for U.S. adults: National Health Interview Survey, 2005. Vital Health Stat 2006:1–153.
14. Annual Estimates of the Population by Selected Age Groups and Sex for the United States: April 1, 2000 to July 1, 2006 (NC-EST2006-02): Population Division, U.S. Census Bureau, 2007.
15. Diaz I, Bamberger DM. Acute sinusitis. Semin Respir infect 1995;10:14–20.
16. Wald ER. Sinusitis in children. N Engl J Med 1992;326:319–323.
17. Wald ER, Guerra N, Byers C. Upper respiratory tract infections in young children: duration of and frequency of complications. Pediatrics 1991;87:129–133.
18. Gwaltney JM Jr. Acute community-acquired sinusitis. Clin Infect Dis 1996;23:1209–1223; quiz 1224–1205.
19. Gwaltney JM Jr, Scheld WM, Sande MA, et al. The microbial etiology and antimicrobial therapy of adults with acute community-acquired sinusitis: a fifteen-year experience at the University of Virginia and review of other selected studies. J Allergy Clin Immunol 1992;90:457–461; discussion 462.
20. Berg O, Carenfelt C, Kronvall G. Bacteriology of maxillary sinusitis in relation to character of inflammation and prior treatment. Scand J Infect Dis 1988;20:511–516.
21. Brook I. Microbiology and management of sinusitis. J Otolaryngol 1996;25:249–256.
22. Brook I. Microbiology and antimicrobial management of sinusitis. J Laryngol Otol 2005;119:251–258.
23. Anon JB, Jacobs MR, Poole MD, et al. Antimicrobial treatment guidelines for acute bacterial rhinosinusitis. Otolaryngol Head Neck Surg 2004;130:1–45.
24. Klossek JM, Chidiac C, Serrano E. Current position of the management of community-acquired acute maxillary sinusitis or rhinosinusitis in France and literature review. Rhinology 2005:4–33.
25. Sande MA, Gwaltney JM. Acute community-acquired bacterial sinusitis: continuing challenges and current management. Clin Infect Dis 2004;39(suppl 3):S151–S158.
26. Huang WH, Fang SY. High prevalence of antibiotic resistance in isolates from the middle meatus of children and adults with acute rhinosinusitis. Am J Rhinol 2004;18:387–391.
27. Bhattacharyya N. Bacterial infection in chronic rhinosinusitis: a controlled paired analysis. Am J Rhinol 2005;19:544–548.
28. Araujo E, Palombini BC, Cantarelli V, et al. Microbiology of middle meatus in chronic rhinosinusitis. Am J Rhinol 2003;17:9–15.
29. Krause HF. Allergy and chronic rhinosinusitis. Otolaryngol Head Neck Surg 2003;128:14–16.
30. Savolainen S. Allergy in patients with acute maxillary sinusitis. Allergy 1989;44:116–122.
31. Emanuel IA, Shah SB. Chronic rhinosinusitis: allergy and sinus computed tomography relationships. Otolaryngol Head Neck Surg 2000;123:687–691.

32. Krouse JH. Computed tomography stage, allergy testing, and quality of life in patients with sinusitis. Otolaryngol Head Neck Surg 2000;123:389–392.
33. Ramadan HH, Fornelli R, Ortiz AO, et al. Correlation of allergy and severity of sinus disease. Am J Rhinol 1999;13:345–347.
34. Karlsson G, Holmberg K. Does allergic rhinitis predispose to sinusitis? Acta Oto-Laryngol 1994;515:26–28; discussion 29.
35. Jani AL, Hamilos DL. Current thinking on the relationship between rhinosinusitis and asthma. J Asthma 2005;42:1–7.
36. Lundback B. Epidemiology of rhinitis and asthma. Clin Exp Allergy 1998;28(suppl 2):3–10.
37. Hamilos DL. Chronic sinusitis. J Allergy Clin Immunol 2000;106:213–227.
38. Settipane GA. Epidemiology of nasal polyps. Allergy Asthma Proc 1996;17:231–236.
39. Bresciani M, Paradis L, Des Roches A, et al. Rhinosinusitis in severe asthma. J Allergy Clin Immunol 2001;107:73–80.
40. Newman LJ, Platts-Mills TA, Phillips CD, et al. Chronic sinusitis. Relationship of computed tomographic findings to allergy, asthma, and eosinophilia. JAMA 1994;271:363–367.
41. Sih T. Correlation between respiratory alterations and respiratory diseases due to urban pollution. Int J Pediatr Otorhinolaryngol 1999;49(suppl 1):S261–S267.
42. Min YG, Jung HW, Kim HS, et al. Prevalence and risk factors of chronic sinusitis in Korea: results of a nationwide survey. Eur Arch Otorhinolaryngol 1996;253:435–439.
43. Wolf C. Urban air pollution and health: an ecological study of chronic rhinosinusitis in Cologne, Germany. Health Place 2002;8:129–139.
44. Pedersen M, Sakakura Y, Winther B, et al. Nasal mucociliary transport, number of ciliated cells, and beating pattern in naturally acquired common colds. Eur J Respir Dis 1983;128 (pt 1):355–365.
45. Hinni ML, McCaffrey TV, Kasperbauer JL. Early mucosal changes in experimental sinusitis. Otolaryngol Head Neck Surg 1992;107:537–548.
46. Aktas D, Kalcioglu MT, Kutlu R, et al. The relationship between the concha bullosa, nasal septal deviation and sinusitis. Rhinology 2003;41:103–106.
47. Cannon CR. Endoscopic management of concha bullosa. Otolaryngol Head Neck Surg 1994;110:449–454.
48. Bolger WE, Butzin CA, Parsons DS. Paranasal sinus bony anatomic variations and mucosal abnormalities: CT analysis for endoscopic sinus surgery. Laryngoscope 1991;101:56–64.
49. Jones NS, Strobl A, Holland I. A study of the CT findings in 100 patients with rhinosinusitis and 100 controls. Clin Otolaryngol Allied Sci 1997;22:47–51.
50. Calhoun KH, Waggenspack GA, Simpson CB, et al. CT evaluation of the paranasal sinuses in symptomatic and asymptomatic populations. Otolaryngol Head Neck Surg 1991;104:480–483.
51. Kayalioglu G, Oyar O, Govsa F. Nasal cavity and paranasal sinus bony variations: a computed tomographic study. Rhinology 2000;38:108–113.
52. Yasan H, Dogru H, Baykal B, et al. What is the relationship between chronic sinus disease and isolated nasal septal deviation? Otolaryngol Head Neck Surg 2005;133:190–193.
53. Holbrook EH, Brown CL, Lyden ER, et al. Lack of significant correlation between rhinosinusitis symptoms and specific regions of sinus computer tomography scans. Am J Rhinol 2005;19:382–387.
54. Chee L, Graham SM, Carothers DG, et al. Immune dysfunction in refractory sinusitis in a tertiary care setting. Laryngoscope 2001;111:233–235.
55. Garcia-Rodriguez JF, Corominas M, Fernandez-Viladrich P, et al. Rhinosinusitis and atopy in patients infected with HIV. Laryngoscope 1999;109:939–944.
56. Savage DG, Taylor P, Blackwell J, et al. Paranasal sinusitis following allogeneic bone marrow transplant. Bone Marrow Transplant 1997;19:55–59.
57. DelGaudio JM. Direct nasopharyngeal reflux of gastric acid is a contributing factor in refractory chronic rhinosinusitis. Laryngoscope 2005;115:946–957.
58. Contencin P, Narcy P. Nasopharyngeal pH monitoring in infants and children with chronic rhinopharyngitis. Int J Pediatr Otorhinolaryngol 1991;22:249–256.

59. Phipps CD, Wood WE, Gibson WS, et al. Gastroesophageal reflux contributing to chronic sinus disease in children: a prospective analysis. Arch Otolaryngol Head Neck Surg 2000;126:831–836.

60. Barbero GJ. Gastroesophageal reflux and upper airway disease. Otolaryngol Clin N Am 1996;29:27–38.

61. Bothwell MR, Parsons DS, Talbot A, et al. Outcome of reflux therapy on pediatric chronic sinusitis. Otolaryngol Head Neck Surg 1999;121:255–262.

62. Dinis PB, Subtil J. *Helicobacter pylori* and laryngopharyngeal reflux in chronic rhinosinusitis. Otolaryngol Head Neck Surg 2006;134:67–72.

63. Sobol SE, Frenkiel S, Nachtigal D, et al. Clinical manifestations of sinonasal pathology during pregnancy. J Otolaryngol 2001;30:24–28.

64. Ray NF, Baraniuk JN, Thamer M, et al. Healthcare expenditures for sinusitis in 1996: contributions of asthma, rhinitis, and other airway disorders. J Allergy Clin Immunol 1999;103: 408–414.

65. Sharp HJ, Denman D, Puumala S, et al. Treatment of acute and chronic rhinosinusitis in the United States, 1999–2002. Arch Otolaryngol Head Neck Surg 2007;133:260–265.

66. Benninger MS, Sedory Holzer SE, Lau J. Diagnosis and treatment of uncomplicated acute bacterial rhinosinusitis: summary of the Agency for Health Care Policy and Research evidence-based report. Otolaryngol Head Neck Surg 2000;122:1–7.

67. Gliklich RE, Metson R. Economic implications of chronic sinusitis. Otolaryngol Head Neck Surg 1998;118:344–349.

68. Murphy MP, Fishman P, Short SO, et al. Health care utilization and cost among adults with chronic rhinosinusitis enrolled in a health maintenance organization. Otolaryngol Head Neck Surg 2002;127:367–376.

69. Gonzales R, Steiner JF, Lum A, et al. Decreasing antibiotic use in ambulatory practice: impact of a multidimensional intervention on the treatment of uncomplicated acute bronchitis in adults. JAMA 1999;281:1512–1519.

70. Gonzales R, Malone DC, Maselli JH, et al. Excessive antibiotic use for acute respiratory infections in the United States. Clin Infect Dis 2001;33:757–762.

71. Dosh SA, Hickner JM, Mainous AG III, et al. Predictors of antibiotic prescribing for nonspecific upper respiratory infections, acute bronchitis, and acute sinusitis. An UPRNet study. Upper Peninsula Research Network. J Fam Pract 2000;49:407–414.

72. Bhattacharyya N. The economic burden and symptom manifestations of chronic rhinosinusitis. Am J Rhinol 2003;17:27–32.

73. Piccirillo JF, Merritt MG Jr, Richards ML. Psychometric and clinimetric validity of the 20-Item Sino-Nasal Outcome Test (SNOT-20). Otolaryngol Head Neck Surg 2002;126:41–47.

74. Gliklich RE, Metson R. Techniques for outcomes research in chronic sinusitis. Laryngoscope 1995;105:387–390.

75. Goetzel RZ, Hawkins K, Ozminkowski RJ, et al. The health and productivity cost burden of the "top 10" physical and mental health conditions affecting six large U.S. employers in 1999. J Occup Environ Med / Am Coll Occup Environ Med 2003;45:5–14.

Chapter 2
Microbiology and Immunology of Rhinosinusitis

Jean Anderson Eloy and Satish Govindaraj

Rhinosinusitis is one of the most common health care problems facing the primary care physician and results in significant heath care costs. With an increasing prevalence and incidence, it is believed that approximately 31 million Americans are affected by this condition annually [1–5]. Rhinosinusitis significantly impacts patients' quality of life and results in marked physical, functional, and emotional impairment. Thus, a good understanding of the pathogenesis, microbiology, and immunology of this illness is needed for accurate diagnosis and proper treatment.

Rhinosinusitis represents a group of disorders characterized by inflammation of the nasal and paranasal sinus mucosa [6]. As such, it is presently thought that rhinosinusitis is initiated with an inflammatory insult (allergic rhinitis exacerbation, viral upper respiratory tract infection, rhinitis medicamentosa, etc.), followed by bacterial or fungal superinfection. Mucociliary clearance is the sinonasal cavity's most powerful protective mechanism through its expeditious removal of offending organisms. Once cleared from the sinonasal cavity, organisms enter the nasopharynx, which is an area devoid of mucociliary clearance, thus resulting in bacterial colonization and the possibility of retrograde sinonasal infection [7]. Bacterial colonization of the nasal vestibule with staphylococcus species (*Staphylococcus epidermidis, Staphylococcus aureus*) is quite common and can affect the quality of sinonasal cultures. Viruses are not considered part of the normal flora of the sinonasal cavity and are considered precursors to bacterial sinusitis. Because specific treatment approaches are crucial for the different types of rhinosinusitis as well as their different pathogens, the microbiology and immunology of rhinosinusitis are now reviewed.

S. Govindaraj
Department of Otolaryngology, Head and Neck Surgery, Mount Sinai School of Medicine, New York, NY, USA

E.R. Thaler, D.W. Kennedy (eds.), *Rhinosinusitis*, DOI: 10.1007/978-0-387-73062-2_2,
© Springer Science+Business Media, LLC 2008

Microbiology

Viral Rhinosinusitis

Viral rhinosinusitis is widespread and is what most people identify as the "common cold." With the exception of herpes simplex and adenoviruses, viruses are not usually part of the normal flora of the nose and paranasal sinuses. Consequently, inoculation of the mucosa of the nose and paranasal sinuses by viruses leads to significant inflammation with subsequent obstruction of the ostiomeatal complex and impaired mucociliary clearance [8,9]. Because of the multitude of viral strains that can cause nasal and paranasal sinus inflammation, viral rhinosinusitis is quite prevalent. Pathogens in viral rhinosinusitis include more than 100 strains of rhinovirus, as well as influenza, parainfluenza, coronavirus, adenovirus, and respiratory syncytial virus. Rhinovirus is the predominant etiology of the common cold and is capable of survival on surfaces for up to 4 days. When inoculation of the nasal cavity occurs with a virus-contaminated finger, infection will result in the majority of cases [7]. Clinically, patients experience a self-limiting illness lasting 3 to 7 days. Treatment is usually supportive with adequate hydration and nasal decongestants. Unfortunately, by creating ostiomeatal complex obstruction, impairing mucociliary clearance, and weakening mucosal integrity, viral rhinosinusitis predisposes patients to invasion of their nasal and paranasal sinus mucosa by trapped facultative aerobic bacteria and the development of acute bacterial rhinosinusitis [10–13].

Acute Bacterial Rhinosinusitis

Acute bacterial rhinosinusitis is a clinical condition characterized by nasal congestion and rhinorrhea for 7 to 14 days, but no more than 4 weeks. This diagnosis is based on symptomatology, clinical signs, and duration of symptoms [13]. Specific diagnostic criteria can be elicited through a detailed history and physical examination without the need for endoscopy or computerized tomography, which are often used as adjuncts in the clinical management. Acute bacterial rhinosinusitis usually starts with marked mucosal inflammation from a viral upper respiratory tract infection or allergic rhinitis exacerbation. The mucosal inflammation, combined with retained secretions, constitutes an ideal medium for bacterial overgrowth. When bacterial superinfection occurs, a diagnosis of bacterial rhinosinusitis is established.

The primary pathogens in acute bacterial rhinosinusitis of the maxillary, ethmoid, and frontal sinuses are *Streptococcus pneumoniae*, *Haemophilus influenzae*, and *Moraxella catarrhalis*. Additional pathogens include other streptococcus species, *Staphylococcus aureus*, and anaerobes (Fig. 2.1) [14]. In contrast to the other sinuses, acute sphenoid sinusitis tends to have *Staphylococcus aureus* as one of its most common pathogens [15]. When patients present with acute maxillary sinusitis of odontogenic origin, the primary pathogens are anaerobic bacteria such as anaerobic streptococci, *Bacteroides*, *Proteus*, and coliform bacilli, and appropriate antibiotic treatment as well as proper dental referral is warranted (Fig. 2.2) [16,17].

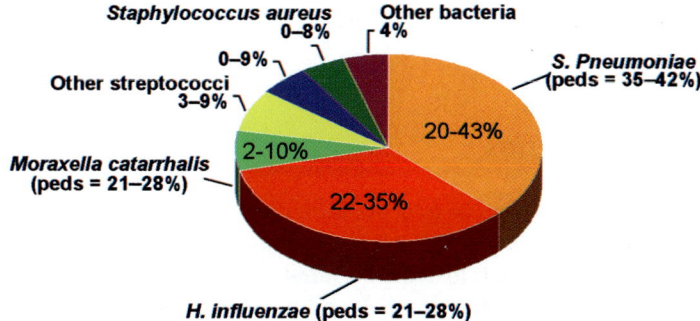

Fig. 2.1 Pathogens in acute bacterial rhinosinusitis. *peds*, pediatric. (Reprinted from James A. Hadley, MD, and David J. Osguthorpe MD. *Rhinosinusitis,* Fifth Edition, 2006, with permission of the American Academy of Otolaryngology–Head and Neck Surgery Foundation, copyright © 2006 [14]. All rights reserved.)

(a)   (b)

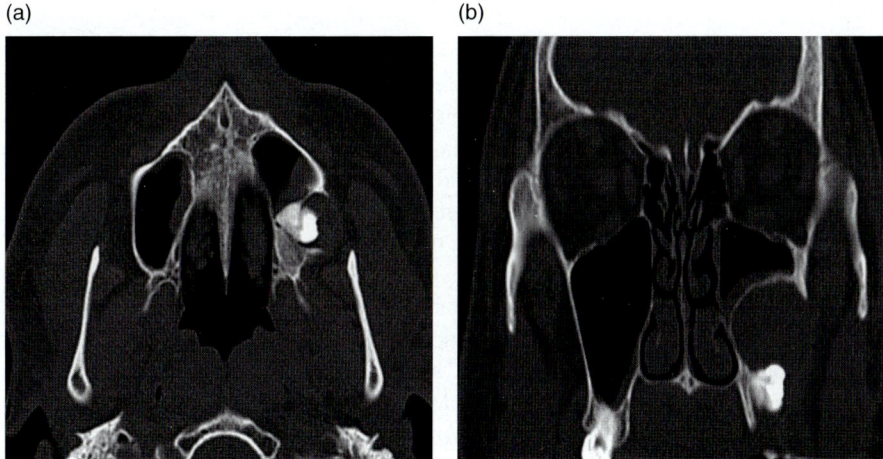

Fig. 2.2 Axial (**a**) and coronal (**b**) computed tomography (CT) scanning of a patient with left maxillary sinusitis from odontogenic origin

Children with acute bacterial rhinosinusitis usually have the same pathogens as previously listed, which tend to parallel those seen in acute otitis media (*Streptococcus pneumoniae, Haemophilus influenzae*, and *Moraxella catarrhalis*) [17].

Treatment of acute bacterial rhinosinusitis is based on restoration of sinus drainage and eradication of the offending organism(s). Most acute bacterial rhinosinusitis patients can be treated medically with topical vasoconstrictors, systemic decongestants, and appropriate antibiotics directed toward the previously listed three most common organisms. It should be noted that those patients with unilateral sinusitis should be appropriately evaluated for an odontogenic source of infection, or, in the case of children, for a foreign-body impaction. Without adequately addressing the underlying cause, these patients will continue to suffer from chronic or repetitive infection.

Subacute Rhinosinusitis

Subacute rhinosinusitis is similar to acute bacterial rhinosinusitis but is present for more than 4 weeks and less than 12 weeks. The microbiology of subacute rhinosinusitis is believed to be similar to acute bacterial rhinosinusitis with the addition of more resistant organisms such as *Staphylococcus aureus* and *Pseudomonas aeruginosa*. Treatment consists of topical vasoconstrictors, systemic decongestants, and adequate antibiotic coverage. Complete and long-term resolution of symptoms is expected after appropriate medical therapy.

Chronic Rhinosinusitis

Chronic rhinosinusitis is defined as rhinosinusitis of at least 12 consecutive weeks duration. Therefore, it represents a group of disorders characterized by inflammation of the nasal and paranasal sinus mucosa for at least 12 consecutive weeks [6]. Chronic rhinosinusitis is typically diagnosed in association with predisposing conditions such as asthma, allergy, dental disease, cystic fibrosis, polyposis, and immunodeficiency syndromes. While there is little debate regarding an association between bacteria and acute rhinosinusitis, the role of bacteria in the pathogenesis of chronic rhinosinusitis is still unclear.

The bacteriology of chronic rhinosinusitis is considerably different than acute bacterial rhinosinusitis [18]. Pathogens such as *Staphylococcus aureus*, coagulase-negative staphylococcus, and anaerobic and gram-negative bacteria replace the pathogens commonly found in acute bacterial rhinosinusitis (*Streptococcus pneumoniae*, *Haemophilus influenzae*, and *Moraxella catarrhalis*). One theory is that prior repeated use of antibiotics in patients with frequent rhinosinusitis accounts for the observed difference in pathogens.

Chronic rhinosinusitis also involves significant osteitis from the prolonged inflammation and remodeling occurring within the bone of the paranasal sinuses. This phenomenon, which seldom occurs in acute bacterial rhinosinusitis, can lead to distal submucosal spread of the infectious process in other parts of the paranasal sinuses and render medical and surgical treatment more difficult [19]. A recent prospective clinicopathological study showed that more than 50% of patients undergoing sinus surgery for chronic rhinosinusitis had pathological evidence of osteitis [20]. Although the direct impact on treatment has not yet been determined, many experts believe that this finding will influence future treatment approaches for chronic rhinosinusitis [19,20].

An important factor in the pathogenesis of chronic rhinosinusitis is the role of bacterial biofilms [21]. Bacterial biofilms are aggregates of bacteria with special properties secondary to their group structures (Fig. 2.3). One of these properties

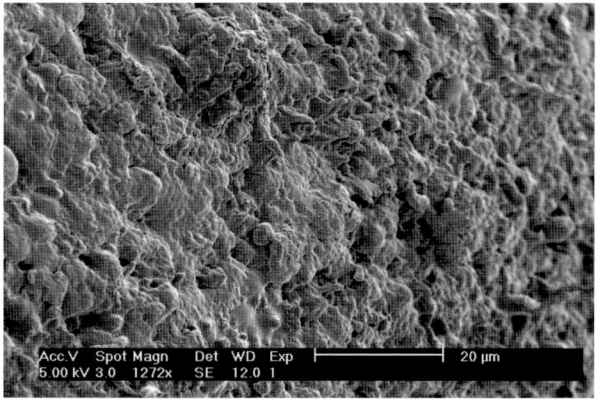

Fig. 2.3 Electron microscopy of *Pseudomonas aeruginosa* biofilms

involves significant increased resistance to antibiotics. Bacterial biofilms have previously been cultured in patients with chronic rhinosinusitis. In fact, strains from two of the most common bacterial isolates in chronic rhinosinusitis (*Pseudomonas aeruginosa* and *Staphylococcus aureus*) have been proven to form biofilms [21]. This finding may explain why a subgroup of patients fails to improve or has frequent recurrence after medical and surgical management for chronic rhinosinusitis [21,22]. Studies are ongoing to determine the utility of topical therapies to penetrate the bacterial biofilms, thus rendering them more susceptible to antibiotic therapy.

Treatment of chronic rhinosinusitis involves the identification and appropriate management of possible underlying conditions causing rhinosinusitis. Intranasal steroid sprays, decongestants, and systemic steroids, with appropriate antibiotic coverage, have all been used with some efficacy. Nevertheless, there are no randomized clinical trials supporting the use of antibiotics in this condition. When medical management fails, surgical intervention is needed to provide sinus drainage and to remove predisposing anatomic obstruction.

Recurrent, Acute Rhinosinusitis

A patient with at least four episodes of acute rhinosinusitis per year—with each episode lasting 7 to 10 days without intervening signs of chronic rhinosinusitis—has, by definition, recurrent acute bacterial rhinosinusitis [13]. These patients tend to have similar pathogens as acute bacterial rhinosinusitis and are usually treated with medical management. Sinonasal culture may be helpful in guiding antibiotic choice in this subgroup of patients (Fig. 2.4).

Acute Exacerbation of Chronic Rhinosinusitis

Acute exacerbations of chronic rhinosinusitis are characterized by sudden worsening of the dull and persistent symptoms of chronic rhinosinusitis. This condition

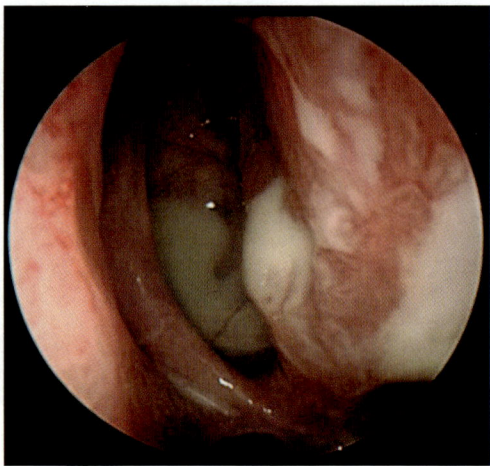

Fig. 2.4 Purulent nasopharyngeal discharge in a patient with recurrent acute rhinosinusitis

may be triggered by factors such as worsening allergic rhinitis or transient decrease in host immune response secondary to a viral upper respiratory infection. The bacteriology is usually similar to chronic rhinosinusitis. Treatment involves topical vasoconstrictors, systemic decongestants, and appropriate antibiotics. After appropriate medical management, these patients typically return to their baseline.

Fungal Rhinosinusitis

Fungi are ubiquitous organisms, and as expected, commonly colonize the nasal cavity and paranasal sinuses in both the normal and disease states. Fungal rhinosinusitis can be classified in five different manifestations: acute invasive, chronic invasive, fungal ball, allergic, and saprophytic. The prognosis and therapy for each histopathological form of fungal rhinosinusitis is different and is primarily based on the immunological status of the host (Table 2.1).

Table 2.1 Classification of fungal rhinosinusitis

Classification	Immunological status	Treatment	Prognosis
Acute invasive	Immunocompromised	Reversal of immunocompromise; surgery; antifungal agents	Guarded/poor
Chronic invasive	Immunocompetent	Surgery; antifungal agents	Fair/good
Fungus ball (mycetoma)	Immunocompetent	Surgery	Good
Allergic	Atopic	Surgery; steroids; immunotherapy	Excellent
Saprophytic	Immunocompetent	Removal	Excellent

Acute invasive fungal rhinosinusitis almost exclusively occurs in immunocompromised patients (organ transplant recipients, diabetic patients, and patients with primary or acquired immunodeficiency), and has a fulminant onset with high mortality. Diagnosis is made by histological evidence of invasive fungal hyphae (within the sinus mucosa, submucosa, blood vessels, or bone) in the nose and paranasal sinuses. Common pathogens causing this condition include aspergillus and fungi of Mucoraceae, of the order Mucorales, including *Rhizopus* and *Mucor* [23,24]. *Aspergillus* species are the most common pathogens identified in acute invasive fungal rhinosinusitis (Fig. 2.5). Although approximately 350 strains of this fungus have been identified, the three strains with pathological significance to humans are *Aspergillus fumigatus*, *Aspergillus flavus*, and *Aspergillus niger*. The strain most commonly responsible for disease in the United States is *A. fumigatus* while *A.flavus* is most often associated with the indolent chronic invasive rhinosinusitis seen in the Sudan. Nonetheless, any of these *Aspergillus* species can cause fatal acute fulminant fungal rhinosinusitis. Treatment involves correction of the immunocompromised state, aggressive surgical debridement, and long-term systemic and topical antifungal agents. Recent reports suggest an increase efficacy of the antifungal posaconazole for fungal sinusitis refractory to standard antifungal therapy [25].

Chronic invasive fungal rhinosinusitis is often divided into granulomatous and nongranulomatous subtypes on the basis of histopathology. However, the diagnosis, management, and prognosis of these two subtypes are comparable. Chronic invasive fungal rhinosinusitis is rare in the United States, with most literature in this condition emanating from the Sudan. This condition usually occurs in immunocompetent or mildly immunocompromised hosts. The overwhelming majority of these cases have *Aspergillus flavus* as the offending organism. Other causative fungi include *Aspergillus fumigatus*, *A. mucor*, *A. alternaria*, *A. curvularia*, *Pseudallescheria*

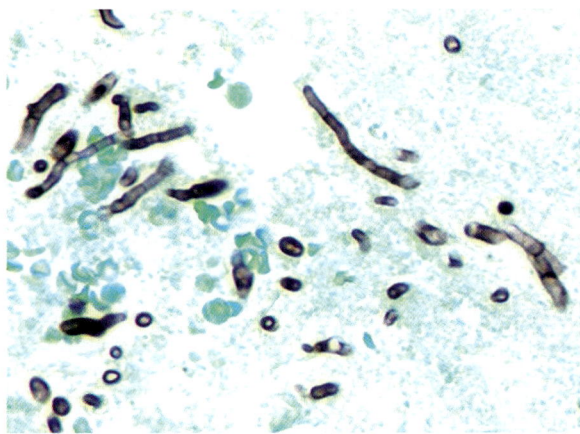

Fig. 2.5 Micrograph of septated hyphae typical of *Aspergillus*. (Grocott–Gomori methenamine-silver nitrate stain; × 400.)

boydii, P. bipolaris, and *Sporothrix schenckii* [26]. Chronic invasive fungal rhinosinusitis is treated with long-term systemic antifungal therapy and surgical debridement.

Mycetomas or fungal balls are common fungal infections found in the immuno-competent host. They can remain asymptomatic for years and be diagnosed inci-dentally, or present with symptoms mimicking chronic bacterial rhinosinusitis. The moist environment of the sinonasal cavity serves as an optimal medium for fungal proliferation. Common pathogens include *Aspergillus fumigatus, A. flavus, A. alternaria*, and *A. mucor* [27,28]. Fungal balls are treated by endoscopic surgical removal alone rather than systemic antifungal therapy. Recurrence is common.

Allergic fungal rhinosinusitis is a noninvasive disease characterized by atopy and a marked inflammatory response to certain fungal antigens. This entity was initially described by Millar et al. in 1981 [29]. The diagnosis of allergic fungal rhinosinusitis is made by histopathological analysis of allergic mucin. In 1994, Bent and Kuhn described five major criteria found in this condition, namely, atopy, nasal polyposis, eosinophilic mucin without fungal invasion into soft tissue, characteristic computed tomographic findings of serpiginous areas of high attenuation in affected sinuses, and positive fungal stain [30]. Organisms commonly found in allergic fungal rhinos-inusitis are primarily dematiaceous and include species of *Alternaria, Bipolaris*, and *Curvularia* [31]. Treatment of allergic fungal rhinosinusitis is mainly endoscopic sinus surgery, as well as systemic and topical corticosteroids. Because of the strong influence of atopy in the development of this condition, immunotherapy has been used with significant success. Recurrence is very common, and patients with allergic fungal rhinosinusitis require long-term follow-up.

Saprophytic fungal infections are commonly seen after sinus surgery and occur when ubiquitous fungal spores land and germinate on mucous crusts and old hematomas. This condition can be prevented with proper office debridement and frequent sinus irrigation after sinus surgery. Treatment consists of simple removal of the crust and hematoma and appropriate nasal irrigation.

Immunology

The immune system plays a vital role in preventing rhinosinusitis, as well as being an integral component to its pathogenicity. The normal sinonasal mucous blanket contains secretory IgA, which serves as a barrier against certain microorganisms and decreases the incidence of infections. Likewise, cell-mediated immune response constitutes a major defense against viruses and fungi. Unfortunately, the numerous cytokines and chemokines released after a potentially self-limiting infection (such as the common cold) is a clear example of the possible deleterious effect of an overly stimulated response. In these cases, the released proinflammatory chemokines cause immunosuppressive effects on neutrophils, macrophages, and lymphocytes, there-fore reducing the efficacy of cell-mediated immune response and raising vulnera-bility to infection by local bacteria.

The immune mechanisms used at the mucosal level in the nose and sinuses can be divided into innate and adaptive immunity. These two immune mechanisms are different in their response time and specificity. While innate immune response is significantly less specific, it has a very short response time and acts as the initial defense mechanism after exposure to a potentially harmful pathogen. Conversely, adaptive immunity is very specific, but has to go through a cascade of cytokine activation before pathogens eradication can occur.

Innate Immunity

The continuous sinonasal mucous flow known as mucociliary clearance represents the primary mechanical innate defense of the sinonasal mucosa. The effectiveness of this process relies on the viscoelastic property of the mucus blanket as well as adequate ciliary beat frequency. When exposed to airborne irritants or bacteria, the Schneiderian epithelium of the sinonasal cavity increases its production of mucus, leading to suppression of bacterial overgrowth from the effects of the secreted antimicrobial products in the mucus, and increases mucociliary flow with the propulsion of trapped irritants and bacteria into the nasopharynx. A healthy and noninflamed sinonasal epithelium is paramount for optimal mucociliary clearance. In fact, many recent studies have demonstrated significant differences in mucociliary clearance between normal subjects and patients with rhinosinusitis [32–34]. In patients with poor mucociliary function, chronic mucous stasis leads to bacterial overgrowth and the development of bacterial rhinosinusitis.

The sinonasal mucous blanket contains numerous antimicrobial products such as immunoglobulins, enzymes (lysozyme, lactoferrin, secretory leukocyte proteinase inhibitor), opsonins, and defensins that help the host defend against pathological bacteria. These molecules, which are secreted by the sinonasal epithelial cells, are responsible for immobilization and destruction of microorganisms and play a vital role in immediate host defense against pathogens entering the body through the sinonasal mucosa. Lysozymes (secreted by macrophages, monocytes, and sinonasal epithelial cells) act against the peptidoglycan cell wall of bacteria and are highly effective against gram-positive bacteria. Lactoferrin (secreted and stored by serous mucosal glands) is a cofactor that enhances lysozyme activity against gram-negative bacteria. This antimicrobial acts as an iron-binding protein that inhibits bacterial growth through iron sequestration. Secretory leukocyte proteinase inhibitor, which is also found in the sinonasal mucous blanket, has been shown to have in vitro activity against gram-positive and gram-negative bacteria, as well as being able to inhibit neutrophil elastase [35–37].

Adaptive Immunity

Similar to other disease processes, the adaptive immunity observed in rhinosinusitis is mediated by T and B lymphocytes and has specificity and memory. CD4$^+$ helper

T cells represent the primary mediator of this process. These T cells are divided into two functionally different phenotypes: "Th1" cells, which are responsible for cell-mediated immune response (phagocytosis and cytotoxic killing), and "Th2" cells, which trigger a humoral response (antibody production). Th1 cells secrete cytokines such as interferon-γ (IFN-γ) and tumor necrosis factor-α (TNF-α), which in turn activate macrophages and cytotoxic T lymphocytes, leading to phagocytosis and cytotoxic cell death. In contrast, Th2 cells secrete the interleukins IL-4, IL-5, IL-9, and IL-13, which promote IgG and IgE secretion, eosinophil production, and proliferation and maturation of mast cells. Each of these two immune pathways exerts an inhibitory effect on the cytokines produced by the other and causes polarization of the immune response [36].

Summary

Rhinosinusitis is a very common medical condition with significant heath care costs. Many different forms of this condition, exist with very distinct microbiology. A thorough understanding of the different forms of rhinosinusitis, as well as their common pathogens, is paramount for appropriate antimicrobial therapy. The most common pathogens in rhinosinusitis are viruses, for which supportive therapy is sufficient. Acute bacterial rhinosinusitis is usually precipitated by viral rhinosinusitis. Antimicrobial therapy for acute bacterial rhinosinusitis should be directed at common pathogens such as *Streptococcus pneumoniae*, *Haemophilus influenzae*, and *Moraxella catarrhalis*. Isolates in chronic rhinosinusitis typically show *Staphylococcus aureus*, coagulase-negative staphylococcus, and anaerobic and gram-negative bacteria. Although antimicrobials are commonly used in chronic rhinosinusitis, no clear role for antibiotic therapy has been determined in this condition. Bacterial biofilms and chronic osteitis are important factors to consider in the patient with chronic rhinosinusitis refractory to medical and surgical management.

References

1. Agency for Health Care Policy and Research. Diagnosis and treatment of acute bacterial rhinosinusitis. Evid Rep Technol Assess (Summ) 1999; 9:1–5.
2. Benninger MS, Holzer SE, Lau J. Diagnosis and treatment of uncomplicated acute bacterial rhinosinusitis: Summary of the Agency for Health Care Policy and Research evidence-based report. Otolaryngol Head Neck Surg 2000; 122:1–7.
3. Gwaltney JM. Acute community acquired sinusitis. Clin Infect Dis 1996;23:1209–1223.
4. Hyattsville, MD: National Ambulatory Medical Care Survey, 1990–1995. National Center for Health Statistics. Series 13 [CD-ROM].
5. Slavin RG. Management of sinusitis. J Am Geriatr Soc 1991; 39:212–217.
6. Benninger MS, Ferguson BJ, Hadley JA, et al. Adult chronic rhinosinusitis: definitions, diagnosis, epidemiology, and pathophysiology. Otolaryngol Head Neck Surg 2003; 129(3 suppl): S1–S32.

7. Winther B, Gwaltney JM Jr. Microbiology of sinusitis. In: Kennedy DW, Bolger WE, Zinreich SJ, eds. Diseases of the Sinuses: Diagnosis and Management. Hamilton, Ontario: Decker, 2001:77–84.

8. Winther B. The effect on the nasal mucosa of respiratory viruses (common cold). Dan Med Bull 1994; 41:193–204.

9. Winther B, Gwaltney JM Jr, Hendley JO. Respiratory virus infection of monolayer cultures of human epithelial cells. Am Rev Respir Dis 1990; 141:839–845.

10. Brook I. Microbiology and antimicrobial management of sinusitis. Otolaryngol Clin N Am 2004; 37:253–266.

11. Gwaltney JM Jr, Sydnor A Jr, Sande MA. Etiology and antimicrobial treatment of acute sinusitis. Ann Otol Rhinol Laryngol Suppl 1981; 90:68–71.

12. Hamory BH, Sande MA, Sydnor A Jr, et al. Etiology and antimicrobial therapy of acute maxillary sinusitis. J Infect Dis 1979; 139:197–202.

13. Lanza DC, Kennedy DW. Adult rhinosinusitis defined. Otolarygol Head Neck Surg 1997; 117(3 pt 2): S1–S7.

14. Hadley JA, Osguthorpe JD. Rhinosinusitis, 5th ed. Alexandria, VA: American Academy of Otolaryngology-Head and Neck Surgery Foundation, Inc., 2006 [CD-ROM].

15. Brook I. Bacteriology of acute and chronic sphenoid sinusitis. Ann Otol Rhinol Laryngol 2002; 111:1002–1004.

16. Brook I, Frazier EH, Gher ME Jr. Microbiology of periapical abscesses and associated maxillary sinusitis. J Periodontol 1996; 67:608–610.

17. Brook I, Friedman EM. Intracranial complications of sinusitis in children. A sequela of periapical abscess. Ann Otol Rhinol Laryngol 1982; 91:41–43.

18. Brook I, Frazier EH, Foote PA. Microbiology of the transition from acute to chronic maxillary sinusitis. J Med Microbiol 1996; 45:372–375.

19. Chiu AG. Osteitis in chronic rhinosinusitis. Otolaryngol Clin N Am 2005; 38:1237–1242.

20. Lee JT, Kennedy DW, Palmer JN, Feldman M, Chiu AG. The incidence of concurrent osteitis in patients with chronic rhinosinusitis: a clinicopathological study. Am J Rhinol 2006; 20:278–282.

21. Palmer J. Bacterial biofilms in chronic rhinosinusitis. Ann Otol Rhinol Laryngol Suppl 2006; 196:35–39.

22. Harvey RJ, Lund VJ. Biofilms and chronic rhinosinusitis: systematic review of evidence, current concepts and directions for research. Rhinology 2007; 45:3–13.

23. de Shazo RD, O' Brien M, Chapin K, et al. A new classification and diagnostic criteria for invasive fungal sinusitis. Arch Otolaryngol Head Neck Surg 1997; 123:1181–1188.

24. Oliveria PJ, Zinreich SJ. Radiology of the nasal cavity and paranasal sinuses. In: Cummings CW, Fredrickson JM, eds. Otolaryngology-Head and Neck Surgery, vol 2, 3rd ed. St. Louis: Mosby-Year Book, 1998:1065–1091.

25. Notheis G, Tarani L, Costantino F, et al. Posaconazole for treatment of refractory fungal disease. Mycoses 2006; 49:37–41.

26. Ferguson BJ. Definitions of fungal rhinosinusitis. Otolaryngol Clin N Am 2000; 33:227–235.

27. Chakrabarti A, Sharma SC, Chandler J. Epidemiology and pathogenesis of paranasal sinus mycoses. Otolaryngol Head Neck Surg 1992; 107:745–750.

28. Henderson LT, Robbins KT, Weitzner S, et al. Benign mucor colonization (fungus ball) associated with chronic sinusitis. South Med J 1988; 81:846–850.

29. Millar JW, Johnston A, Lamb D. Allergic aspergillosis of the maxillary sinuses. Thorax 1981; 36:710 (abstract).

30. Bent JP, Kuhn FA. Diagnosis of allergic fungal sinusitis. Otolaryngol Head Neck Surg 1994; 111:580–588.

31. Manning SC, Schaefer SD, Close LG, et al. Culture-positive allergic fungal sinusitis. Arch Otolaryngol Head Neck Surg 1991; 117:174–178.

32. Antunes MB, Cohen NA. Mucociliary clearance–a critical upper airway host defense mechanism and methods of assessment. Curr Opin Allergy Clin Immunol 2007; 7:5–10.

33. Chen B, Shaari J, Claire SE, et al. Altered sinonasal ciliary dynamics in chronic rhinosinusitis. Am J Rhinol 2006; 20:325–329.
34. Cohen NA. Sinonasal mucociliary clearance in health and disease. Ann Otol Rhinol Laryngol Suppl 2006; 196:20–26.
35. Lane AP, Truong-Tran QA, Schleimer RP. Altered expression of genes associated with innate immunity and inflammation in recalcitrant rhinosinusitis with polyps. Am J Rhinol 2006; 20:138–144.
36. Ramanathan M Jr, Lane AP. Innate immunity of the sinonasal cavity and its role in chronic rhinosinusitis. Otolaryngol Head Neck Surg 2007; 136:348–356.
37. Schleimer RP, Lane AP, Kim J. Innate and acquired immunity and epithelial cell function in chronic rhinosinusitis. Clin Allergy Immunol 2007; 20:51–78.

Chapter 3
Diagnosis and Management
of Acute Rhinosinusitis

Karen A. Kölln and Brent A. Senior

Acute rhinosinusitis is a major health concern in the United States; and patients are cared for by a diverse group of physicians and physician extenders whose specialties range from internal medicine and family practice to pulmonology, immunology, pediatrics, and otolaryngology. The wide variety among treating health care professionals makes standardization of the diagnosis a challenge. The aim of this chapter is to review the definition and diagnosis of acute rhinosinusitis in adults and to discuss the associated controversies.

Definition

In 1997 the Rhinosinusitis Task Force published the first definitions and guidelines for the diagnosis of rhinosinusitis in the otolaryngological literature. In general, rhinosinusitis was defined as a manifestation of an inflammatory response involving the mucous membranes of the sinonasal cavities with or without involvement of the underlying bone. As such, it manifests with symptoms and physical findings over a particular timeframe. To establish a consistent definition among all health care professionals treating patients, major and minor criteria incorporating these symptoms and physical findings were established (see Chapter 1, Table 1.1). A time factor was thought necessary to distinguish various forms of rhinosinusitis including acute, subacute, and chronic. Therefore, acute rhinosinusitis was defined by a sudden onset with symptoms lasting no more than 4 weeks, while subacute rhinosinusitis encompassed symptoms lasting for 4 to 12 weeks (thought to reflect acute rhinosinusitis that had not completely resolved itself). Finally, chronic rhinosinusitis was defined by symptoms lasting more than 12 weeks with either two or more major factors or one major and two minor factors [1].

Notable in these criteria is that fever and/or facial pressure/pain without other nasal factors do not by themselves constitute a diagnosis of rhinosinusitis.

B.A. Senior
Department of Otorhinolaryngology – Head and Neck Surgery, University of North Carolina at Chapel Hill, Chapel Hill, NC, USA
e-mail: brent_senior@med.unc.edu

E.R. Thaler, D.W. Kennedy (eds.), *Rhinosinusitis*, DOI: 10.1007/978-0-387-73062-2_3,
© Springer Science+Business Media, LLC 2008

Additionally, in contrast to acute rhinosinusitis, fever is not a major factor in subacute rhinosinusitis as the symptoms overall are less severe in nature. Since the original attempt to clinically define rhinosinusitis in 1997, the guidelines have been enhanced to make them more useful. In the 2007 clinical practice guidelines, acute rhinosinusitis was further subdivided—based on symptom pattern—into acute bacterial rhinosinusitis (ABRS) and viral rhinosinusitis (VRS), which are further discussed under "Presenting Symptoms and Signs [2]. "

In the 2005 position paper by the European Academy of Allergology and Clinical Immunology, the definition of acute rhinosinusitis is symptom based. Acute rhinosinusitis is defined as the sudden onset of two or more of the following symptoms for less than 12 weeks: blockage/congestion, rhinorrhea/postnasal drip, facial pressure/pain, and reduction/loss of sense of smell. Symptom-free intervals must also exist if the problem is intermittent in nature. Acute viral rhinosinusitis is further defined as symptoms lasting less than 10 days, whereas a worsening of symptoms after 5 days or with persistence of symptoms after 10 days (but less than 12 weeks) constitutes acute nonviral rhinosinusitis [3].

Pathophysiology

Acute rhinosinusitis begins with a viral upper respiratory tract infection (URI). Predisposing factors such as allergy, trauma, dental infection, nasal anatomy, and systemic diseases (e.g., vasculitis, granulomatous disease, or immunodeficient states) contribute to the frequency and severity of symptoms. The most common virus implicated in acute rhinosinusitis is human rhinovirus, followed by coronavirus, influenza A and B viruses, parainfluenza virus, respiratory syncytial virus, adenovirus, and enterovirus. Once the virus attaches to epithelial cells, there is an upregulation of inflammatory pathways resulting in the production of histamine,

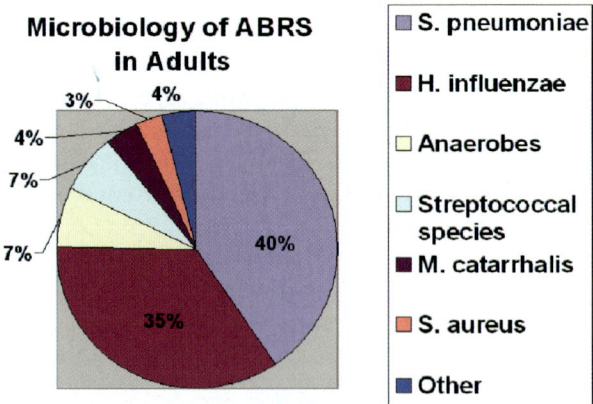

Fig. 3.1 Microbiology of acute bacterial rhinosinusitis in adults

bradykinin, and various cytokines. A downstream effect of this inflammation is the suppression of macrophage and lymphocyte function, which creates a milieu susceptible to bacterial infection and overgrowth [4,5].

Bacteria subsequently superinfect the sinonasal mucosa, as shown by repeated sinus aspiration studies demonstrating that 60% of adults with URI symptoms for 10 days or more have significant bacterial growth in sinus cultures. Isolates from maxillary sinus aspirates show that the most common pathogens are *Streptococcus pneumoniae* and *Haemophilus influenzae*, together comprising more than half of the bacterial isolates. Figure 3.1 displays the incidence of bacterial pathogens in acute maxillary rhinosinusitis in an adult population [6].

Epidemiology

Acute rhinosinusitis, either viral or bacterial, carries a significant health burden in the United States even with the most conservative estimates. The most recent data from the National Health Interview Study showed that rhinosinusitis is the most common respiratory disease among Americans, with 13% having been told by a doctor that they have rhinosinusitis in the last year. Female respondents were nearly twice as likely to have the diagnosis; and it was also more common in the South than in other regions of the country [7]. There is a significant cost associated with acute rhinosinusitis, both in health care as well as in the workforce. Rhinosinusitis also ranks in the top 10 most costly physical health conditions affecting U.S. employers [8].

Given that acute rhinosinusitis has such a high prevalence, it is imperative that health care providers are able to accurately diagnose the condition and appropriately prescribe antibiotics. As one recent study illustrated, 81% of patients diagnosed with acute rhinosinusitis have received antibiotics [9]. Appropriate use of antibiotics is vital to avoid a further increase in antibiotic resistance [10]. Prescribing patterns can change the prevalence of specific drug resistance. In Finland, macrolide-resistant group A streptococcal isolates decreased by 50% (from 16.5% to 8.6% of isolates) when new practice guidelines recommended a decrease in macrolide consumption [11].

Presenting Symptoms and Signs

Fever, Nasal Obstruction, Pain, Headache, Purulent Rhinorrhea

Because a diversity of health care professionals are diagnosing and treating acute rhinosinusitis, the bulk of the diagnosis rests on an individual patient's symptoms and findings on physical examination: purulent nasal drainage, nasal obstruction, and facial pain/pressure/fullness. Although early consensus reports used the major and minor criteria discussed, the more recent reports have strayed from this concept and focused instead on only major symptoms [1–3].

The time-course of the symptoms then becomes the next most important factor in distinguishing VRS from ABRS. VRS tends to be self-limited, with symptoms peaking at day 2 to 3 and then waning with resolution of symptoms between 10 and 14 days after onset. If symptoms initially improve and then subsequently worsen, or if symptoms persist beyond 10 days, the probability of bacterial infection is increased and the diagnosis of ABRS can be made [2,6,12].

On physical examination, anterior rhinoscopy reveals hyperemia of the nasal mucosa and nasal congestion. If purulence is visualized the diagnosis is secured; pain on palpation over the individual sinuses may aid in the diagnosis. Pharyngeal irritation or purulence in the posterior or lateral pharynx can also be used to aid in the proper diagnosis.

Associated Factors

During evaluation for acute rhinosinusitis, associated factors must be considered. The European Academy of Allergology and Clinical Immunology (EAACI) recommends a query for allergic symptoms such as sneezing, watery rhinorrhea, nasal itching, and itchy watery eyes [3]. Although there are limited data, it does appear that individuals with baseline allergic symptoms may be at increased risk for bacterial rhinosinusitis. Alho and colleagues examined 48 individuals during the first days of a viral upper respiratory infection [13]. Evaluation included a paranasal sinus computed tomography (CT) scan at the initial evaluation and then again after 21 days. The individuals with allergic rhinitis (19%) had significantly poorer CT scan results when compared with nonallergic subjects both initially and at follow-up. These results may indicate impairment in mucociliary clearance with a subsequent predisposition to the development of ABRS [13].

Other factors that must be considered include unilateral symptoms (foreign body, tumor), history of trauma or prior surgery, presence of immunosuppression or systemic disease (Wegener's granulomatosis, sarcoidosis), or impairments in mucociliary clearance (cystic fibrosis, primary ciliary dyskinesia).

Sinonasal Endoscopy

Examination with a 0° endoscope reveals hyperemia, congestion, crusting, and purulence emanating from the sinuses. The location of the purulence can help in localizing the infection, as purulence in the middle meatus streaming anterior to the eustachian tube orifice originates from the maxillary, anterior ethmoid, and frontal sinuses whereas purulence seen in the sphenoethmoid recess and above the eustachian tube orifice comes from the sphenoid and posterior ethmoid sinuses. Endoscopy yielded a sensitivity of 80% and specificity of 94% in one retrospective review, which was an improvement from the standard used in this study, which was standard X-ray [14]. Although sinonasal endoscopy is considered standard in an otolaryngological practice, this is not the case for most practitioners who are confronted with the challenge of diagnosing ARS. Therefore, sinonasal endoscopy is not considered necessary for an accurate diagnosis, although it should be utilized if available as this enables the practitioner to culture any purulence that is visualized.

Sinonasal Culture

The gold standard for sinus culture has been the maxillary sinus tap via a trocar through the canine fossa or with a needle through the inferior meatus [15]. Although this method is considered the standard for pharmaceutical trials, it is impractical in the clinical realm. Patients are unlikely to agree to the procedure secondary to real or perceived discomfort, and most practitioners treating acute bacterial rhinosinusitis (ABRS) are not skilled in performing the procedure. Nasal cavity swabs, although easily performed, have not been shown to reliably identify a causative organism without endoscopic guidance, as these cultures have only a 65% concordance rate with maxillary antral cultures [16].

With the advent of sinonasal endoscopy, a more directed and less invasive culture technique was introduced. One of the early studies evaluating endoscopic middle meatal cultures (EMMC) was performed by Vogan and colleagues in 2000 [17]. EMMC and antral puncture were performed on 16 individuals presenting with symptoms of acute rhinosinusitis and maxillary sinus air-fluid levels on CT. This group reported a concordance rate of 93.8% for aerobic culture and 87.4% for anaerobic culture [17]. Further support for the validity of EMMC was demonstrated by two meta-analyses, the first in 2005 by Dubin et al., that revealed accuracy of 82% per isolate when compared with maxillary sinus aspirates [18]. Benninger and colleagues then described a sensitivity of 80.9% and specificity of 90.5%, a positive predictive value of 82.6%, a negative predictive value of 89.4%, and an overall accuracy of 87% of EMMC [19].

Culture-directed therapy, although ideal, has remained elusive in the majority of cases of acute rhinosinusitis. The majority of practitioners treating ABRS do not have endoscopic tools at their disposal and, therefore, cultures are reserved for complex and recalcitrant cases necessitating specialty care.

Laboratory Data

Although not routine, serologic markers for inflammation may be helpful in the diagnosis of ABRS. In 1995, Hansen et al. reported on a cohort of 174 patients with physician suspected rhinosinusitis, and the diagnosis was confirmed with maxillary antral puncture in 92 (53%) [20]. The diagnosis was then correlated with CT imaging, physical signs and symptoms, and erythrocyte sedimentation rate (ESR) and C-reactive protein (CRP). Only an ESR more than 20 mm/h in females and more than 10 mm/h in males, as well as a CRP more than 10 mg/l, were significantly associated with the correct diagnosis [20]. Other groups have also supported the use of ESR for increasing the positive predictive value of the diagnosis, but this has not been supported as being cost-effective by others [3,21].

Imaging

Ultrasound

As a cost-effective means for aiding in the diagnosis of acute maxillary rhinos-inusitis, ultrasound has been recommended. Although rapid and noninvasive, the technology is operator dependent and, therefore, has not gained support for standard diagnosis. In one study of 197 adults with symptoms of the common cold, ultra-sonography and Waters' view were performed, and magnetic resonance imaging (MRI) was performed randomly on 40 participants on day 7 of the study [22]. The calculated sensitivity of ultrasonography for the diagnosis of maxillary rhinos-inusitis was 64% with a specificity of 95% in this study,[22] which would indicate that a positive ultrasound could be used to diagnose acute rhinosinusitis. However, a negative exam would have little value.

X-Ray

Plain X-ray has been used to evaluate the presence of air-fluid levels or mucosal thickening in the paranasal sinuses. Waters' (occipitomental) view, where the X-ray beam is oriented through the chin, is used to obtain views of the maxillary and frontal sinuses. In the Caldwell view, the X-ray beam is oriented directly through the forehead and is used to evaluate the frontal sinus. In one report, the sensitivity and specificity are somewhat modest at 76% and 79%, respectively [23]. When evaluating the efficacy of using a single Waters' view for diagnosing acute maxil-lary versus frontal rhinosinusitis, the accuracy has been shown to be even worse. When evaluating the maxillary sinus, a single Waters' view has a false-negative rate of 32% and a mean negative predictive value of 76.9%; and the sensitivity for evaluating the frontal sinus is only 14.6% when compared to CT. Radiologists in this study also could not commit to a diagnosis when evaluating the ethmoid and sphenoid sinuses, indicating that this modality is not adequate for the evaluation of these sinuses [24,25]. Figures 3.2 and 3.3 are plain X-rays of Caldwell and Waters views demonstrating mucosal thickening. These images reveal how the diagnosis of acute rhinosinusitis from X-ray can be difficult. Structural overlapping can lead to the impression of edematous mucosa, a hypoplastic sinus can be misinterpreted as pathological opacification, and infection can be difficult to distinguish from tumor and polyp.

Computed Tomography

Computed tomography (CT) in acute rhinosinusitis demonstrates partial or complete opacification, air-fluid levels, and air bubbles within fluid levels in the paranasal sinuses (Fig. 3.4). This finding contrasts to chronic rhinosinusitis that may show mucosal thickening in addition to complete opacification (Figs. 3.5, 3.6, 3.7). CT, although more sensitive than plain films, is not specific, as demonstrated by partial opacification noted on up to 42% of head CTs performed for various reasons, and

(a)   (b)

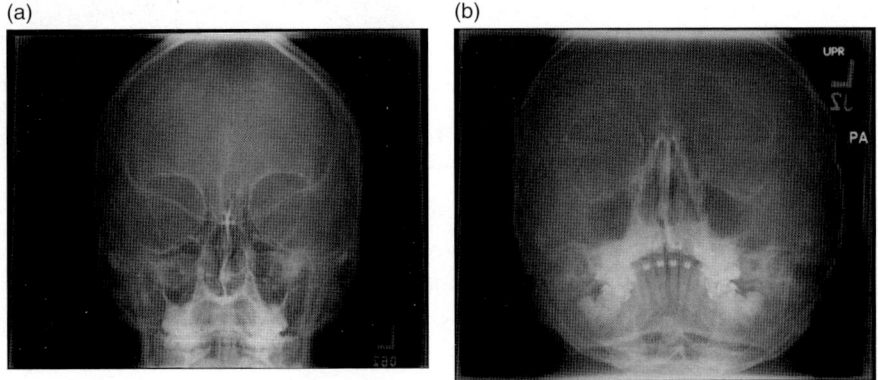

Fig. 3.2 Caldwell view of the sinuses demonstrating well-pneumatized paranasal sinuses (**A**) versus chronic mucosal thickening (**B**)

Fig. 3.3 Waters' view demonstrating chronic mucosal thickening

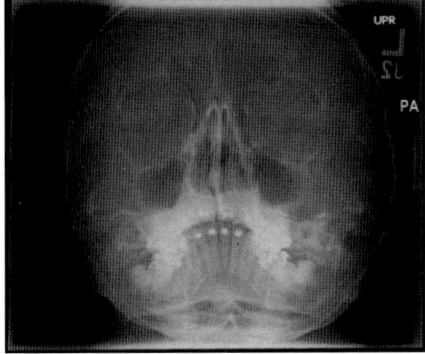

Fig. 3.4 Coronal computed tomography (CT) demonstrating acute maxillary rhinosinusitis

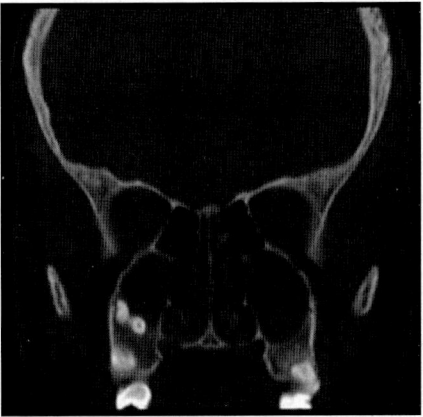

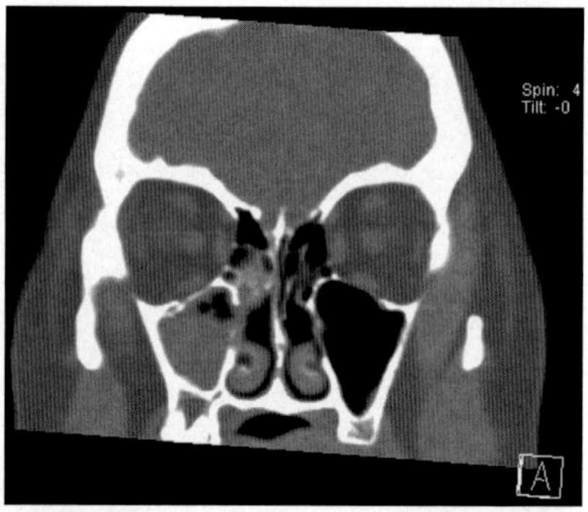

Fig. 3.5 Coronal CT demonstrating acute maxillary and ethmoid rhinosinusitis with air bubbles within fluid density, indicating purulence in the right maxillary sinus

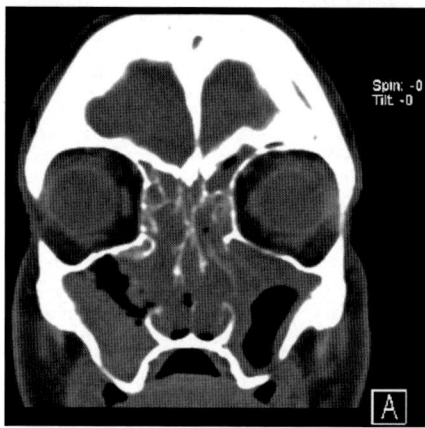

Fig. 3.6 Coronal CT demonstrating acute on chronic rhinosinusitis with complete opacification of bilateral ethmoid sinuses, left maxillary sinus mucosal thickening, and air bubbles within the right maxillary sinus indicating purulence

Fig. 3.7 Coronal CT demonstrating changes associated with chronic rhinosinusitis, including mucosal thickening of bilateral maxillary sinuses

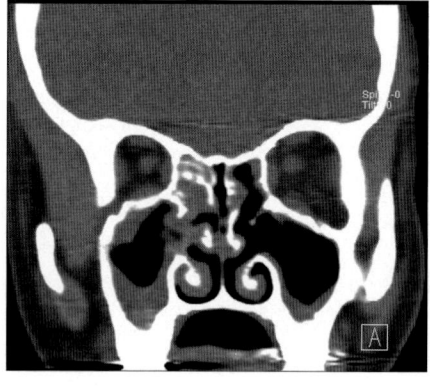

unrelated to the paranasal sinuses [26]. In addition, CT cannot distinguish between viral and bacterial rhinosinusitis, as opacification of the infundibulum and paranasal sinuses can be seen on CT scan 48 h after the onset of cold-type symptoms [27]. CT radiography has also shown to have no effect on outcome [28].

Imaging, independent of the modality, is neither sensitive nor specific when striving to make the diagnosis of acute rhinosinusitis. Therefore, imaging is not recommended as a first-line procedure when evaluating a patient. CT should be reserved for the diagnosis of complicated acute rhinosinusitis, which is discussed in detail below.

Diagnosis of Complicated Acute Rhinosinusitis

Most episodes of acute rhinosinusitis are self-limited and resolve without further sequelae. However, complicated acute rhinosinusitis involves intracranial and intra-orbital spread of infection and must be accurately diagnosed for immediate intervention. Orbital extension is demonstrated by periorbital edema, erythema, conjunctival injection, chemosis, proptosis, diplopia, ophthalmoplegia, and/or decreased visual acuity. Orbital complications are thought to be secondary to extension of infection from osteitis of the thin lamina papyracea or via thrombophlebitis of communicating veins [29,30]. Diagnosis is best performed by a team including an ophthalmologist and otolaryngologist and should include CT scan of the orbit and sinuses to evaluate the extent of the infection, and complete ophthalmologic examination, as well as endoscopic evaluation.

Intracranial complications of rhinosinusitis include subdural empyema, intracere-bral abscess, extradural abscess, and meningitis. Infection spreads most commonly from the frontal sinus through direct spread from osteomyelitis of the skull, by retro-grade thrombophlebitis through the small diploic veins of the sinus to the small vessels traversing the dura, or via a defect (surgical or traumatic) that directly connects the sinus to the cranial vault. Adolescent and young males are at highest risk for intracranial complications, which is thought to be secondary to an abundant valve-less diploic system providing a good conduit for bacterial infection [31]. Individuals most commonly present with altered mental status, headache, fever, seizure, vomiting, hemiparesis, or a cranial neuropathy; CT and MRI are used to confirm the diagnosis.

Controversy

The subjective nature of symptoms-based criteria for the diagnosis of rhinosinusitis presents many challenges. First, interpretation and standardization in the literature are difficult as there is no true "gold standard" with which to compare the various modalities. This problem has been extensively discussed in regard to chronic rhinos-inusitis (CRS), as there has been poor correlation between symptoms and findings on CT imaging. For example, Hwang et al. found that 35% of patients with symp-toms of CRS had negative CT imaging [32]. In 2002, Stankiewicz and Chow sought to determine the relationship between symptoms (as defined by the 1997 Rhinology task force), nasal endoscopy, and CT scan [33]. They found that neither endoscopy nor CT scanning correlated with the symptoms-based criteria for CRS, as more than 50% and 68% of patients who met the criteria for CRS had negative CT scans and normal endoscopic examinations. However, they did find that if purulence, polyps, or polypoid congested mucosa were present on endoscopy, sinus disease was usually present on the CT scan and that a negative endoscopic exam was a relatively good predictor of a negative CT scan [33].

This observation then brings into question the importance of clinical symptoms, imaging, and nasal endoscopy in acute rhinosinusitis. Given the diversity of health care professionals who are involved with diagnosing ARS, and lack of better noninvasive physical examination techniques, we support the symptoms-based schemes that have been discussed. We also believe that, given the poor sensitivity and specificity of diagnostic imaging, there is little role for this modality in the diagnosis of uncomplicated rhinosinusitis. Endoscopic evaluation on the other hand, if available, should be used as an adjunct in the diagnosis of rhinosinusitis and should be considered before imaging. Endoscopy may aid greatly in the diagnosis of acute rhinosinusitis, especially in two scenarios: when negative, it may help to avoid antibiotic use; and further, for the patient who is not responding to therapy, endoscopically obtained cultures may provide guidance in antibiotic choice.

References

1. Lanza DC, Kennedy DW. Adult rhinosinusitis defined. Otolaryngol Head Neck Surg 1997:117;S1–S7.
2. Rosenfeld RM. Clinical practice guideline on adult sinusitis. Otolaryngol Head Neck Surg 2007;137:365–377.
3. Fokkens W, Lund V, Bachert C, et al. EAACI position paper on rhinosinusitis and nasal polyps executive summary. Allergy 2005;60:583–601.
4. Makela MJ, Puhakka T, Ruuskanen O, et al. Viruses and bacteria in the etiology of the common cold. J Clin Microbiol 1998;36:539–542.
5. Winther B, Gwaltney JM Jr, Mygind N, et al. Viral induced rhinitis. Am J Rhinol 1998;12: 17–20.
6. Gwaltney JM, Scheld WM, Sande MA, et al. The microbial etiology and antimicrobial therapy of adults with acute community-acquired sinusitis: a fifteen year experience at the University of Virginia and review of other selected studies. J Allergy Clin Immunol 1992;90:457–462.
7. Pleis JR, Lethbridge-Çejku M. Summary health statistics for U.S. adults: National health interview survey, 2005. National Center for Health Statistics. Vital Health Stat 2006;10(232).
8. Goetzel RZ, Hawkins K, Ozmikowski RJ, et al. The health and productivity cost burden of the "Top 10" physical and mental health conditions affecting six large U.S. employers in 1999. J Occup Environ Med 2003;45:5–14.
9. Gill JM, Fleischut P, Haas S, et al. Use of antibiotics for adult upper respiratory infections in outpatient settings: a national ambulatory network study. Fam Med 2006;38(5):349–354.
10. Dowell SF, Schwartz B. Resistant pneumococci: protecting patients through judicious use of antibiotics. Am Fam Physician 1997;55:1647–1658.
11. Seppala H, Klaukka T, Vuopio-Varkila J, et al. The effect of changes in the consumption of macrolide antibiotics on erythromycin resistance in group A streptococci in Finland. N Engl J Med 1997;337:441–446.
12. Gwaltney JM, Hendley JO, Simon G, et al. Rhinovirus infections in an industrial population. II. Characteristics of illness and antibody response. JAMA 1967;202:494–500.
13. Alho OP, Karttunen TJ, Karttunen R, et al. Subjects with allergic rhinitis show signs of more severely impaired paranasal sinus functioning during viral colds than nonallergic subjects. Allergy 2003;58:767–771.

14. Berger G, Steinberg DM, Popovtzer A, et al. Endoscopy versus radiography for the diagnosis of acute bacterial rhinosinusitis. Eur Arch Otorhinolaryngol 2005;262:416–422.
15. Carenfelt C, Lundberg C, Nord CE, et al. Bacteriology of maxillary sinusitis in relation to quality of the retained secretion. Acta Otolaryngol 1978;86:298–302.
16. Axelsson A, Brorson JE. The correlation between bacterial findings in the nose and maxillary sinus in acute maxillary sinusitis. Laryngoscope 1973;83:2003–2011.
17. Vogan JC, Bolger WE, Keyes AS. Endoscopically guided sinonasal cultures: a direct comparison with maxillary sinus aspirate cultures. Otolaryngol Head Neck Surg 2000;122:370–373.
18. Dubin MG, Ebert CS, Coffey CS, et al. Concordance of middle meatal swab and maxillary sinus aspirate in acute and chronic sinusitis: a meta-analysis. Am J Rhinol 2005;19:462–470.
19. Benninger MS, Payne SC, Ferguson BJ, et al. Endoscopically directed middle meatal cultures versus maxillary sinus taps in acute bacterial maxillary rhinosinusitis: a meta-analysis. Otolaryngol Head Neck Surg 2006;134:3–9.
20. Hansen JG, Schmidt H, Rosborg J, et al. Predicting acute maxillary sinusitis in a general practice population. BMJ 1995;311:233–236.
21. Lindbaek M, Hjortdahl P. The clinical diagnosis of acute purulent sinusitis in general practice: a review. Br J Gen Pract 2002;52:491–495.
22. Puhakka T, Heikkinen T, Mäkelä MJ, et al. Validity of ultrasonography in diagnosis of acute maxillary sinusitis. Arch Otolaryngol Head Neck Surg 2000;126:1482–1486.
23. Lau J, Zucker D, Engels EA, et al. Diagnosis and treatment of acute bacterial rhinosinusitis. Evidence Report/Technology Assessment No. 9. Agency for Health Care Policy and Research, Rockville, MD. Publication no. 99-E016.
24. Konen E, Faibel M, Kleinbaum Y, et al. The value of the occipitomental (Waters') view in diagnosis of sinusitis: a comparative study with computed tomography. Clin Radiol 2000;55:856–860.
25. Aalokken TM, Hagtvedt T, Dalen I, et al. Conventional sinus radiography compared with CT in the diagnosis of acute sinusitis. Dentomaxillofac Radiol 2003;32:60–62.
26. Havas TE, Motbey JA, Gullane PJ. Prevalence of incidental abnormalities on computed tomographic scans of the paranasal sinuses. Arch Otolaryngol Head Neck Surg 1998;114:856–859.
27. Gwaltney JM Jr, Phillips CD, Miller RD, et al. Computed tomographic study of the common cold. N Engl J Med 1994;330:25–30.
28. van Buchem FL, Knottnerus JA, Schrijnemaekers VJJ, et al. Primary-care-based randomised placebo-controlled trial of antibiotic treatment in acute maxillary sinusitis. Lancet 1997;349:683–687.
29. Chandler JR, Langenbruner DJ, Stevens ER. The pathogenesis of orbital complications in acute sinusitis. Laryngoscope 1970;80:141–148.
30. Krohel GB, Krauss HR, Winnick J. Orbital abscess: presentation diagnosis, therapy, and sequalae. Ophthalmology 1982;89:492–498.
31. Kaplan RJ. Neurological complications of infections of the head and neck. Otolaryngol Clin N Am 1976;9:729–749.
32. Hwang PH, Irwin SB, Griest SE, et al. Radiologic correlates of symptom-based diagnostic criteria for chronic rhinosinusitis. Otolaryngol Head Neck Surg 2003; 128:489–496.
33. Stankiewicz JA, Chow JM. Nasal endoscopy and the definition and diagnosis of chronic rhinosinusitis. Otolaryngol Head Neck Surg 2002;126:623–627.

Chapter 4
Diagnosis of Chronic Rhinosinusitis

Rodney J. Schlosser and Richard J. Harvey

Chronic mucosal inflammation of the nose and paranasal sinuses is common. The symptoms of chronic rhinosinusitis (CRS) are thought to affect 16%, or 30 million, Americans in population-based studies [1,2]. While these surveys are questionnaire based and may overdiagnose the condition, even physician-diagnosed incidences are reported as 2% to 4% [3,4], which still represents an enormous disease burden. No solid data have been published on the duration of episodes, whether treated or from natural resolution. CRS affects an increasing proportion of the adult population until the sixth decade, then declines [3]. The quality-of-life impact of the disease, as measured by SF-36 scores, is comparable or worse to other chronic conditions such as chronic obstructive pulmonary disease (COPD), congestive heart failure (CHF), and back pain [5].

Identifying CRS patients correctly, from other sinonasal conditions, and providing health care interventions can greatly reduce the burden of disease within this group. We discuss the following concepts for the diagnosis of CRS:

- Defining CRS
- Presenting symptoms and differential diagnoses
- Other significant patient history
- Primary and secondary investigations
- Diagnostic schemes and clinical workup

This chapter discusses the current concepts of CRS with or without nasal polyps and an evidence-based review of the diagnostic methods.

Defining CRS

Defining the condition of chronic rhinosinusitis (CRS) has been one of the greatest challenges for otolaryngology. Patients with chronic nasal symptoms have been collectively diagnosed as CRS without further inclusive features. This situation has

R.J. Schlosser
Department of Otolaryngology, Medical University of South Carolina, Charleston, SC, USA
e-mail: schlossr@musc.edu

E.R. Thaler, D.W. Kennedy (eds.), *Rhinosinusitis*, DOI: 10.1007/978-0-387-73062-2_4,
© Springer Science+Business Media, LLC 2008

led to a heterogeneous group of pathological processes defined as either rhinitis or rhinosinusitis. The diagnosis of rhinosinusitis is made by a wide variety of practitioners, including primary care physicians, otolaryngologists, allergy specialists, and pulmonologists. The defining CRS patient, for each of these groups, has traditionally been subtly, but importantly, different. A more structured diagnostic process for the patient with chronic nasal symptoms will often lead to greater accuracy in classification and less ambiguity in treatment decisions.

Rhinitis Versus Rhinosinusitis

Rhinosinusitis is a more accurate term to discuss the pathophysiological changes within a common physiological unit.

Rhinosinusitis is an inflammatory condition of the respiratory mucosa of the nasal cavity proper and paranasal sinuses. The traditional discussion of rhinitis and rhinosinusitis as separate entities is rarely applied in modern otolaryngology practice. The mucosa of both the nasal cavity and paranasal sinuses are exposed to common inflammatory triggers, have a similar histology, and represent a single physiological unit. Thus, the term rhinitis is commonly replaced by rhinosinusitis to define this pathophysiological unit [6]. A continuum also exists between the common mucosa of the upper and lower respiratory tracts. This continuum accounts for the high prevalence of lower respiratory tract pathology, such as asthma, within chronic rhinosinusitis suffers [7]. Current concepts of rhinosinusitis define the difference between perennial intermittent rhinosinusitis, or allergic rhinitis, and CRS by the evidence of persistent inflammation of the nasal cavity and paranasal sinus mucosa. While histopathological assessment of the respiratory mucosa from these areas may represent the definitive test for chronic inflammatory changes, these are usually inferred by computed tomography (CT) or nasal endoscopy in the clinical setting. Those patients without chronic mucosal changes, despite chronic symptomatology, are not considered to have CRS but may have other forms of allergic (extrinsic), vasomotor (intrinsic), and occupational rhinosinusitis or even a nonsinogenic origin of their symptoms.

CRS as a Multifactorial Disease

The inflammatory changes of CRS (including nasal polyps) represent a common endpoint of several, potentially coexisting, pathological factors.

What mediates this prolonged inflammatory mucosal response? Even though allergy has always been implicated, evidence that atopy predisposes to chronic or acute rhinosinusitis is still lacking [8,9]. Other pathological etiologies in chronic rhinosinusitis include ciliary dysfunction, immune deficiency, ostial obstruction, bacteria, fungi, superantigens (i.e., exotoxins), leukotriene abnormalities, biofilms [10], osteitis, and environmental factors [8,11]. The concept of a single unifying pathological process is unlikely. There is significant heterogeneity between individual immune responses. The clinical spectrum of disease may partly be the result of individual diversity in the CD4$^+$ helper T-cell response to antigens [12], the Th1- and Th2-mediated immune responses [12]. CRS, as a clinical entity, defining a common chronic inflammatory endpoint from a range of pathogenic mechanisms, is a popular concept [11].

The Sinonasal Symptoms

Nasal obstruction and discharge are the defining symptoms of CRS.

Local Symptoms

Many symptoms have been attributed to CRS (Table 4.1). Chronic mucosal edema and inflammatory exudate often accompany the inflammatory changes that define CRS. Thus, obstruction and discharge are considered to be the cardinal symptoms of CRS. The symptoms of facial pain, pressure, or headache along with reduction or loss of smell are considered less consistent. These complaints constitute the four major symptoms of CRS. Questions on allergic symptoms (i.e., sneezing, watery rhinorrhea, nasal itching, and itchy watery eyes), although not diagnostic for CRS, should be included to identify concurrent pathological processes. Nasal symptoms may be secondary to CRS, but the physician must keep in mind the differential diagnoses for these common symptoms, as discussed later in this chapter.

Table 4.1 Local, regional, and systemic symptoms of chronic rhinosinusitis (CRS)

Local
    Nasal obstruction and congestion
    Nasal discharge: anterior or posterior
    Facial pain
    Facial fullness
    Headache
    Smell dysfunction
    Anosmia (loss of smell)
Regional
    Sore throat
    Dysphonia
    Cough
    Halitosis
    Bronchospasm
    Ear fullness or pain
    Eustachian tube dysfunction
    Dental pain
Systemic
    Fatigue
    Malaise
    Fever
    Anorexia

Regional and Systemic Symptoms

There is great variation in the intensity and pattern of symptoms of CRS. For some patients, extensive mucosal changes in the nasal cavity or paranasal sinuses can progress largely unnoticed until later in the disease process. Large asymptomatic nasal polyps are not an uncommon finding. A subgroup of these patients may present with regional or systemic symptoms as their chief complaint (see Table 4.1). Regional symptoms, such as cough, may have a sinonasal origin. Laryngeal inlet irritation from inflammatory postnasal discharge has some merit, and subsequent bronchospasm may even occur. The medical management of CRS in asthma patients is often associated with an improvement in these symptoms [13]. At these regional areas, other pathological etiologies, such as laryngopharyngeal reflux, may also be contributory. Careful evaluation as to the significance of CRS in the etiology of these regional symptoms should be undertaken.

Duration of Symptoms

Symptoms that have been present more than 12 weeks define CRS as chronic.

The symptom duration for CRS has been arbitrarily established at 12 weeks. It is unlikely that inflammation from an acute infective rhinosinusitis will still be present at this stage without other predisposing factors. There is typically a variable clinical course in CRS over those 12 weeks to many years. CRS is often characterized by incomplete resolution of symptoms with intermittent exacerbations (Fig. 4.1).

CRS with Polyps

Nasal polyps represent the "ballooning" of inflamed mucosa at discrete areas within the nose (Fig. 4.2). They commonly arise from the lateral nasal wall and middle meatus and are present in up to 4% of the population [14]. The mechanisms as to why the mucosa degenerates into polyps in some individuals and not others

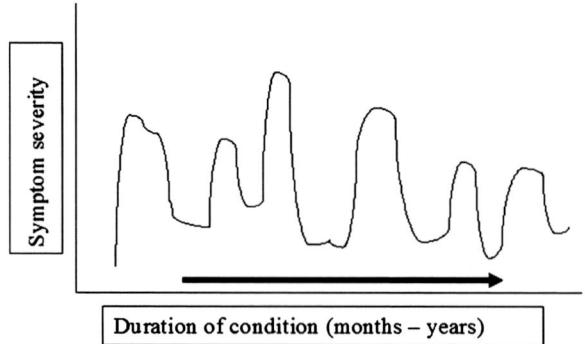

Fig. 4.1 The classic symptom course for chronic rhinosinusitis (CRS). Exacerbations with more acute infective features, such as purulent discharge, are common

Fig. 4.2 Nasal inflammatory polyps

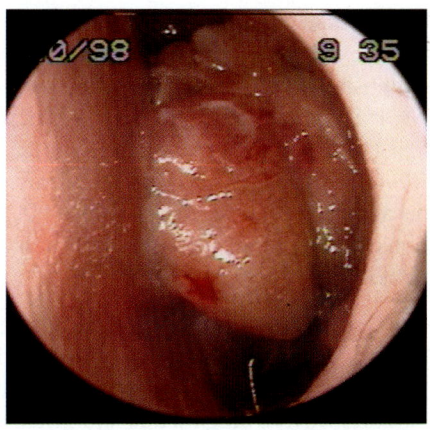

are unknown. Much research has speculated that individual variations in epithelial structure, inflammatory mediators, and immune responses account for the development of polyps [15–17]. Patients with asthma have a 7% to 15% prevalence of polyps and may represent a group with a predisposition to a strong panrespiratory inflammatory response [18]. Nasal polyps are considered to represent a form of chronic focal inflammatory change and are defined as a subgroup within CRS (Fig. 4.3). Although not all CRS patients have polyps, all polyp patients have CRS even if the symptomatology is very mild. Separating CRS patients based on the presence of polyps has previously been popular but does reflect different etiologic events [19,20]. However, the management of a CRS patient with nasal polyps is often more aggressive and may be reflective of a more exuberant inflammatory/immune response in that individual person [19].

Current Concepts

Rhinosinusitis is a group of disorders characterized by inflammation of the mucosa of the nose and paranasal sinuses. *Chronic rhinosinusitis* is rhinosinusitis of at least 12 consecutive weeks duration. Therefore, *chronic rhinosinusitis* is a group

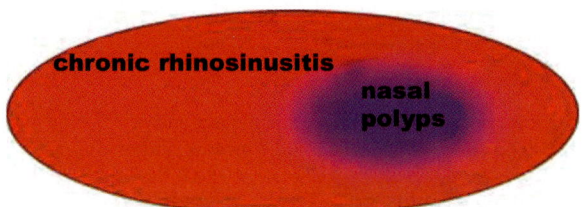

Fig. 4.3 The spectrum of chronic rhinosinusitis and nasal polyps [59]. (Reproduced with permission from Fokkens W, Lund VJ, Mullol J. European position paper on rhinosinusitis and nasal polyps. Rhinology Journal, June 2007 [19].)

of disorders characterized by inflammation of the mucosa of the nose and paranasal sinuses of at least 12 consecutive weeks duration [11]. This early definition by the Rhinosinusitis Task Force of the American Academy of Otolaryngology-Head and Neck Surgery is commonly accepted. However, such a definition has limited clinical utility for the practicing physician. Recently, the *European Position Paper on Rhinosinusitis and Nasal Polyps* clinically defined chronic rhinosinusitis, including nasal polyps, as listed in Table 4.2. Those patients with the following conditions are generally considered to have sinonasal manifestations of a broader pathology:

1. Cystic fibrosis based on positive sweat test or DNA alleles
2. Gross immunodeficiency (congenital or acquired)
3. Congenital mucociliary problems, i.e., primary ciliary dyskinesia (PCD)
4. Noninvasive fungal balls and invasive fungal disease
5. Systemic vasculitis and granulomatous diseases
6. Cocaine abuse
7. Neoplasia

Although these patients may have chronic sinonasal symptoms that are similar to CRS, the treatment will often be directed toward the management of global condition and will not follow classic CRS management paradigms.

The clarification of CRS as a disease from other sinonasal complaints has tremendous benefit both clinically and for research. Sinonasal conditions too broadly defined can lead to a heterogeneous group of patients who clinically may respond poorly to initial treatment and be an unrepresentative group academically. Adoption of the *European Position Paper on Rhinosinusitis and Nasal Polyps* definition for CRS within clinical practice has the potential to better direct treatment, enhancing patient care, and will help provide a greater understanding of the origins of CRS through better defined research populations.

Table 4.2 The current working definition of CRS (as defined by EPOS [19])

Inflammation of the nose and the paranasal sinuses characterized by two or more symptoms, one of which should be either nasal blockage/obstruction/congestion or nasal discharge (anterior/posterior nasal drip):
± facial pain/pressure
± reduction or loss of smell
and either
• endoscopic signs of:
polyps and/or
mucopurulent discharge primarily from middle meatus and/or
edema/mucosal obstruction primarily in middle meatus, and/or
• CT changes:
mucosal changes within the ostiomeatal complex and/or sinuses.
These criteria must be combined with:
more than 12 weeks symptoms without complete resolution of symptoms.

Presenting Symptoms and Differential Diagnoses

CRS can present with significant variability in symptom pattern and intensity. The course of CRS is often characterized by fluctuating symptoms and acute exacerbations. Patient presentations that are dominated by pain or headache, without corresponding nasal obstruction or discharge of similar significance, rarely lead to a diagnosis of CRS as the underlying cause of the presenting complaint. This is true even if there is supporting CT or endoscopic findings of mucosal thickening. Chronic mucosal inflammation is not a classical generator of significant pain. This section describes sinonasal symptoms commonly send in clinical practice and brief differential diagnoses that physicians should keep in mind when evaluating the CRS patient.

Nasal Obstruction/Congestion/Blockage/Stuffiness

Clinical Basis

Nasal obstruction and congestion has a broad interpretability and may encompass a sensation of true mechanical obstruction of airflow to a midfacial fullness. This symptom may be variable and even cyclical. Defining patterns of nasal obstruction with time of day, posture (lying down), during work, or on contact with possible allergens can greatly assist with identifying causes. Chronic inflammation leading to vascular dilatation and narrowed airspace (Fig. 4.4) is likely to account for loss of airflow. Nasal polyps (see Fig. 4.2) and mucosal sensory dysfunction may also be causes.

(a)   (b)

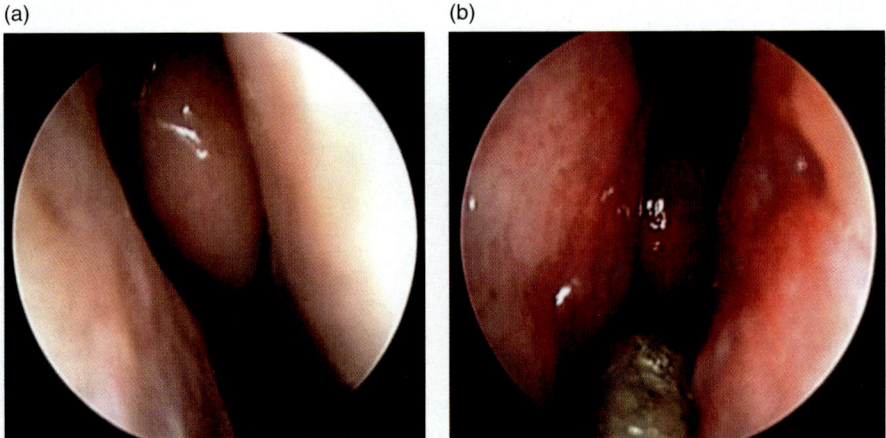

Fig. 4.4 Endoscopic assessment of inflamed mucosa (**a**) compared to normal mucosa (**b**). Photographs were taken of the middle meatus with the same endoscopic, lighting, and recording equipment from one patient with a chronic left maxillary and ethmoid rhinosinusitis and a normal right paranasal sinus system

Fig. 4.5 Septal deviation to
the right. Endoscopic view of
the right nasal cavity

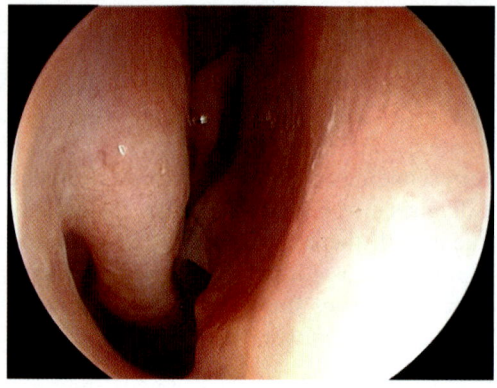

Differential Diagnoses for Nasal Obstruction

1. Septal deviation (Fig. 4.5)
2. Turbinate hypertrophy (Fig. 4.6)
3. Neoplasm (Figs. 4.7, 4.8)
4. Adenoid hypertrophy
5. Rhinitis medicamentosa
6. Nasal valve dysfunction

Objective Evaluation of Nasal Obstruction

Individual perception of nasal obstruction is likely to be highly variable [19]. Thus,
intrapatient assessment of airflow generally has a good correlation with subjective

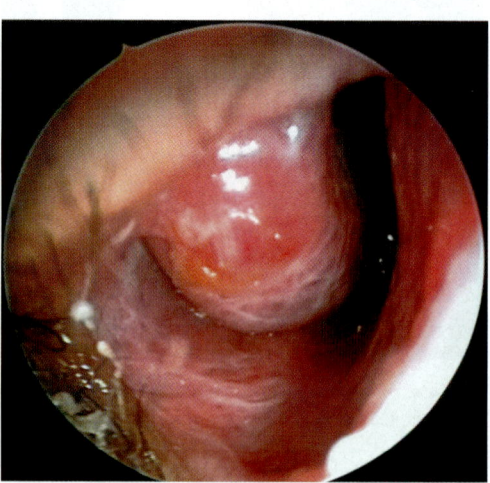

Fig. 4.6 Hypertrophy of the
right inferior turbinate

Fig. 4.7 Nasal tumor. An olfactory neuroblastoma in the left nasal cavity

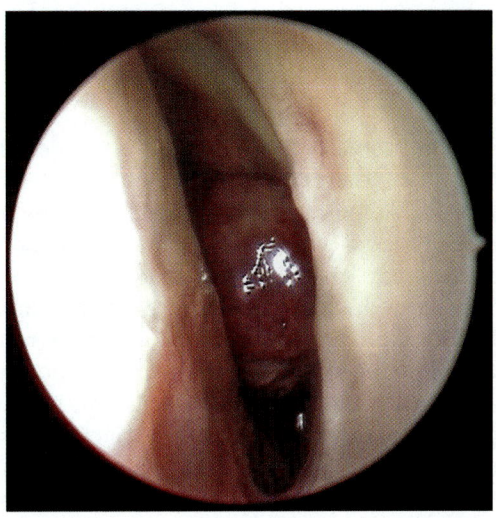

Fig. 4.8 Computed tomography (CT) scan of the nasal tumor in Fig. 4.7

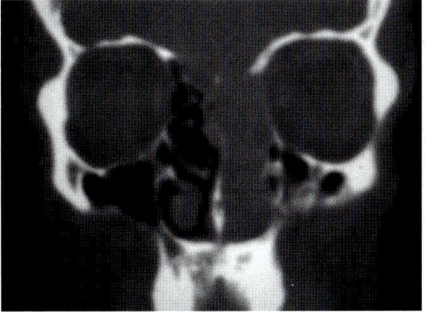

assessment but has limited value in comparison between patients [21,22]. Nasal peak inspiratory flow (NPIF) is a simple and easily performed measurement. It allows "at home" recordings, and patients can create logs of their flow rate in a similar fashion to peak expiratory flow measurements in asthmatics. It is effort dependent and may give large test–retest variability if not performed correctly. Normal NPIF rates for men are 143 L/min (SD48.6) and 121.9 L/min (SD36) for women [23]. Other measurements of airflow, such as rhinomanometry, show good correlations with patient-recorded symptoms but, due to complexity in use, are reserved for research and academic units only. Measurements of nasal air space or cross-sectional area, while providing a sensitive objective measurement, do not closely correlate with the symptom of nasal obstruction [24,25]. Acoustic rhinometry and rhinosterometry are examples of these investigations.

Nasal Discharge and Postnasal Drip

Clinical Basis

The inflammatory mucus that is produced in CRS is commonly discolored (Fig. 4.9). The exudate can be either an eosinophilic- or neutrophilic-dominated process. A constant anterior nasal discharge may be evident by local excoriations around the nasal vestibule from contact and constant nose blowing. Dorsal nasal creases may have also formed from years of handkerchief use and nasal rubbing. There may be a perception of discharge draining posteriorly or "postnasal drip." Examination of the oropharynx may demonstrate purulent secretions on the lateral and posterior walls. True purulent secretions can produce this symptom, but it can also be a manifestation of changes in mucous rheology with hydration or local pharyngeal inflammation with irritants such as laryngopharyngeal reflux. Unilateral and very malodorous secretions should prompt further investigation for dental infection or a foreign body. Similarly, watery unilateral discharge should raise suspicion of a cerebrospinal fluid (CSF) leak. Examination for the beta-2 transferrin protein will identify CSF.

Differential Diagnoses for Nasal Discharge

Foreign body
Allergic rhinosinusitis
Nonallergic rhinosinusitis
CSF leak
Rheological changes to normal mucus production with hydration
Laryngopharyngeal reflux

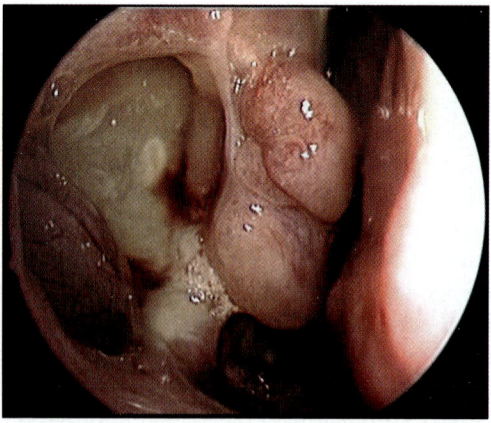

Fig. 4.9 Typical thick eosinophilic mucin of chronic rhinosinusitis (CRS). There is also cystic degeneration of the right maxillary sinus mucosa

Objective Evaluation

Measurements of the amount of nasal discharge are extremely difficult. Subjective recording alone is likely to produce very wide interpatient assessments. Counting tissues or handkerchiefs along with weighing tissues have been used in studies but this method remains of limited use clinically [26]. A sample may be produced for demonstration of color. However, if culture or collection is required, then a direct endoscopic collection from the middle meatus is required. This is currently the gold standard for collecting mucopurulent discharge and replaces previous puncture and aspiration of the maxillary sinus [27].

Facial Pain, Ache, Headache, and Pressure

Clinical Basis

A patient with facial pain alone or as the dominating symptom in the presenting complaint is rarely a consequence of CRS. Minimal production of nociceptive products in CRS has brought the concept of chronic facial pain as a symptom of CRS into question [28]. Discriminative facial pain in response to sinus mucosal stimulation is also unlikely [29]. However, facial pain parameters within disease-specific quality-of-life measures show good content validity and correlation with global changes in health status [30]. Questions that determine the influence of pain on social, professional, and family activities will assist in evaluating the impact of pain on the presenting profile.

Differential Diagnoses for "Sinus" Pain

> Dental infection
> Migraine
> Atypical migraine/midfacial headache
> TMJ disorders including bruxism
> Trigeminal neuralgia
> Obstructive sleep apnoea

Objective Evaluation of Pain

In acute rhinosinusitis, pain may have a good correlation with the presence and site of disease [31]. However, for patients with CRS, pain is neither a good localizing symptom nor a predictive factor [29,32–34]. Subjective recording of pain on visual analogue scales or as Likert scores may be helpful in assessing a cyclical pattern to the symptom or in measuring a response to treatment.

Reduction or Loss (Anosmia) of Smell

Clinical Basis

Reduction or loss of smell is a common complaint among CRS sufferers and may be the strongest predictor of disease when present [35]. Dysfunction of olfactory epithelium and obstruction of airflow with odorants to the olfactory cleft are both likely to be causes. Appetite is often affected as a significant component of flavor. Questions regarding food, appetite, and weight loss are important. Loss of smell can be a potential health hazard. Failure to detect gas or smoke may have significant consequences for those living alone or responsible for others at home or in the workplace.

Differential Diagnoses for Loss of Smell

    Viral upper respiratory tract infection
    Previous head trauma
    Chemical or toxin exposure
    Adverse drug reaction
    Early degenerative brain disease
    Anterior cranial fossa pathology (meningioma)

Objective Evaluation of Smell (Olfaction)

Perhaps the simplest technique to identify smell dysfunction is to use perfume as a screening test. The use of alcohol wipes may be misleading as they may stimulate part of the trigeminal system, which is not involved in odorant detection. Of the variety of semiquantitative and validated objective measures for olfaction, The University of Pennsylvania Smell Identification Test (UPSIT) is perhaps the most well known [36]. It consists of identification of 40 encapsulated odors, each released by a scratch-and-sniff technique; this is followed by a questionnaire. Interpatient correlations and tests for malingering can be made.

Regional Symptoms

Cough

Clinical Basis

Cough is often attributed to chronic postnasal drip. The concept of draining mucopurulent secretions causing a local inflammatory response near the larynx, while lacking an evidence basis, is popular. Exclusion of purulent posterior nasal secretions may be needed to "rule out" a sinus origin in chronic cough of unknown cause. However, the majority of patients with purulent secretions do not complain of cough [37].

Differential Diagnoses for Cough

> Laryngopharyngeal reflux
> Asthma
> Bronchitis (pulmonary infection)
> Aspiration
> Laryngitis
> Laryngeal tumors and masses

Objective Evaluation of Cough

Pulmonary function tests and associated bronchodilator challenge is mandatory for patients with chronic cough. A 15% improvement in FEV_1 combined with clinical features is strongly suggestive of underlying bronchospasm or asthma. Esophageal endoscopy may reveal changes related to gastroesophageal reflux disease. Intrapharyngeal pH probe testing can help to confirm incompetence of the upper esophageal sphincter. Chest radiographs and bronchoscopy may be required to rule out pulmonary causes. Identification of a pharyngeal pouch on barium studies is also useful in the elderly.

Halitosis

Clinical Basis

Strong halitosis, such as cacosmia, should warrant an exclusion of dental pathology or retained foreign body. Exclusion of purulent nasal secretions often forms part of a screening process for those with both subjective and objective halitosis.

Differential Diagnoses for Halitosis

> Periodontal disease
> Gastroesophageal reflux
> Upper aerodigestive tract tumor
> Pharyngeal pouch
> Chronic lingual tonsillitis
> Chronic palatine tonsillitis and tonsilith formation

Objective Evaluation of Halitosis

Apart from confirming with the partner or family member for the presence of objective halitosis, examinations are aimed at excluding other causes. Thorough endoscopy and dental examination form the basis for this. Exclusion of necrotic tumor within the upper aerodigestive tract is essential. Evaluation of reflux and pharyngeal pouch is the same as above.

Warnings and Pitfalls

CRS is often characterized by a long clinical course with fluctuating symptoms. Treatment may be initiated on clinical grounds alone within a primary care setting with follow-up often after many weeks. The potential for delayed diagnosis of significant pathology is great. Sinonasal neoplasms may present with pseudo-CRS symptoms. Careful history usually identifies unilateral symptoms, even if only at the initial onset of complaints. Bleeding can be attributed to aggressive nose blowing; but persistent blood, especially unilaterally, should herald a prompt referral for specialist review. Cacosmia, or offensive smell, which may be evident to the patient and/or others, is often a marker of retained foreign body, dental infection, or neoplasm. There is good correlation between these pathologies on CT and the predominance of cacosmia on history [38] (Fig. 4.10). Table 4.3 highlights some simple clinical flags for non-CRS pathology in patients with chronic sinonasal symptoms.

(a)   (b)

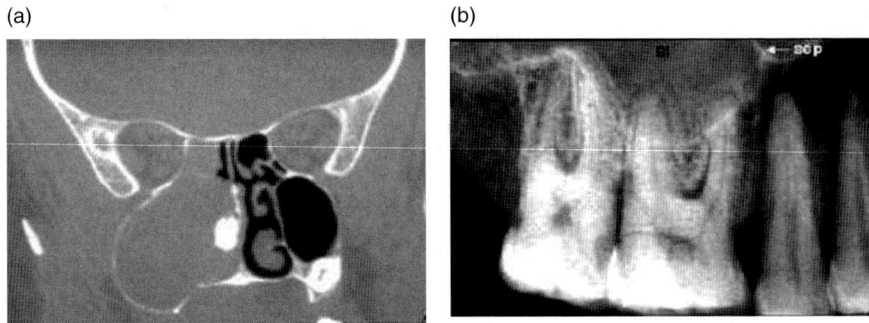

Fig. 4.10 Dental pathology can cause chronic sinonasal symptoms as is evident in (**a**) a CT scan of the maxillary and ethmoid sinuses, showing opacification of both, with a tooth remnant in the maxillary sinus; and (**b**) a plain film demonstrating that the dental roots are closely associated with the maxillary sinus floor

Table 4.3 Clinical features warning of possible non-CRS origin for sinonasal complaints

Sinonasal:
    Unilateral symptoms
    Bleeding
    Crusting
    Cacosmia
Orbital:
    Periorbital edema
    Displacement of the globe
    Dipolpia
    Decreased visual acuity
    Opthalmoplegia (reduced eye movements)
Cranial:
    Severe frontal headache
    Meningism
    Focal neurological deficits
Significant systemic signs

Other Significant Patient History

Medications

Chronic use of nasal decongestants such as oxymetazoline (Afrin®) can produce mucosal hypertrophy and rebound vascular dilation resulting in nasal obstruction. The resulting state is referred to as "rhinitis medicamentosa." This scenario may mimic CRS and should be excluded in all patients. Loss of smell can be the result of adverse drug reactions to a variety of medications. Zinc-containing homeopathic nasal sprays have also been linked to smell dysfunction [39,40].

Past Medical History

Immune deficiency is perhaps an underreported factor in many chronic conditions. Careful evaluation of prior lower respiratory tract disease and childhood infections will help elucidate subtle abnormalities. Low immunoglobulin (Ig)G, IgA, and IgM titers were found in 18%, 17%, and 5% of refractory CRS patients, respectively. Common variable immunodeficiency and selective IgA have also been diagnosed in 10% and 6% of patients within this group [41].

Allergy has always been implicated in CRS, but there is little direct evidence to suggest a strong link in large epidemiologic studies [19]. Asthma and bronchospasm have a very close association with CRS, both with and without nasal polyps. The clinical course of either disease can be significantly altered by addressing each condition [7].

Cyclical changes with menstruation, hormonal abnormalities (such as hypothyroidism), and pregnancy can have an impact on sinonasal symptoms. Up to 20% of pregnant women will experience nasal obstruction [42]. The underlying pathophysiology of these changes has not been widely investigated.

Social History

Direct and second-hand cigarette smoke may have a deleterious effect on the respiratory mucosa in CRS and is currently under investigation [43]. Work environments can provide a significant exposure to occupational antigens and induce contact hypersensitivity or occupational rhinosinusitis. Home environments that are both damp and poorly ventilated may present high volumes of fungus; this may play a role in variety of chronic sinonasal conditions. Cocaine-induced rhinosinusitis should also elicited.

Family History

A strong family history, especially in nasal polyp patients, has provided speculation for a genetic predisposition to CRS. In the families of CRS patients, there is an affected member in 14% to 53% of cases [44,45]. However, this possible genetic relationship has not been demonstrated in monozygotic twin studies [46].

Primary and Secondary Investigations

Nasal endoscopy and CT scans of paranasal sinuses form the foundation of CRS investigation

Endoscopy

Visual assessment of the nasal cavity is an invaluable tool in determining underlying pathological processes. Evaluation can be made with or without decongestion of the nasal mucosa. Oxymetazoline (Afrin®) is commonly used. A local anesthetic spray is usually added but may have little added benefit as mucosal drag is thought to account for any discomfort [47–49]. Assessment can be performed with a 0° or 30° rigid endoscope (Fig. 4.11) or a flexible endoscope (Fig. 4.12).

Mucosal edema (see Fig. 4.4), polyps (see Fig. 4.2), discharge (Fig. 4.13; see also Fig. 4.9), and crusting (Fig. 4.14) form the cardinal endoscopic features of CRS. Mucosal edema and erythema can be somewhat subjective due to differences in lighting, endoscope optics, or camera quality, but are identifiable to an expe-

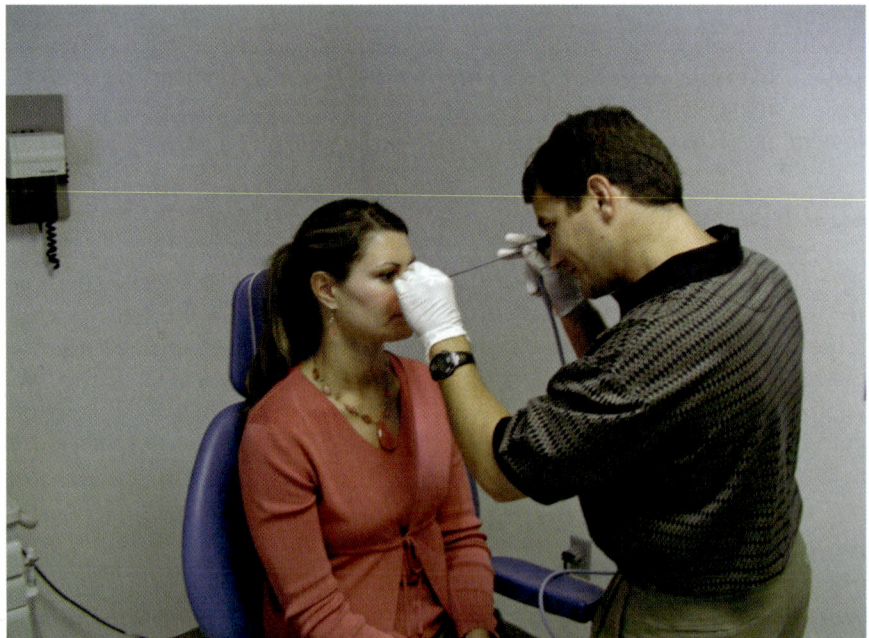

Fig. 4.11 Rigid endoscopy of the nose under topical anesthesia

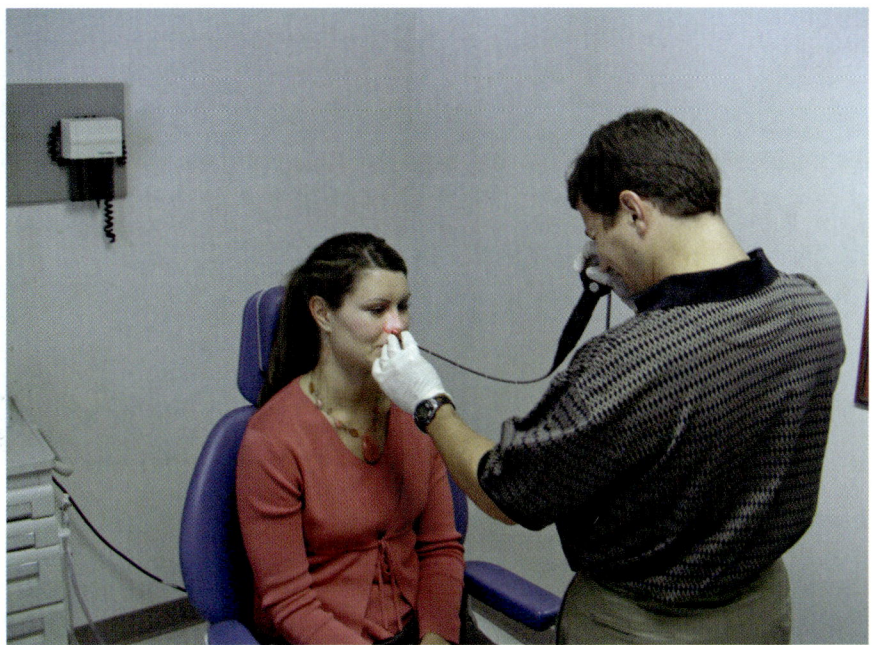

Fig. 4.12 Flexible endoscopy of the nose under topical anesthesia

Fig. 4.13 Purulent discharge
from the left middle meatus
may accompany an acute
exacerbation in CRS

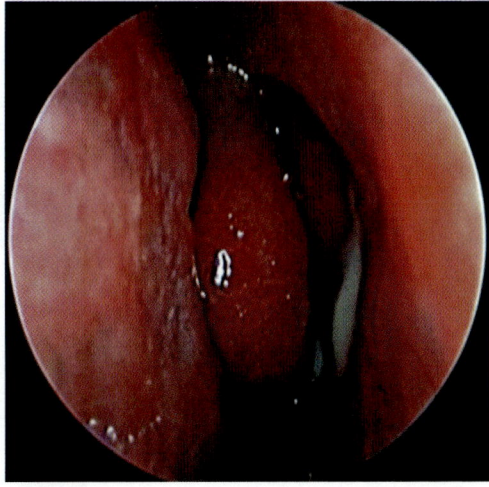

rienced endoscopist. Positive endoscopic findings have a strong correlation with positive CT findings in CRS [50]. However, for negative endoscopic assessments only 71% of patients had negative CT scans in those with chronic nasal complaints without previous sinus operations [50]. Nasal endoscopy has a 67% to 78% negative predictive value (NPV) but offers an excellent positive predictive value [51].

Fig. 4.14 Crusting in the
right nasal cavity

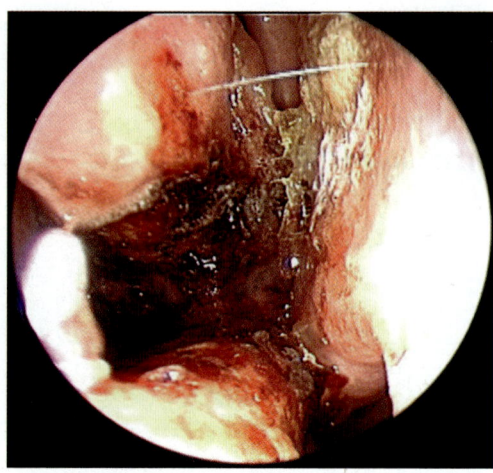

Anterior Rhinoscopy

Anterior rhinoscopy has little role in the diagnosis of CRS. However, it should be
performed on patients examined for CRS for its simplicity and ease in which to
exclude obvious septal deviation (see Fig. 4.5), gross polyposis, or intranasal masses
(Fig. 4.15).

CT Scan

Paranasal sinus computed tomography is performed without intravenous contrast in
the axial position. Modern spiral or helical CT scanners will perform 1- to 3-mm

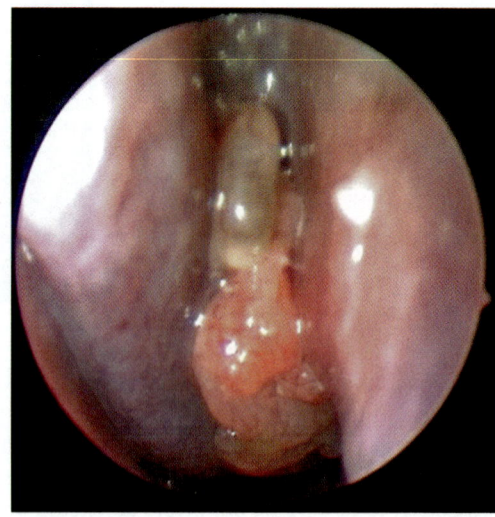

Fig. 4.15 Benign nasal
tumors such as papilloma
may mimic the appearance of
inflammatory polyps.
Unilateral findings should
always prompt referral to a
specialist

axial slices and reconstruct images in the coronal plane. This has several advantages over traditional direct coronal assessment. Dental artefacts, from amalgam or other metal implants, can be avoided in the coronal reconstructions. Patients find a neutral neck position more comfortable, and spiral CT allows scanning of those with cervical arthropathy. Finally, helical or spiral axial imaging is very quick, and many centers may have "in-office" CT scanners dedicated to this process.

CT scans demonstrate mucosal thickening and secretions well (Fig. 4.16). The scans provide an excellent assessment for mucosal thickening but little insight into the nature of the histopathological correlate. Thus, CT scans bear little relevance to the state or severity of the CRS. Neither symptom scores or disease-specific quality-of-life measures correlate with the distribution or degree of CT opacification [52,53].

Even with some minor mucosal thickening taken to be within normal limits (Lund Mackay score below 4), the CT remains a highly sensitive test (94%), although the specificity remains low at 41% [54]. Incidental mucosal cysts can be present in up to 17% and mucosal thickening in 30% of the normal population [55]. Despite some shortcomings in specificity, CT remains an invaluable tool for diagnosing CRS. Symptom-based diagnosis alone is 89% sensitive but only 2% specific [56]. The positive predictive value of symptoms alone, as a diagnostic tool for CRS, is 73% for otolaryngologists and 58% for other physicians when compared to a diagnosis based on combined CT and clinical symptoms [56].

X-Ray

In general, plain sinus X-rays are insensitive and limited in their utility in modern CRS evaluation. False positives and false negatives are high with plain X-rays [57,58]. Underdiagnosis of disease in the anterior ethmoid sinuses and overdiagnosis of maxillary sinus disease are the most common findings in comparative studies [57,58]. Plain sinus radiographs (Water's view) revealing mucous membrane thickening of 5 mm or complete opacification of one or more sinuses are no longer recommended in either the European[19] or American guidelines [11], except for research purposes.

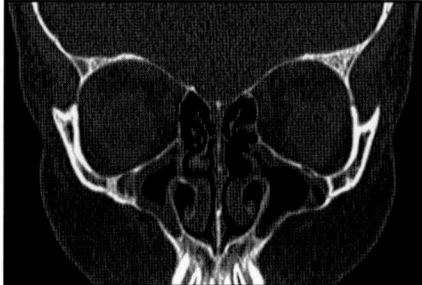

Fig. 4.16 Typical appearances of mucosal thickening in CRS as seen by CT

Secondary Investigations

The majority of additional sinonasal investigations are of limited use in general clinical practice. Some of these tests for olfaction and the nasal airway have already been discussed. These tests are rarely performed routinely outside of speciality practice. It is important for the reader to be aware that objective measures of many of the sinonasal symptoms do exist. The majority of these are used for research, academic, and medicolegal purposes.

Mucociliary dysfunction is often discussed in the context of CRS. Mucociliary transport (MCT) times can be measured. The saccharine clearance time is an often quoted test of MCT. A standard saccharine sweetener tablet is placed 1 cm from the head of the inferior turbinate, and the elapsed time until perception of a sweet taste is recorded. Any time within 20 min is considered within normal limits. Ciliary beat frequency can also be measured under light microscopy after nasal mucosa brushings have been taken. Nasal nitric oxide levels also reflect mucosal inflammatory response and are extremely low in primary ciliary dysfunction. In addition, nasal inflammation can be measured by biopsy, electron microscopy, cytology, bacteriology, and nasal lavage. Peripheral blood leukocyte levels and C-reactive protein have little diagnostic value in the CRS patient.

Diagnostic Schemes

The following diagnostic schemes and clinical workups are currently endorsed by the European Academy of Allergology and Clinical Immunology (EAACI) [19]. These diagnostic pathways combine simple management with evaluation in the

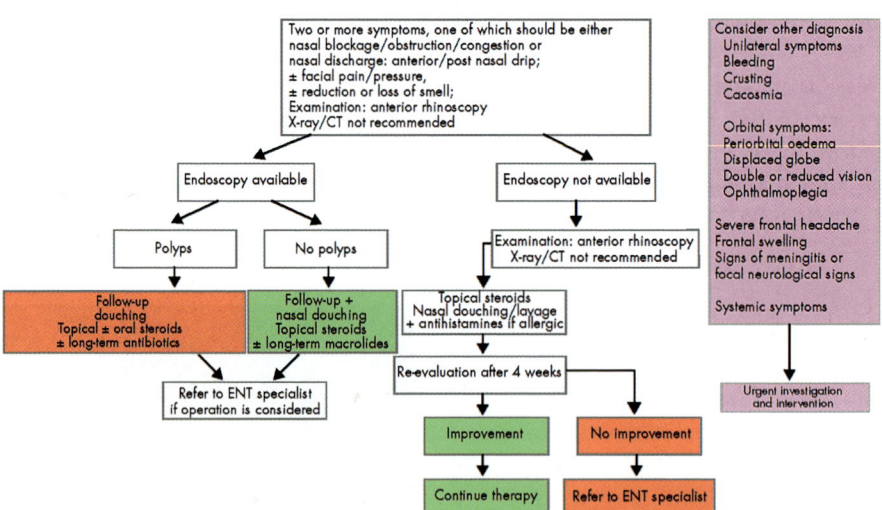

Fig. 4.17 Diagnostic flow chart for adult CRS as recommended by the European position paper on CRS. Simplified management schemes have been provided. (Reproduced with permission from Fokkens W, Lund VJ, Mullol J. European position paper on rhinosinusitis and nasal polyps. Rhinology Journal, June 2007 [19].)

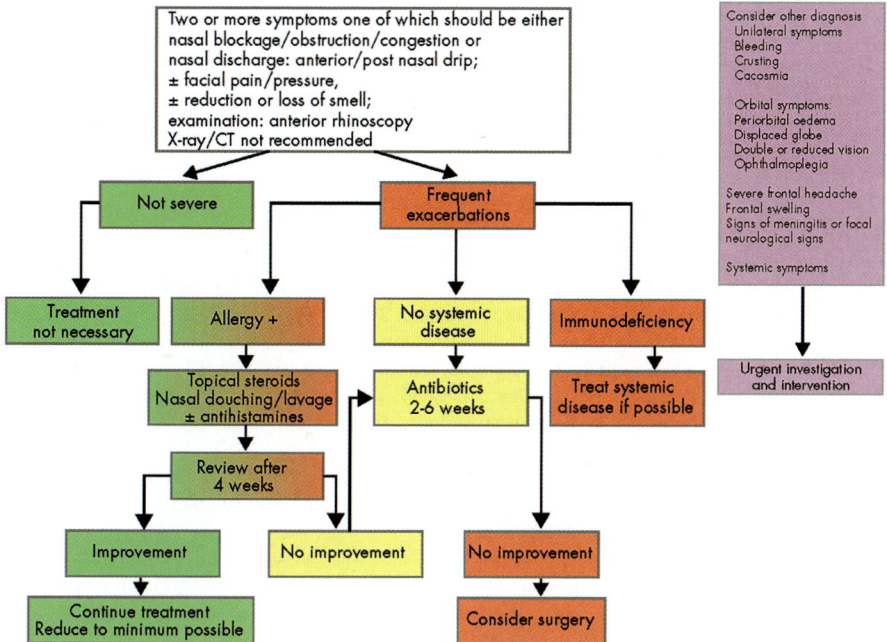

Two or more symptoms one of which should be either
nasal blockage/obstruction/congestion or
nasal discharge: anterior/post nasal drip;
± facial pain/pressure,
± reduction or loss of smell;
examination: anterior rhinoscopy
X-ray/CT not recommended

Consider other diagnosis
Unilateral symptoms
Bleeding
Crusting
Cacosmia

Orbital symptoms:
Periorbital oedema
Displaced globe
Double or reduced vision
Ophthalmoplegia

Severe frontal headache
Frontal swelling
Signs of meningitis or focal
neurological signs

Systemic symptoms

Not severe

Frequent
exacerbations

Treatment
not necessary

Allergy +

No systemic
disease

Immunodeficiency

Urgent investigation
and intervention

Topical steroids
Nasal douching/lavage
± antihistamines

Antibiotics
2-6 weeks

Treat systemic
disease if possible

Review after
4 weeks

Improvement

No improvement

No improvement

Continue treatment
Reduce to minimum possible

Consider surgery

Fig. 4.18 Diagnostic flow chart for pediatric CRS as recommended by the European position paper on CRS. *ENT*, ear-nose-throat. (Reproduced with permission from Fokkens W, Lund VJ, Mullol J. European position paper on rhinosinusitis and nasal polyps. Rhinology Journal, June 2007 [19].)

workup of the CRS patient. They represent good clinical practice founded on the current evidence-based diagnosis and management.

Adult CRS

See Fig. 4.17.

Pediatric CRS

See Fig. 4.18.

References

1. Blackwell DL, Collins JG, Coles R. Summary health statistics for U.S. adults: National Health Interview Survey, 1997. Vital & Health Statistics. Series 10: Data From the National Health Survey. 2002(205): 1–109.
2. Collins JG. Prevalence of selected chronic conditions: United States, 1990–1992. Vital & Health Statistics. Series 10: Data From the National Health Survey. 1997(194): 1–89.
3. Chen Y, Dales R, Lin M. The epidemiology of chronic rhinosinusitis in Canadians. Laryngoscope 2003;113(7):1199–1205.

4. Shashy RG, Moore EJ, Weaver A. Prevalence of the chronic sinusitis diagnosis in Olmsted County, Minnesota. Arch Otolaryngol Head Neck Surg 2004;130(3):320–323.

5. Metson RB, Gliklich RE. Clinical outcomes in patients with chronic sinusitis. Laryngoscope 2000;110(3 pt 3):24–28.

6. Lanza DC, Kennedy DW. Adult rhinosinusitis defined. Otolaryngol Head Neck Surg. 1997;117(3 pt 2):S1–S7.

7. Bousquet J, Van Cauwenberge P, Khaltaev N, et al. Allergic rhinitis and its impact on asthma. J Allergy Clin Immunol. 2001;108(5 suppl):S147–S334.

8. Fokkens W, Lund V, Bachert C, et al. European position paper on rhinosinusitis and nasal polyps. Rhinology Suppl 2005 (18): 1–87.

9. Karlsson G, Holmberg K. Does allergic rhinitis predispose to sinusitis? Acta Oto-Laryngologica Suppl 1994;515:26–28; discussion 29.

10. Harvey RJ, Lund VJ. Biofilms and chronic rhinosinusitis: systematic review of evidence, current concepts and directions for research. Rhinology 2007;45(1):3–13.

11. Benninger MS, Ferguson BJ, Hadley JA, et al. Adult chronic rhinosinusitis: definitions, diagnosis, epidemiology, and pathophysiology. Otolaryngol Head Neck Surg 2003;129 (3 suppl):S1–S32.

12. Roitt IM, Brostoff J, Male DK. Immunology, 5th ed. London: Mosby, 1998.

13. Ragab S, Scadding GK, Lund VJ, et al. Treatment of chronic rhinosinusitis and its effects on asthma. Eur Respir J 2006;28(1):68–74.

14. Hedman J, Kaprio J, Poussa T, et al. Prevalence of asthma, aspirin intolerance, nasal polyposis and chronic obstructive pulmonary disease in a population-based study. Int J Epidemiol 1999;28(4):717–722.

15. Berger G, Kattan A, Bernheim J, et al. Polypoid mucosa with eosinophilia and glandular hyperplasia in chronic sinusitis: a histopathological and immunohistochemical study. Laryngoscope 2002;112(4):738–745.

16. Rudack C, Stoll W, Bachert C. Cytokines in nasal polyposis, acute and chronic sinusitis. Am J Rhinol 1998;12(6):383–388.

17. Hamilos DL, Leung DY, Wood R, et al. Eosinophil infiltration in nonallergic chronic hyperplastic sinusitis with nasal polyposis (CHS/NP) is associated with endothelial VCAM-1 upregulation and expression of TNF-alpha. Am J Respir Cell Mol Biol 1996;15(4):443–450.

18. Larsen K. The clinical relationship of nasal polyps to asthma. Allergy Asthma Proc 1996;17(5):243–249.

19. Fokkens W, Lund VJ, Mullol J. European Academy of Allergology and Clinical I. European position paper on rhinosinusitis and nasal polyps. Rhinology Suppl 2007 (18): 1–87.

20. Dykewicz MS. 7. Rhinitis and sinusitis. J Allergy Clin Immunol 2003;111(2 suppl): S520–S529.

21. Fairley JW, Durham LH, Ell SR. Correlation of subjective sensation of nasal patency with nasal inspiratory peak flow rate. Clin Otolaryngol Allied Sci 1993;18(1):19–22.

22. Simola M, Malmberg H. Sensation of nasal airflow compared with nasal airway resistance in patients with rhinitis. Clin Otolaryngol Allied Sci 1997;22(3):260–262.

23. Ottaviano G, Scadding GK, Coles S, et al. Peak nasal inspiratory flow; normal range in adult population. Rhinology 2006;44(1):32–35.

24. Hirschberg A, Rezek O. Correlation between objective and subjective assessments of nasal patency. J Oto-Rhino-Laryngol Relat Spec 1998;60(4):206–211.

25. Numminen J, Ahtinen M, Huhtala H, et al. Comparison of rhinometric measurements methods in intranasal pathology. Rhinology 2003;41(2):65–68.

26. Ostberg B, Winther B, Borum P, et al. Common cold and high-dose ipratropium bromide: use of anticholinergic medication as an indicator of reflex-mediated hypersecretion. Rhinology 1997;35(2):58–62.

27. Benninger MS, Payne SC, Ferguson BJ, et al. Endoscopically directed middle meatal cultures versus maxillary sinus taps in acute bacterial maxillary rhinosinusitis: a meta-analysis. Otolaryngol Head Neck Surg 2006;134(1):3–9.

28. Jones NS, Cooney TR. Facial pain and sinonasal surgery. Rhinology 2003;41(4):193–200.
29. Abu-Bakra M, Jones NS. Does stimulation of nasal mucosa cause referred pain to the face? Clin Otolaryngol Allied Sci 2001;26(5):430–432.
30. Piccirillo JF, Merritt MG, Jr., Richards ML. Psychometric and clinimetric validity of the 20-Item Sino-Nasal Outcome Test (SNOT-20). Otolaryngol Head Neck Surg 2002;126(1):41–47.
31. Williams JW Jr, Roberts L Jr, Distell B, et al. Diagnosing sinusitis by X-ray: is a single Waters view adequate? [see comment]. J Gen Intern Med 1992;7(5):481–485.
32. Mudgil SP, Wise SW, Hopper KD, et al. Correlation between presumed sinusitis-induced pain and paranasal sinus computed tomographic findings. Ann Allergy Asthma Immunol 2002;88(2):223–226.
33. Daudia AT, Jones NS. Facial migraine in a rhinological setting. Clin Otolaryngol Allied Sci 2002;27(6):521–525.
34. Jones NS. Sinogenic facial pain: diagnosis and management. Otolaryngol Clin N Am 2005;38(6):1311–1325.
35. Bhattacharyya N. Clinical and symptom criteria for the accurate diagnosis of chronic rhinosinusitis. Laryngoscope 2006;116(7 suppl 2):1–22.
36. Doty RL, Shaman P, Dann M. Development of the University of Pennsylvania Smell Identification Test: a standardized microencapsulated test of olfactory function. Physiol Behav 1984;32(3):489–502.
37. O'Hara J, Jones NS. "Post-nasal drip syndrome": most patients with purulent nasal secretions do not complain of chronic cough. Rhinology 2006;44(4):270–273.
38. Bonfils P, Halimi P, Le Bihan C, et al. Correlation between nasosinusal symptoms and topographic diagnosis in chronic rhinosinusitis. Ann Otol Rhinol Laryngol 2005;114(1 pt 1):74–83.
39. Anonymous. Zicam: safe cold cure? Consum Rep 2007;72(1):47.
40. Alexander TH, Davidson TM. Intranasal zinc and anosmia: the zinc-induced anosmia syndrome.[see comment]. Laryngoscope 2006;116(2):217–220.
41. Chee L, Graham SM, Carothers DG, et al. Immune dysfunction in refractory sinusitis in a tertiary care setting. Laryngoscope 2001;111(2):233–235.
42. Ellegard EK. The etiology and management of pregnancy rhinitis. Am J Respir Med 2003; 2(6):469–475.
43. Samet JM. Adverse effects of smoke exposure on the upper airway. Tobacco Control 2004; 13(suppl 1):i57–i60.
44. Greisner WA III, Settipane GA. Hereditary factor for nasal polyps. Allergy Asthma Proc 1996;17(5):283–286.
45. Rugina M, Serrano E, Klossek JM, et al. Epidemiological and clinical aspects of nasal polyposis in France; the ORLI group experience. Rhinology 2002;40(2):75–79.
46. Lockey RF, Rucknagel DL, Vanselow NA. Familial occurrence of asthma, nasal polyps and aspirin intolerance. Ann Intern Med 1973;78(1):57–63.
47. Georgalas C, Sandhu G, Frosh A, et al. Cophenylcaine spray vs. placebo in flexible nasendoscopy: a prospective double-blind randomised controlled trial. Int J Clin Pract 2005;59(2):130–133.
48. Cain AJ, Murray DP, McClymont LG, et al. The use of topical nasal anaesthesia before flexible nasendoscopy: a double-blind, randomized controlled trial comparing cophenylcaine with placebo. Clin Otolaryngol Allied Sci 2002;27(6):485–488.
49. Sadek SA, De R, Scott A, et al. The efficacy of topical anaesthesia in flexible nasendoscopy: a double-blind randomised controlled trial. Clin Otolaryngol Allied Sci 2001;26(1):25–28.
50. Stankiewicz JA, Chow JM. Nasal endoscopy and the definition and diagnosis of chronic rhinosinusitis. Otolaryngol Head Neck Surg 2002;126(6):623–627.
51. Casiano RR. Correlation of clinical examination with computer tomography in paranasal sinus disease. Am J Rhinol 1997;11(3):193–196.
52. Bhattacharyya T, Piccirillo J, Wippold FJ II. Relationship between patient-based descriptions of sinusitis and paranasal sinus computed tomographic findings. Arch Otolaryngol Head Neck Surg 1997;123(11):1189–1192.

53. Kenny TJ, Duncavage J, Bracikowski J, et al. Prospective analysis of sinus symptoms and correlation with paranasal computed tomography scan. Otolaryngol Head Neck Surg 2001;125(1):40–43.
54. Bhattacharyya N, Fried MP. The accuracy of computed tomography in the diagnosis of chronic rhinosinusitis. Laryngoscope 2003;113(1):125–129.
55. Jones NS. CT of the paranasal sinuses: a review of the correlation with clinical, surgical and histopathological findings. Clin Otolaryngol Allied Sci 2002;27(1):11–17.
56. Hwang PH, Irwin SB, Griest SE, et al. Radiologic correlates of symptom-based diagnostic criteria for chronic rhinosinusitis. Otolaryngol Head Neck Surg 2003;128(4):489–496.
57. Iinuma T, Hirota Y, Kase Y. Radio-opacity of the paranasal sinuses. Conventional views and CT. Rhinology 1994;32(3):134–136.
58. McAlister WH, Lusk R, Muntz HR. Comparison of plain radiographs and coronal CT scans in infants and children with recurrent sinusitis [see comment]. AJR Am J Roentgenol 1989;153(6):1259–1264.

Chapter 5
Medical Management of Acute Rhinosinusitis

Richard R. Orlandi

Broadly defined, acute rhinosinusitis is an inflammatory condition of the nose and paranasal sinuses lasting up to 4 weeks [1]. This straightforward definition does not take into account etiology, which is typically, but not always, infectious. Viruses and bacteria are the most common causes of acute rhinosinusitis, with both resulting from, as well as causing, mucosal thickening and trapped mucous secretions. As a result of the upper and lower airways typically reacting in concert, lower airway inflammation may also be a feature of acute upper airway inflammation. Treatment of acute rhinosinusitis, therefore, is aimed not only at causative organisms, but also at the associated inflammation and resulting symptoms.

Chronic rhinosinusitis, defined as symptoms lasting longer than 12 weeks, is a condition separate from acute rhinosinusitis in etiology and pathophysiology. The syndrome of chronic rhinosinusitis appears to be a primarily inflammatory condition, with intermittent acute exacerbations primarily caused by bacteria. The treatments of uncomplicated acute rhinosinusitis and of acute exacerbation of chronic rhinosinusitis both emphasize antimicrobials as the primary modality. Medications to treat the underlying chronic inflammatory condition play a much more important and sustained role in acute exacerbations of chronic rhinosinusitis.

This chapter focuses on treatment of uncomplicated acute bacterial rhinosinusitis (ABRS). Acute viral rhinosinusitis is discussed inasmuch as it may lead to ABRS and its treatment is similar to ABRS, with the exception of the use of antimicrobials. Acute fungal rhinosinusitis, typically invasive and often fatal, affects immunocompromised individuals. It is a rare entity and is not discussed herein [2].

Treatment Strategy

As mentioned previously, inflammation is the hallmark of acute rhinosinusitis, regardless of the etiology. Allergy and trauma may contribute to nasal and sinus inflammation and result in ABRS. Dental infections may directly seed the sinuses

R.R. Orlandi
Division of Otolaryngology – Head and Neck Surgery, University of Utah School of Medicine, Salt Lake City, UT, USA
e-mail: richard.orlandi@hsc.utah.edu

E.R. Thaler, D.W. Kennedy (eds.), *Rhinosinusitis*, DOI: 10.1007/978-0-387-73062-2_5,   65
© Springer Science+Business Media, LLC 2008

with bacteria. Viruses are thought to play a significant role in the pathogenesis of ABRS, with viral upper respiratory tract infections (URIs) commonly preceding episodes of ABRS. Nevertheless, ABRS is an uncommon sequela of viral URIs, complicating less than 2% of them [3]. The exact mechanism by which viral infection can lead to a bacterial one is not entirely clear, although impaired mucociliary clearance through inflammation with colonization from nasal and nasopharyngeal sources is the likely pathogenesis. Cilial transport of secreted mucus can be impaired by viral mucosal injury directly, especially in adenovirus and influenza virus infections. Mucous secretion increases and thickens during inflammation of the respiratory mucosa, further inhibiting transport. Edema may narrow or completely obstruct the sinus drainage pathways, resulting in mucus stasis and favoring bacterial growth [4]. Interestingly, reflux of nasal secretions into the sinuses from nose blowing has recently been demonstrated during a viral URI and may play a prominent role as well [5].

Treatment of acute rhinosinusitis, therefore, is targeted at reducing inflammation and its associated mucociliary transport impairment, in addition to treating causative bacteria. Antiinflammatory agents, decongestants, mucolytics, and other agents therefore may complement antimicrobials in treating ABRS.

Antiinflammatory Therapy

Corticosteroids are effective inhibitors of the inflammatory response in the nasal cavity and sinuses. They are typically delivered as topical nasal sprays and are FDA approved for allergic rhinitis and for some nasal polyps. They are a mainstay of treatment for chronic rhinosinusitis, yet a number of studies have examined their role in the treatment of acute bacterial rhinosinusitis. Previously thought to have too slow an onset of action to be effective in acute rhinosinusitis, recent placebo-controlled trials have demonstrated their efficacy when given with oral antibiotics.

Steroid nasal sprays (SNSs) result in a greater reduction in total symptoms compared to placebo sprays when given with an oral antibiotic [6]. When similar administration was studied specifically in children, earlier reductions in cough and postnasal drip were seen [7,8]. In patients with recurring acute rhinosinusitis, SNSs have been shown to improve the global symptoms of acute episodes, especially those related to "obstruction" such as headache, congestion, and facial pain [9]. Patients with acute exacerbations of chronic rhinosinusitis also have improved outcomes, similar to those with recurring episodes [10]. An interesting study compared double-dosing of an SNS to a standard dose of amoxicillin (500 mg three times a day) in uncomplicated acute rhinosinusitis. The SNS without antibiotic showed a greater improvement in total and major symptoms than the antibiotic alone, raising the question of the relative importance of antimicrobial as compared to antiinflammatory treatment [11].

These studies have used radiologic or symptomatic criteria for inclusion and may, therefore, include some patients with viral or other nonbacterial etiologies. Additionally, the treatment effect is rather small, although the sprays have been well tolerated. These medications are rather expensive, so the more rapid and greater degree of reduction in symptoms must be weighed against their expense. Nevertheless, evidence of sustained improvement after initial resolution and even superiority over traditional antibiotic therapy are compelling arguments for their inclusion in the treatment of ABRS.

Topical delivery of corticosteroids, especially short-term use, results in a minuscule and clinically irrelevant absorption of the drug. Systemic short-term delivery of oral corticosteroids, however, results in much greater systemic levels with numerous potential side effects; these include immunosuppression, impaired wound healing, peptic ulcer, easy bruising, elevation of blood glucose, elevation of blood pressure, elevation of intraocular pressure, water retention, potassium and calcium loss, and emotional lability. Rarely, short-term use has been associated with aseptic necrosis of the hip or shoulder or even psychosis, which appear to be rare idiosyncratic reactions. Because of the severity of these side effects, oral corticosteroids should be used cautiously in cases of acute rhinosinusitis and as infrequently as possible. Typical clinical scenarios for their use might include refractoriness to appropriate antibiotic therapy or the presence of accompanying lower airway symptoms.

Macrolide antibiotics (erythromycin, clarithromycin, and azithromycin) have a unique place in the treatment of acute rhinosinusitis. In addition to their antimicrobial effects, these agents have shown evidence of modulating the inflammatory response, separate from their effect on bacteria. They inhibit eosinophilic inflammation, alter cytokine production, influence the rheology of mucus, reduce goblet cell secretion, and increase mucociliary transport [12]. Numerous studies have demonstrated their antiinflammatory effect in chronic sinus and pulmonary conditions [13]. The mechanism of these actions is not entirely clear, but may involve inhibition at the transcriptional level, similar to that seen with corticosteroids [14,15]. Their antiinflammatory effects have been postulated to diminish symptoms in acute infections as well [16]. The antiinflammatory effects of macrolide antibiotics may augment their clinical efficacy in ABRS.

Other antiinflammatory agents, such as leukotriene inhibitors, have not been examined in acute rhinosinusitis.

Decongestant Therapy

Mucosal edema appears to play a significant role in the pathogenesis and symptomatology of ABRS. Nasal congestion, pressure, and obstruction result from swelling of the respiratory mucosa. Decongestants are common components of over-the-counter sinus medications, and many patients report symptomatic relief with either topical or systemic use. These alpha-adrenergic agents, delivered either topically or systemically, act on smooth muscle in the mucosal vasculature, decreasing blood flow and thereby reducing mucosal edema.

Very little objective work has been done to investigate the efficacy of decongestant therapy in ABRS. A few early studies centered on the usefulness of phenylpropanolamine, use of which has since been discontinued in the United States due to concerns over its association with cerebral hemorrhage. One study found phenylpropanolamine inferior to amoxicillin in resolving acute rhinosinusitis [17]. Another found no improvement with the addition of phenylpropanolamine and an antihistamine to antibiotic therapy in children [18]. No other efficacy studies with oral decongestants in acute rhinosinusitis have been published. With regard to topical decongestants, histological examination of rabbits with induced ABRS found increased inflammation on the sides treated with oxymetazoline. The investigators postulated that this finding may be due to decreased blood flow caused by the decongestant [19]. Nevertheless, one group has found a salutary effect of decongestants, finding improved mucociliary clearance in acute rhinosinusitis following topical treatment with oxymetazoline. This effect was greater than that seen with topical nasal corticosteroids [20].

Decongestants, therefore, lack clear objective evidence to support their efficacy, notwithstanding their widespread use in acute rhinosinusitis and their theoretical benefit in promoting sinus drainage patency. In fact, one study in rabbits calls decongestant use in ABRS into question. The alpha-adrenergic effects of decongestants can worsen hypertension and can cause urinary obstruction in men with prostatic hypertrophy. Topical therapy lasting longer than 3 to 5 days can result in rebound edema, known as rhinitis medicamentosa. Prolonged topical use can lead to atrophic rhinitis as well.

In patients without contraindications to their use, however, decongestants may provide significant symptomatic relief during episodes of ABRS. Their judicious use may be indicated in ABRS absent strong clinical evidence to the contrary.

Antihistamine Therapy

Antihistamines are frequently combined with decongestants in over-the-counter sinus preparations. Although the inflammation from inhalant allergies predisposes individuals to ABRS, there is little evidence that treatment of ABRS with antihistamines is effective. Some have argued against the use of antihistamines, particularly first-generation drugs, postulating that their anticholinergic effects may thicken mucus and inhibit its transportation. No evidence exists to support this claim either, although an anticholinergic-induced decrease in mucous production may yield significant symptomatic relief. The sedative effects of first-generation antihistamines likely counteract the stimulation caused by decongestants, thereby legitimizing their combination.

Anticholinergic Therapy

Ipratropium bromide nasal spray is effective in reducing nasal discharge. Its anticholinergic properties act directly on mucous glands, diminishing their production. Historically, experts have argued against the use of antihistamines because of the potential for anticholinergic thickening of secretions. No studies have evaluated the effect of anticholinergic therapy in ABRS. Ipratropium bromide has the potential to provide symptomatic relief of nasal discharge during ABRS, although it also may worsen or prolong the condition by possible inhibition of mucus transportation. In the absence of any evidence, it is difficult to weigh the risks and benefits of its use in ABRS.

Mucous Transport Therapies

Mucolytics and saline spray or irrigation have been recommended for the treatment of ABRS to assist with the transport of mucus from the sinuses. Little or no evidence exists to either support or refute these recommendations. Mucolytics such as guaifenesin are common ingredients in sinus preparations and theoretically may enhance the transport of mucus out of the sinuses, although no studies evaluate their use in ABRS. Nevertheless, guaifenesin has a very favorable risk–benefit profile, encouraging its use in the absence of evidence to the contrary.

Saline, either isotonic or hypertonic, may be delivered into the nasal cavity by spray, irrigation, or nebulization. Little, if any, of the saline enters the sinuses, instead affecting the anterior nasal cavity [21]. Evidence for or against nasal saline treatment in ABRS is scant and contradictory. Inasmuch as these treatments are typically inexpensive and low in risk, any potential benefit weighs in favor of their use.

Antimicrobial Therapy

ABRS is the fifth most common diagnosis for which antibiotics are prescribed in the United States, accounting for 9% of pediatric and 21% of adult antibiotic prescriptions [22]. The specific aim of antibiotic treatment is, of course, to eliminate the causative pathogen. Clinically, the goal is to provide quicker relief of symptoms. ABRS, proven by positive cultures, still has a relatively high spontaneous recovery rate, estimated at about 50% for both adults and children [22]. Roughly one-third of patients suspected of ABRS who undergo sinus puncture and culture have negative culture results. Sinus puncture and culture is rarely done outside a clinical research setting, so that nearly all patients with community-acquired suspected ABRS are diagnosed based on clinical signs and symptoms alone. When these additional culture-negative patients, likely with viral URIs, are included in the overall analysis, the spontaneous resolution rate in a clinical setting climbs even higher, closer to 60% to 65% [22].

There is little evidence that untreated or poorly treated acute bacterial rhinosinusitis becomes chronic rhinosinusitis. Instead, chronic rhinosinusitis appears to be primarily an inflammatory disorder. While the cause or causes of chronic rhinosinusitis have not yet been elucidated, clinical experience indicates this condition is more insidious in onset and not typically associated with a persistent acute infection. Treatment of ABRS should therefore not be initiated as a strategy to prevent development of chronic rhinosinusitis.

Similarly, antimicrobial treatment of ABRS to prevent intracranial or orbital complications of sinus bacterial infections has little evidence to support it. Although these complications of ABRS are potentially very serious, they are extremely rare and there is no evidence that antimicrobial agents prevent them. Instead, host factors (such as age and gender) and individual pathogen virulence properties appear to play a more prominent role.

Differentiating viral from bacterial rhinosinusitis can be challenging, as previously discussed in Chapter 3. Combining this diagnostic dilemma with the high spontaneous resolution rate and low rate of complications of ABRS, it becomes obvious that many antibiotics are unnecessarily prescribed and consumed. This overprescribing results in a selection of nasal and nasopharyngeal flora resistant to these agents. The health care provider must therefore make every effort to determine the likelihood of bacterial rhinosinusitis and treat the patient accordingly. When there is a question about viral versus bacterial etiology, the patient's symptoms are relatively mild, and there are no comorbidities such as immunocompromise that make an untreated ABRS intolerable, withholding antimicrobials is a reasonable strategy [23]. In these patients, use of nonantimicrobial therapies outlined previously, combined with patient education, may be the best treatment strategy. On the other hand, when symptoms are moderate to severe or comorbidities require quick resolution and the clinical suspicion of bacterial etiology is high, antimicrobial agents should be employed.

Making the difficult decision of whether to prescribe antibiotics is only the first half of the battle. Making an objective choice as to which one, or even which class, can be equally troublesome. Community-acquired ABRS is predominantly caused by *Streptococcus pneumoniae* or *Haemophilus influenzae* in adults. These organisms, combined with *Moraxella catarrhalis*, cause most cases in children. In acute exacerbations of chronic rhinosinusitis, *Staphylococcus aureus* and other staphylococcal species, as well as gram-negative organisms, are more commonly cultured.

Numerous guidelines and analyses have examined antimicrobial therapies in ABRS and have made recommendations based on predicted efficacy [22–28]. These estimates take into account in vitro bacteriostatic and bacteriocidal activity, pharmacokinetic and pharmacodynamic parameters, pathogen prevalence, resistance patterns, and other indices [22]. Sophisticated mathematical modeling has been used to weigh these factors objectively [29]. These mathematical models do not, however, take into account other factors that affect antibiotic efficacy, such as patient compliance, side effects, cost, and safety. Compliance plays a large role in real world efficacy, so that an antibiotic that is dosed once or twice a day may be much more effective than an antibiotic dosed four times a day, regardless of in vitro data. Similarly, a drug with a bitter aftertaste or one associated with objectionable side effects may lead the patient to prematurely terminate the course of therapy, leading to failure and potential antibiotic resistance. Other factors not taken into account in guidelines based solely on in vitro data are the potential *positive* side effects, such as the antiinflammatory effects of macrolide antibiotics discussed earlier.

A final consideration in evaluating guideline recommendations is the numerous clinical studies comparing antibiotics. Statistically, these studies are almost always insufficiently powered to demonstrate superiority, but rather typically demonstrate equivalency between the two antibiotics being considered. While this practice does raise a statistically relevant concern, one must question whether this problem is clinically relevant. In other words, if a study must accumulate hundreds more patients to show statistical superiority, is such a difference *clinically* important?

Taking all these factors into consideration, what antibiotic should be prescribed to patients with moderate to severe ABRS? Most guidelines recommend high-dose amoxicillin, up to 4000 mg per day for adults. Despite recent concerns over resistance, especially among *S. pneumoniae*, this strategy appears to remain effective. This drug can be dosed twice a day and is well tolerated, enhancing compliance. Moreover, it is relatively inexpensive. In regions or in patients with high predicted rates of resistance, addition of clavulanate to the amoxicillin appears to improve the symptom resolution rate, but this is associated with increased gastrointestinal side effects. Second-line therapy for amoxicillin failures or patients with penicillin allergies may include any of a number of antibiotics. Respiratory quinolones and ketolides appear to have superior in vitro results, but macrolides may have dosing and antiinflammatory advantages. Cephalosporins are another alternative with poor in vitro results, but with moderately favorable dosing regimens for second- and third-generation agents.

Length of therapy is another consideration where there is little solid evidence to guide treatment. Most ABRS antibiotic regimens aim for maintaining serum or tissue levels above minimal inhibitory concentrations for 7 to 10 days. Such treatment is typically sufficient. Shorter regimens have been introduced for some agents, again based on studies powered to show equivalence. Thus, there are limited clinical data to support these shorter regimens.

Patients with acute exacerbations of chronic rhinosinusitis have a much higher chance of having gram-negative or resistant bacteria. These patients are best treated based on culture results, when possible. In the absence of these, amoxicillin-clavulanate, respiratory quinolones, or ketolides may have the best chance of effectively resolving a patient's symptom flare. The antiinflammatory and rheological effects of macrolide antibiotics make them another possible choice. The underlying inflammation and impaired mucociliary clearance in these patients suggests a longer course of therapy is likely needed regardless of the antibiotic chosen.

For patients who fail antibiotic therapy, a culture to determine the causative bacterium and to what agents it is sensitive can be helpful. Blind swabbing of the nasal cavity is not effective in determining the bacteriology of the sinuses, yet swabbing of the middle meatus under direct visualization, typically with a nasal endoscope, appears to correlate well with samples obtained from maxillary sinus puncture [30,31]. Similar to antral puncture, nasal endoscopy with culture of the middle meatus is not necessary for uncomplicated cases of acute bacterial

Fig. 5.1 View of the left
nasal cavity using a 0°,
4.0-mm nasal telescope,
demonstrating purulence in
the middle meatus, lateral to
the middle turbinate

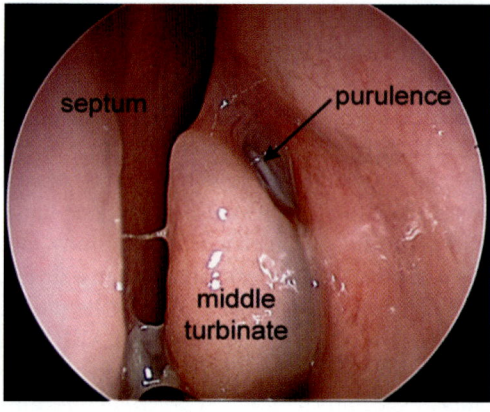

rhinosinusitis, but can be quite helpful in conditions that persist despite effective
first- or second-line therapy (Fig. 5.1).

Conclusion

Acute bacterial rhinosinusitis has inflammatory as well as microbial components.
Treatments aimed at controlling the inflammatory edema and impaired mucociliary
clearance, in combination with eradicating the causative bacteria, are likely to be
most effective. There are limited data for many interventions—such as decongestants, antihistamines, and mucolytics—yet they are typically safe and may provide
salutary effects in ABRS. Limited data support the use of nasal steroids, but there is
significant cost associated with this therapy, limiting its application. Antibiotics may
be withheld in patients with mild symptoms or in cases where a bacterial etiology
remains questionable. Many of these cases will resolve spontaneously, even where
bacteria are present. In moderate to severe cases of ABRS, the practitioner must take
into account in vitro data, local resistance patterns, cost, compliance, side effects,
and safety in choosing an antibiotic. Numerous guidelines support the use of amoxicillin as a first-line therapy, although few data exist to differentiate second-line
antimicrobials.

References

1. Benninger MS, Ferguson BJ, Hadley JA, et al. Adult chronic rhinosinusitis: definitions,
   diagnosis, epidemiology, and pathophysiology. Otolaryngol Head Neck Surg 2003;129(3
   suppl):S1–S32.
2. Ferguson BJ. Definitions of fungal rhinosinusitis. Otolaryngol Clin N Am 2000;33(2):
   227–235.
3. Gwaltney JM Jr. Acute community-acquired sinusitis. Clin Infect Dis 1996;23(6):1209–1223;
   quiz 1224–1225.

4. Orlandi RR, Kennedy DW. Surgical management of rhinosinusitis. Am J Med Sci 1998; 316(1):29–38.
5. Gwaltney JM Jr, Hendley JO, Phillips CD, et al. Nose blowing propels nasal fluid into the paranasal sinuses. Clin Infect Dis 2000;30(2):387–391.
6. Nayak AS, Settipane GA, Pedinoff A, et al. Effective dose range of mometasone furoate nasal spray in the treatment of acute rhinosinusitis. Ann Allergy Asthma Immunol 2002;89(3): 271–278.
7. Meltzer EO, Orgel HA, Backhaus JW, et al. Intranasal flunisolide spray as an adjunct to oral antibiotic therapy for sinusitis. J Allergy Clin Immunol 1993;92(6):812–823.
8. Yilmaz G, Varan B, Yilmaz T, et al. Intranasal budesonide spray as an adjunct to oral antibiotic therapy for acute sinusitis in children. Eur Arch Otorhinolaryngol 2000;257(5):256–259.
9. Meltzer EO, Charous BL, Busse WW, et al. Added relief in the treatment of acute recurrent sinusitis with adjunctive mometasone furoate nasal spray. The Nasonex Sinusitis Group. J Allergy Clin Immunol 2000;106(4):630–637.
10. Dolor RJ, Witsell DL, Hellkamp AS, et al. Comparison of cefuroxime with or without intranasal fluticasone for the treatment of rhinosinusitis. The CAFFS Trial: a randomized controlled trial. JAMA 2001;286(24):3097–3105.
11. Meltzer EO, Bachert C, Staudinger H. Treating acute rhinosinusitis: comparing efficacy and safety of mometasone furoate nasal spray, amoxicillin, and placebo. J Allergy Clin Immunol 2005;116(6):1289–1295.
12. Rhee CS, Majima Y, Arima S, et al. Effects of clarithromycin on rheological properties of nasal mucus in patients with chronic sinusitis. Ann Otol Rhinol Laryngol 2000;109(5): 484–487.
13. Gotfried MH. Macrolides for the treatment of chronic sinusitis, asthma, and COPD. Chest 2004;125(2 suppl):52S–60S; quiz 60S–61S.
14. Wallwork B, Coman W, Mackay-Sim A, et al. Effect of clarithromycin on nuclear factor-kappa B and transforming growth factor-beta in chronic rhinosinusitis. Laryngoscope 2004;114(2):286–290.
15 Wallwork B, Coman W, Feron F, et al. Clarithromycin and prednisolone inhibit cytokine production in chronic rhinosinusitis. Laryngoscope 2002;112:1827–1830.
16. Bishai WR. Macrolide immunomodulatory effects and symptom resolution in acute exacerbation of chronic bronchitis and acute maxillary sinusitis: a focus on clarithromycin. Expert Rev Anti Infect Ther 2006;4(3):405–416.
17. Axelsson A, Jensen C, Melin O, et al. Treatment of acute maxillary sinusitis. V. Amoxicillin azidocillin, phenylpropanolamine and pivampicillin. Acta Otolaryngol 1981;91(3-4): 313–318.
18. McCormick DP, John SD, Swischuk LE, et al. A double-blind, placebo-controlled trial of decongestant-antihistamine for the treatment of sinusitis in children. Clin Pediatr (Phila) 1996;35(9):457–460.
19. Bende M, Fukami M, Arfors KE, et al. Effect of oxymetazoline nose drops on acute sinusitis in the rabbit. Ann Otol Rhinol Laryngol 1996;105(3):222–225.
20. Inanli S, Ozturk O, Korkmaz M, et al. The effects of topical agents of fluticasone propionate, oxymetazoline, and 3% and 0.9% sodium chloride solutions on mucociliary clearance in the therapy of acute bacterial rhinosinusitis in vivo. Laryngoscope 2002;112(2): 320–325.
21. Orlandi RR. Biopsy and specimen collection in chronic rhinosinusitis. Ann Otol Rhinol Laryngol Suppl 2004;193:24–6.
22. Anon JB, Jacobs MR, Poole MD, et al. Antimicrobial treatment guidelines for acute bacterial rhinosinusitis. Otolaryngol Head Neck Surg 2004;130(1 suppl):1–45.
23. Acute rhinosinusitis in adults. 2005 [cited 2007]. Available from: http://cme.med.umich.edu/pdf/guideline/rhino05.pdf.
24. Marple BF, Brunton S, Ferguson BJ. Acute bacterial rhinosinusitis: a review of U.S. treatment guidelines. Otolaryngol Head Neck Surg 2006;135(3):341–348.

25. Respiratory Illness in Children and Adults (Guideline). 2007 [cited 2007]. Available from: http://www.icsi.org/guidelines_and_more/guidelines__order_sets___protocols/respiratory/ respiratory_illness_in_children_and_adults__guideline_/respiratory_illness_in_children_and_ adults__guideline__13110.html.
26. Acute Bacterial Sinusitis Guideline Team CCsHMC. Evidence-based care guideline for management of acute bacterial sinusitis in children 1–17 years of age. 2006 [cited]. Available from: http://www.cincinnatichildrens.org/svc/alpha/h/health-policy/ev-based/sinus.htm.
27. Snow V, Mottur-Pilson C, Hickner JM. Principles of appropriate antibiotic use for acute sinusitis in adults. Ann Intern Med 2001;134(6):495–497.
28. Ip S, Fu L, Balk E, et al. Update on Acute Bacterial Rhinosinusitis. Evidence Report/ Technology Assessment No. 124. (Prepared by Tufts-New England Medical Center Evidence-based Practice Center under Contract No. 290-02-0022). AHRQ Publication No. 05-E020-2. 2005. Agency for Healthcare Research and Quality, Rockville, MD.
29. Poole MD. A mathematical therapeutic outcomes model for sinusitis. Otolaryngol Head Neck Surg 2004;130(1 suppl):46–50.
30. Vogan JC, Bolger WE, Keyes AS. Endoscopically guided sinonasal cultures: a direct comparison with maxillary sinus aspirate cultures. Otolaryngol Head Neck Surg 2002;122(3): 370–373.
31. Meltzer EO, Hamilos DL, Hadley JA, et al. Rhinosinusitis: developing guidance for clinical trials. Otolaryngol Head Neck Surg 2006;135(5 suppl):S31–S80

Chapter 6
Medical Management of Chronic Rhinosinusitis

Rakesh K. Chandra

Appropriate medical management of chronic rhinosinusitis (CRS) requires a thorough understanding of the dynamics of the disease process, which is often multifactorial. Furthermore, the spectrum of factors at work in any individual patient varies depending on medical comorbidities, atopic status, whether the patient has had sinus surgery, and regional geographic variations. As for any other local or systemic inflammatory disease, treatment outcomes in CRS certainly depend on the patient's general medical condition. This aspect mandates diagnosis and management of diabetes and any immunodeficiency, as well as control of air quality and smoking cessation. Unfortunately, however, the dominant driving force behind the chronic inflammatory process is often idiopathic, and a final common biochemical pathway is yet to be elucidated. Nonetheless, it is clear that the pathophysiology is far more complex than merely representing a prolonged bacterial infection or a simple allergic phenomenon.

CRS as a pathological process is better understood as a chronic inflammatory disease rather than an infectious disease, although microorganisms do play a significant role in the progression and exacerbation of the condition. The clinical syndrome of CRS, as has been defined elsewhere in this text, may be further described according to phenotypic presentation as CRS with nasal polyps (CRSwNP) or CRS without nasal polyps (CRSsNP). Prevailing thought is that these entities represent distinct disease processes, whereby CRSwNP tends to demonstrate a T-helper 2 (Th2) cytokine profile [interleukin (IL)-4, IL-5, IL-13] and eosinophilic inflammation, while CRSsNP tends to exhibit a T-helper 1 cytokine profile and neutrophilic inflammation. This distinction may also have therapeutic implications.

A number of metabolic, genetic, or inflammatory disease states may be associated with the syndrome of CRS, including various immunodeficiencies, cystic fibrosis (CF), aspirin sensitivity triad (asthma, aspirin allergy, and rhinosinusitis/nasal polyposis), ciliary diskinesia, and allergic fungal sinusitis (AFS). Phenotypic

R.K. Chandra
Department of Otolaryngology – Head and Neck Surgery, Northwestern University Feinberg School of Medicine, Chicago, IL, USA
e-mail: RickChandra@hotmail.com

characterization, as well as recognition of underlying disease processes, is critical in the selection of appropriate medical therapy.

Multiple theories have been proposed for the development of CRS (with or without nasal polyps) in the absence of definable underlying conditions. These ideas address the roles of atopy, osteitis [1], bacterial biofilms [2], bacterial superantigens [3], and defects in innate immunity [4]. Others have even demonstrated that fungi may stimulate the cascade immune responses seen in some patients with CRS, in the absence of florid AFS. In any individual patient, one or more of these processes may be at work. The present chapter addresses medical management of the CRS patient, with or without polyps, in the context of known and hypothesized pathophysiologies of the disease process. Although a standardized algorithm or a "one size fits all" approach cannot be applied in the management of CRS, our state of knowledge to date does permit definition of key treatment principles. Medical treatments can broadly be divided into agents that address the target of the inflammatory reaction (particularly antimicrobial therapy) and agents which modulate the inflammatory reaction itself (immunomodulatory therapies).

Microbiology and Antibiotic Selection

Selection of Routine Antibiotic Therapy

The bacteria isolated in CRS differ significantly from those observed in acute rhinosinusitis [5]. In the latter condition, the most commonly isolated organisms include pneumococcus, *Haemophilus influenzae*, and *Moraxella catarrhalis*. In contrast, CRS often exhibits *Staphylococcus aureus* and gram-negative rods, particularly *Pseudomonas aeruginosa*. Coagulase-negative staphylococci are also frequently isolated [6], although the pathogenic role of this organism may be questionable as it is a known normal inhabitant of the nasal vestibule. Cultures in the setting of CRS (and acute exacerbations of CRS) may also reveal the same organisms observed in acute rhinosinusitis, enteric gram-negatives, and anaerobes. Polymicrobial infections are often observed, with one study demonstrating a mean of 2.5 organisms per cultured specimen [7]. The pattern of bacteria isolated also varies between pre- and postsurgical CRS patients in that the latter are even more likely to exhibit gram-negative organisms, particularly pseudomonas. Greater than one-third of specimens in one study revealed a mixture of aerobic and anaerobic organisms, and the overall prevalence of beta-lactamase production was more than 50% [7]. Antibiotic resistance is an increasing concern, particularly in settings where broad-spectrum antibiotics are overprescribed, and where antibiotics are utilized for likely viral upper respiratory infections. Resistance of *Pseudomonas* to quinolones is also a mounting problem.

The unique bacterial milieu encountered in CRS underscores the importance of culture-directed therapy. One study even demonstrated that data from cultures result in modification of the antibiotic selection in more than 50% of cases [8]. Before the endoscopic era, paranasal sinus culture required antral puncture with aspiration of

Fig. 6.1 Nasal endoscopy with culture swab of the right middle meatus. Note the presence of purulent material admixed with polypoid mucosal changes

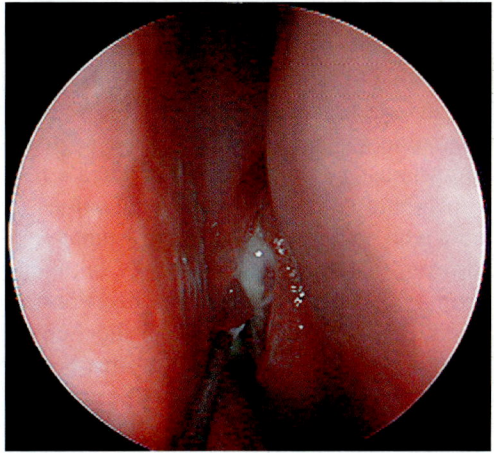

the maxillary sinus through the bone of either the canine fossa or lateral nasal wall. Recent studies suggest, however, that swab or aspiration of middle meatal secretions via endoscopic guidance (Fig. 6.1) provides an accurate assessment. Furthermore, this technique has the advantages of being less invasive and better tolerated than antral puncture [9]. Long-term medical management of CRS patients who have undergone prior functional endoscopic sinus surgery (FESS) includes regular endoscopic evaluations, where purulent material can be visualized and cultured (Fig. 6.2), thus permitting medical treatment prior to a full-blown symptomatic exacerbation.

In cases where empiric choices are required, broad-spectrum therapy should be selected, which may include the use of amoxicillin/clavulanate, respiratory quinolones (i.e., levofloxacin), or combination therapy such as clindamycin plus trimethoprim/sulfamethoxazole. There is no consensus regarding the exact length of antibiotic treatment for CRS, although a systemic course of at least 3 weeks is

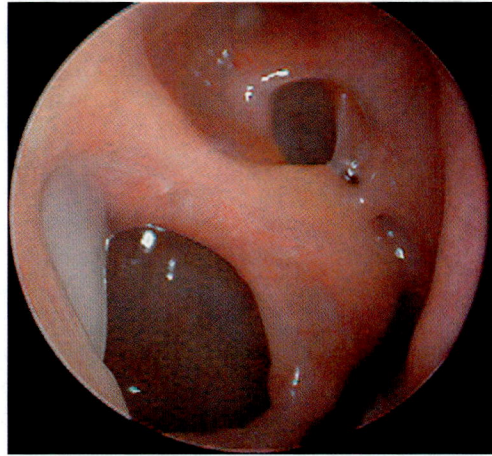

Fig. 6.2 Nasal endoscopy in a patient who has undergone prior functional endoscopic sinus surgery (FESS). Purulent discharge is observed in the region of natural outflow from a patent right maxillary antrostomy

recommended [10]. Although there is no randomized controlled evidence to validate this practice, rationale for such prolonged therapy can be inferred post hoc from studies that have demonstrated the unique mechanisms of bacterial pathogenicity at play in CRS (described below) compared to those observed in acute rhinosinusitis.

Antibiotic therapy, as discussed up to this point, implies oral administration. Intravenous (IV) antibiotics may have a role in selected cases, such as in patients with orbital or intracranial complications (or pending complications), as well as those who manifest organisms resistant to oral antibiotics. It should be underscored, however, that a clear benefit of IV antibiotics in the management of routine CRS has not been demonstrated. The decision to select IV antibiotics must therefore be based on the patient's overall medical condition and the organisms cultured [11]. This choice must be weighed against consideration of costs and complications of IV therapy; particularly because the use of IV antibiotics does not preclude relapse, and most oral antibiotics penetrate the paranasal sinus mucosa at levels exceeding the minimum inhibitory concentration of target bacteria.

Unique Roles of Bacteria in CRS

The treatment of *S. aureus* is particularly important in light of recent data suggesting that this organism may drive the chronic inflammatory process by mechanisms that are distinct from traditional inflammatory pathways. A growing body of research has implicated exotoxins liberated by *S. aureus* as being capable of activating diverse populations of T lymphocytes by directly linking the major histocompatibility II marker on antigen-presenting cells to the beta chain of the T-cell receptor. This linkage results in a localized response consisting of various cytokines and polyclonal IgE, ultimately leading to eosinophil recruitment and polyp formation. This pathway has been suggested as a relevant mechanism, or at least a disease modifier, in the development of CRSwNP in some patients [3,12]. Why other patients with CRSwNP do not exhibit evidence of this pathophysiology remains unknown. Nonetheless, this exciting area of investigation provides provocative support for including empiric treatment for *S. aureus* in the medical management of CRSwNP, irrespective of culture results.

Rabbit models of experimentally induced rhinosinusitis, using both *S. aureus* and *P. aeruginosa*, have revealed extension of inflammation through the Haversion canal system, suggesting the condition may reflect a form of osteomyelitis [1]. The need for prolonged antibiotic treatment, as well as higher doses, is also supported by the observation that many of the bacteria implicated in CRS may exist in the form of a biofilm. Bacterial biofilms represent three-dimensional aggregates of bacteria that have been demonstrated on both inanimate and biological surfaces, including mucosa of the middle ear and sinonasal tract. Bacteria that exist as biofilms may exhibit increased antibiotic resistance secondary to their group properties, thus necessitating increased antibiotic exposure for bacteriocidal effect that is required for planktonic bacterial forms. Whether this can even be achieved with conventional oral or IV antibiotic therapy is presently unknown, and this is an area of active investigation [2].

Novel Antibiotic Delivery Methods

Recent trends have explored the role of various topical delivery methods for antibiotics, including nebulization and irrigation. In theory, this approach may allow use of antibiotics such as aminoglycosides that cannot be administered orally, but without necessitating IV therapy. Topical treatment may also theoretically achieve antibiotic concentrations at the mucosal surface that are not achievable by systemic administration and may spare the systemic side effects of oral or IV antibiotics. Most studies reporting experience with topical antibiotic preparations have utilized this modality in patients who have undergone prior FESS; this is an important caveat given that penetration of topical medications is minimal into sinuses that have not been surgically opened [13]. Thus, topical antibiotic administration is not considered a substitute for systemic therapy in patients whose sinuses have not been opened surgically.

Nebulized antibiotics are often utilized in the management of pulmonary infections in CF patients, and limited studies have shown potential benefit of nebulized antibiotics in CRS. One investigation suggested that CRS patients who underwent prior FESS achieved a prolonged infection-free period after the addition of nebulized antibiotics to their therapeutic regimen [14]. These data must be interpreted with caution, because there is a paucity of controlled studies with extended followup to validate the efficacy of nebulized antibiotics in CRS [15]. In addition, there are studies demonstrating that nebulized materials are less likely than topical irrigants to penetrate the sinus lumen, even in patients who have undergone surgery [16].

Use of a nebulizer requires the patient to obtain special equipment. In contrast, topical irrigation can be accomplished with a bulb syringe, turkey baster, or any one of several commercially available bottles. Various antibiotic solutions have been described, but as with nebulized antibiotics, the majority of studies report clinical outcomes with limited follow-up, and little is known regarding exact drug levels within the sinus lumen, mucosal lining, or the underlying bone. An initial report in this area described the use of tobramycin irrigations in CF patients with nasal polyposis who underwent FESS. Those who utilized postoperative irrigations had a significantly lower rate of revision surgery than those managed without irrigations (27% vs. 88%) [17]. Tobramycin is typically utilized at a concentration of 80 mg per liter of normal saline, and the patient is instructed to irrigate each nostril with 50 mL twice daily. Gentamicin irrigations may also be utilized at this same concentration and volume. It is hypothesized that far greater concentrations (approximately four times the concentrations described above) may be necessary to disrupt bacterial biofilms [2]. It should be noted, however, that studies have demonstrated systemic absorption and even potential ototoxicity with aminoglycoside sinus irrigations even at 80 mg/L [18], so that elevated concentrations cannot be used with impunity. This is an area of active ongoing investigation.

Another topical antibiotic irrigation that has been described, which averts the concern of aminoglycoside toxicity, is ceftazidime (0.6 mg/mL) irrigated at 50 mL to each nostril three times daily [19]. Aminoglycosides and ceftazidime are utilized to target gram-negative bacilli, particularly *Pseudomonas*, which may not be sensitive to oral medications. Anecdotally, this may avert the need for IV therapy in selected patients, particularly those whose sinus cavities have been well opened surgically.

Methicillin-resistant *Staphylococcus aureus* (MRSA) can also be a difficult organism to manage with conventional oral therapies. When this bacterium is isolated, patients may be treated with mupirocin irrigations. Mupirocin is available as an ointment prepared in a water-miscible base. One-third of a 22.5-g tube is added to 1 L normal saline, and the patient is instructed to irrigate each nostril with 50 mL twice daily. One study has suggested that this agent may help to avert the need for IV antibiotics in patients with MRSA when combined with appropriate oral antibiotics [20]. Again, it should be noted that drug levels delivered to the sinus lumen, as well as to the mucosa and underlying bone, are unknown. MRSA and many strains of enterococcus can even be controlled by irrigation with a solution of 10 mL providine-iodine per liter of normal saline. Each nostril is irrigated with 50 mL twice daily. The advantage of this preparation is that it is broad spectrum and nonspecific in its microbicidal activity; thus, resistance is not a concern. However, further study is necessary to determine the effects of providine-iodine on the normal biology of paranasal sinus mucosa, including mucociliary function.

In summary, many patients with CRS, particularly following FESS, are treated with saline nasal irrigations for ongoing mechanical debridement of irritants, pollen, bacteria, and fungi. Antibiotic solutions, such as those described above, are a useful adjunct when the patient exhibits persistent purulent accumulations by office endoscopy. It should be noted, however, that there are no controlled studies to date demonstrating the efficacy of antibiotic-containing irrigations compared to saline alone. Nonetheless, augmenting the efficacy of topical medical therapy is an important frontier inspired by the identification of paranasal sinus biofilms. High-dose topical antibiotics may avert the need for IV therapy in selected patients. Ongoing investigation has even explored the role of various detergents for disruption of biofilms.

Role of Fungi and Antifungal Therapy

Another area of intense investigation has been the role of fungi in CRS. Recent data have demonstrated that fungi are ubiquitous within the nose in normal subjects as well as in patients with CRS. The fungal hypothesis of CRS suggests that affected individuals may manifest an abnormal or exaggerated immune response to fungi. The mechanism of this exaggerated response may relate to IgE-mediated responses, but there is a significant body of evidence to support a role for non-IgE-dependent pathways. In the latter scheme, fungal antigens are able to directly stimulate Th2-type inflammatory cascades, which results in eosinophil influx, eventually leading to the clinical syndrome of CRS with possible polyp formation. Among the fungi evaluated, *Alternaria* was implicated as the most vigorous trigger of T-helper cytokines (particularly IL-5 and IL-13) and eosinophil degranulation [21,22]. Some have hypothesized that this is the underlying mechanism of all forms of eosinophilic CRS and that classic AFS merely reflects the end stage of the disease process [23]. This matter of great debate has inspired investigation of the role of antifungal antibiotics in the management of CRS.

Initial studies exhibited favorable subjective and objective results using amphotericin B irrigation in patients with CRS [24]. Objective improvement was established by changes seen by computed tomography (CT), but it should be noted that the use of amphotericin B was not associated with decrease in *Alternaria* antigen load within the nose, which calls into speculation whether the improvement was secondary to specific fungicidal effect or secondary to mechanical effects of irrigation. Another much larger multicenter, double-blind, placebo-controlled investigation of the therapeutic value of amphotericin irrigations revealed no benefit in any of the subjective or objective parameters studied [25]. Similar findings were observed in a randomized placebo-controlled trial with oral turbinafine [26], where no improvement was seen in any of the subjective or objective (radiologic) parameters after 6 weeks of therapy. Even in patients who had positive fungal cultures, no benefit was demonstrated. The authors hypothesized that either fungi were not a major pathophysiological force in the development of CRS or that the drug may have failed to reach therapeutic levels in the mucus. The preponderance of the data reviewed here does not support a role for antifungals in the routine management of CRS, with or without polyps. These data also call into question the exact role of fungi in the pathophysiology of typical CRS. Antifungals may be considered in refractory cases where other conventional therapies have failed, but the use of these medications must be weighed against issues such as cost, drug toxicity (e.g., hepatotoxicity), and the ubiquitous nature of fungi in the environment and the sinonasal tract. It should be noted, however, that some retrospective noncontrolled data suggest that oral antifungal therapy (itraconazole) may reduce need for revision FESS in patients with classic AFS [27], and thus it may be more strongly considered in this disease process.

Immunomodulatory Therapies

Intranasal Corticosteroids

As CRS can best be considered an inflammatory disease, it is not surprising that corticosteroids have become a cornerstone of management. By reducing the underlying inflammation, corticosteroids decrease obstruction of nasal airflow and sinus drainage and thus may facilitate mucociliary clearance of allergens, irritants, bacteria, and fungi. These medications may be administered topically or locally, as well as systemically. The advantage of topical preparations is that they avert concerns associated with systemic effect, such as elevation of blood glucose and suppression of the hypothalamic-pituitary-adrenal axis [28]. Furthermore, effect on growth velocity in children appears to be negligible [29]. Topical corticosteroid administration is most commonly achieved using one of many commercially available intranasal steroid sprays; and none of the currently available products is thought to induce significant systemic hormonal effects at prescribed doses.

The primary effect of intranasal corticosteroids is to reduce obstructive symptoms secondary to mucosal inflammatory disease from underlying chronic rhinitis or allergic rhinitis, but decreases in the size of nasal polyps and prevention of postoperative polyp recurrence have been observed as well [30]. Intranasal corticosteroids have also been shown to reduce epithelial and subepithelial eosinophilia in patients with allergic rhinitis when comparing mucosal biopsies before and after treatment during pollen season [31]. It remains unclear how and to what degree intranasal corticosteroids may modulate these responses in the setting of CRS, particularly because studies have shown that penetration into the sinus cavity using a metered-dose spray bottle is poor, even in patients who have had prior surgery [13]. Weighing the risks and benefits, however, intranasal corticosteroids are considered a mainstay of long-term medical therapy in CRS patients with or without nasal polyps.

The technique of administration of intranasal corticosteroids has been explored in the literature [32]. To optimize distribution and reduce complications (such as septal erosion or epistaxis), a cross-handed technique is recommended. Patients are instructed to use the right hand to spray the left nostril and the left hand to spray the right nostril; this maximizes delivery to the inferior turbinate, a key structure in the development of congestive symptoms, and also increases the chance of the medication reaching the middle meatus. Various other administration techniques have been explored, and, in selected cases, patients may benefit from steroid instillation with the vertex in a dependent position, such as the "Mecca" position. This technique augments delivery to the middle meatus, frontal recess, or olfactory cleft and may be useful when the endoscopist observes persistent chronic inflammatory disease in these regions. Other head-dependent positions have been described, such as the Mygind position (Fig. 6.3), where the patient lies supine and hangs the head off the edge of the bed. This method appears to be associated with less discomfort than the Mecca position [33]. Other methods of topical steroid application include nasal irrigation with steroid-containing solutions, nebulized steroids, and catheter-assisted steroid instillation.

Various off-label compounded mixtures have been described for irrigation, including mixtures of budesonide with saline at various concentrations. Nebulized steroids, similar to nebulized antibiotics, are administered via specialized commercially available cannulas. Catheter-assisted instillation involves serial infusions of steroid-containing solution through a cannula placed via a surgical sinusotomy. One study examined subjective and objective outcomes of daily infusion of budesonide in postsurgical patients with both CRS and dust mite allergy. After 3 weeks of therapy, data revealed improved symptom scores as well as decreases in eosinophilia and Th2 cytokines compared to placebo controls [34]. In summary, topical nasal steroids can accomplish significant antiinflammatory effect, while

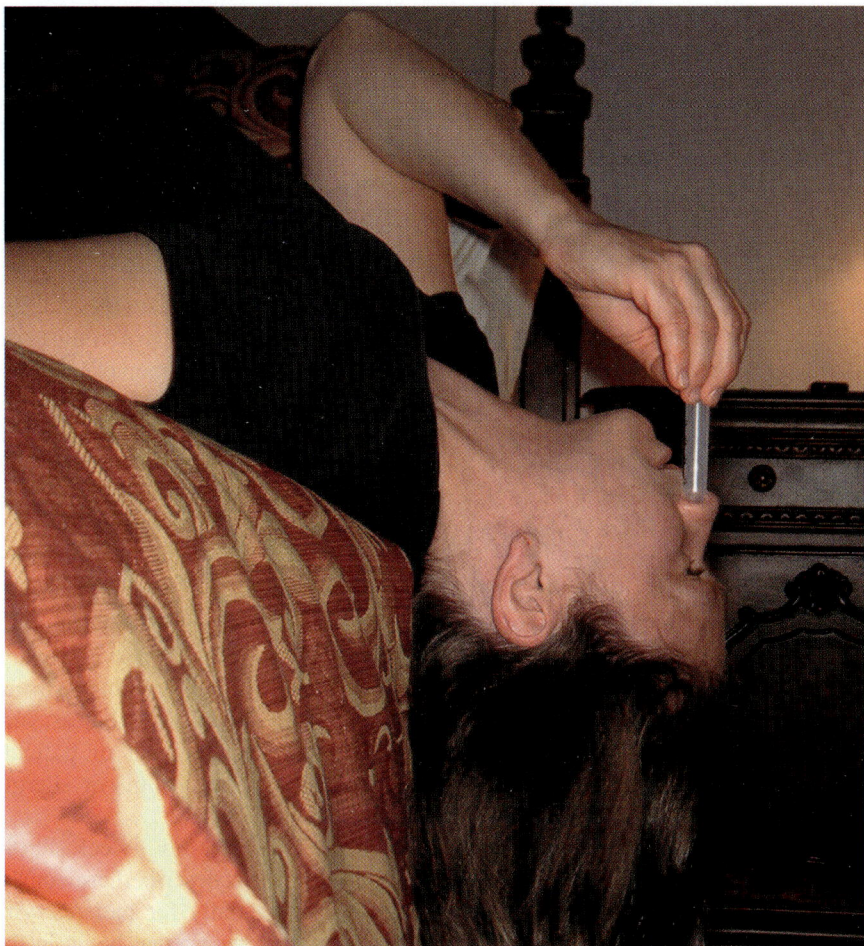

Fig. 6.3 Mygind's position

sparing the patient from side effects and the toxicities of systemic steroids. These medications, therefore, have a vital role in the long-term management of the CRS patient, particularly in postsurgical patients. At the very least, patients with CRS should be treated with intranasal corticosteroid sprays on a long-term basis. Patients should also be monitored regularly by an otolaryngologist for development of complications associated with corticosteroid sprays, such as epistaxis and septal erosion.

For the sake of completeness, intranasal steroid injection deserves note. In this procedure, performed by an otolaryngologist under endoscopic visualization, triamcinolone is injected directly into polyps or persistent/recurrent foci of polypoid change. Some studies have demonstrated a possible reduction in the need for further sinus surgery when patients underwent close endoscopic follow-up with serial injections [35]. Patients should be counseled, however, that blindness is a reported, although remote, risk of this procedure.

Systemic Steroids

The value of systemic steroids in the management of chronic inflammatory respiratory disease is well known, particularly in the treatment of asthma and acute exacerbations of asthma. CRS is often described as "asthma of the nose," and it therefore follows that systemic steroids may take on a similar role in this disease process. In the management of CRS, systemic steroids are typically administered orally in one of the following clinical scenarios: (1) as part of a regimen of maximal medical therapy before considering a patient a candidate for surgery, (2) for use in the perioperative period to reduce the inflammatory burden intraoperatively and to augment optimal healing postoperatively, (3) during exacerbations of CRS, and (4) in management of comorbidities such as asthma or other allergic/inflammatory conditions. Occasionally, IV therapy is needed, such as if the patient suffers an asthma exacerbation or is unable to take oral medications.

Unfortunately, there is no uniform algorithm regarding exactly when steroids are indicated and what the appropriate dosage and length of therapy may be. This clinical judgment is based on balancing the risks and benefits in any individual patient. Systemic steroids must be used with caution in patients with gastrointestinal ulcers, diabetes, cataracts, glaucoma, and osteoporosis. Nonetheless, oral steroids are considered an integral component in the management of patients with CRSwNP or AFS and in selected patients with comorbid asthma or allergic conditions [36].

Before considering surgery, patients may be treated with a 2- to 3-week steroid taper in conjunction with a prolonged course of antibiotics, as described previously. Initial doses of steroids may begin at 30 mg prednisone daily for patients with CRSsNP. In contrast, patients with CRSwNP may require tapers that begin in the range of 60 to 80 mg per day. Responses may be significant (Fig. 6.4), and these regimens will avert the need for surgery in a subset of patients. However, it remains unclear why some patients do not respond adequately or experience rapid recurrence of symptoms after therapy is discontinued. Suggested oral steroid regimens are outlined in Table 6.1.

Patients who fail maximal medical therapy, and those with diffuse sinonasal polyposis or AFS, are typically considered candidates for surgery. Oral steroids may be initiated from a few days to several weeks preoperatively and then continued postoperatively until resolution of mucosal inflammatory disease is observed endoscopically. Patients with AFS may anticipate prolonged courses (up to several months) and higher dosages. Exacerbations of CRS can be treated using tapers such as those described in Table 6.1. Some patients require chronic low-dose steroid therapy, such as prednisone 5 mg daily or 10 mg every other day. Dosages utilized in chronic low-dose therapy are often lower than that which induces axis suppression. Furthermore, the exact mechanism of action of chronic low-dose oral steroids is largely unknown.

(a)

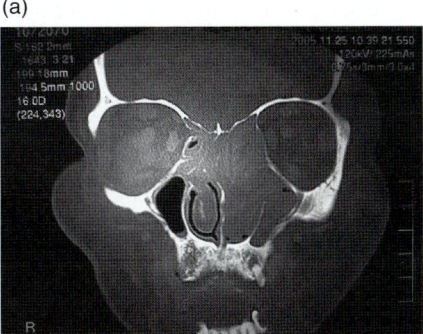

(b)

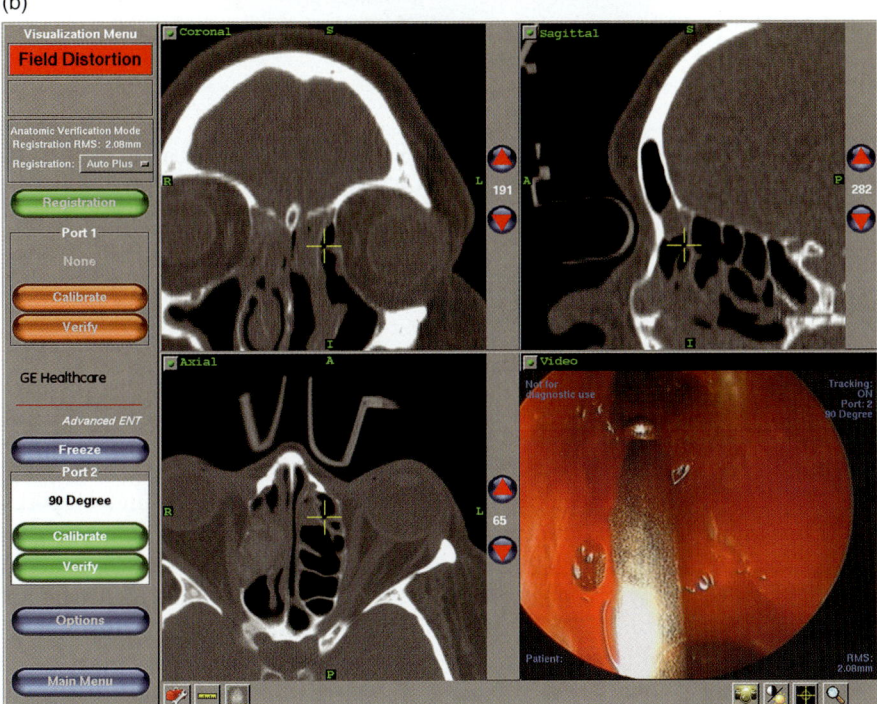

Fig. 6.4 (**a**) Coronal computed tomography (CT) in a patient with allergic fungal sinusitis (AFS). Note the marked paranasal sinus opacification, more pronounced on the patient's left side. (**b**) The patient underwent repeat CT with triplanar reconstruction (for intraoperative navigation) after 4 weeks of oral steroid therapy. Note the significant decrease in sinus opacification, particularly when comparing the coronal projection (*upper left panel*) to the preoperative image

It should be noted that these dosing schemes may require modification based on the patient's body mass index and comorbidities. Patients who require long-term therapy or frequent tapers should undergo frequent monitoring of blood sugar, bone density, and ophthalmologic status.

Table 6.1 Suggested steroid regimens for various clinical scenarios

Scenario	CRSsNP	CRSwNP	AFS
Presurgical treatment trial	30 mg po qD × 3 20 mg po qD × 3 10 mg po qD × 3 10 mg po qOD × 3	30 mg po qD × 3 20 mg po qD × 3 10 mg po qD × 3 10 mg po qOD × 3	30 mg po BID × 3 20 mg po BID × 3 10 mg po BID × 3 10 mg po qD × 3
Perioperative treatment, preoperatively	Steroid use not routine	30 mg po qD × 3 20 mg po qD × 3 Start 6 days preoperatively	30 mg po BID × 7 20 mg po BID × 7 30 mg po qD × 7 Start 3 weeks preoperatively
Perioperative treatment, postoperatively	Steroid use not routine	30 mg po qD continued until endoscopic resolution of disease Then tapered to off over 1 week	30 mg po qD continued until endoscopic resolution of disease Then tapered to off over 1 week
Acute exacerbation	30 mg po qD × 3 20 mg po qD × 3 10 mg po qD × 3 10 mg po qOD × 3	30 mg po qD × 3 20 mg po qD × 3 10 mg po qD × 3 10 mg po qOD × 3	30 mg po qD × 3 20 mg po qD × 3 10 mg po qD × 3 10 mg po qOD × 3

CRS, chronic rhinosinusitis; CRSwNP, CRS with nasal polyps; CRSsNP, CRS without nasal polyps; AFS, allergic fungal sinusitis.

Allergy Management

The exact role of allergic rhinitis in the pathophysiology of CRS remains a matter of some controversy, but incidence of allergic rhinitis does exhibit some correlation with CRS. One review summarized that the prevalence of allergic rhinitis reported in patients with CRS ranges from 25% to 84%, with higher prevalence observed in children and in patients undergoing FESS. This review also suggested that mucosal disease, as measured by CT, is greater in patients with inhalant allergies, and that allergen exposure worsens CRS in most patients with both conditions. Additionally, comorbid allergic rhinitis decreases success rates of FESS [5].

Inhalant allergy induces a Th2 cytokine response, with IgE-mediated histamine release in the early phase and inflammatory cell (e.g., eosinophil) influx in the late phase. In addition to histamine, other preformed mediators, as well as synthesized mediators such as leukotrienes, are also involved. The inflammatory milieu observed in allergic rhinitis leads to intuitive links between this disease and CRS and provides a rationale for incorporating allergy management into the management of CRS. There is no consensus regarding the exact roles of antihistamines or leukotriene inhibitors in therapy for CRS, but long-term use of these medications appears rational in patients with suspected inhalant allergies, and particularly those with positive allergy testing. It should be noted that antihistamines appear to be most beneficial in controlling symptoms of nasal pruritis and rhinorrhea, whereas congestive and obstructive symptoms are more responsive to intranasal corticosteroids. However, relief of obstructive symptoms appears comparable to intranasal steroid when antihistamine is combined with an oral decongestant [37]. Newer-generation, less-sedating antihistamines (loratidine, desloratidine, fexofenadine, cetirizine) should be prescribed, as older-generation, sedating medications (e.g., diphenhydramine) have been associated with significant impairment of alertness and memory [38].

Mucolytics and oral decongestants are potentially useful for symptomatic relief for acute exacerbations of CRS and, occasionally, as long-term therapy. Care must be taken with oral decongestants secondary to potential cardiovascular sympathomimetic side effects. Additionally, extreme care must be taken with the use of topical decongestant nasal sprays, because prolonged (more than 3 to 5 days) use is associated with rebound vasocongestion, or rhinitis medicamentosa. New frontiers in the medical management of allergic rhinitis include also use of omalizumab (Xolair), an anti-IgE monoclonal antibody administered subcutaneously every 2 to 4 weeks. Although omalizumab has been demonstrated to reduce symptoms of allergic rhinitis and asthma, its role in CRS remains unclear. Cost–benefit analysis is an important component to elucidating this issue.

The role of immunotherapy in long-term management of CRS has been the subject of investigation as well. This issue is of particular importance in patients with allergic rhinitis and CRS who undergo FESS, where data has suggested improved outcomes in those who received immunotherapy, except in the presence of nasal polyps [39]. It is possible this lack of observed benefit is secondary to inherent differences in the pathophysiology of CRSwNP, as other studies have demonstrated a higher incidence of polyps in nonallergic patients [40]. Patients with AFS, in contrast, appear to benefit from postoperative immunotherapy [41]. Overall, immunotherapy should be a strong consideration in CRS patients, with or without polyps, who exhibit significant allergies. However, further outcome data are necessary to quantify the benefit of immunotherapy in CRS and in CRS patients who undergo FESS.

Other Immunomodulatory Considerations

Aspirin Desensitization

Patients with CRS in the setting of polyposis, asthma, and aspirin sensitivity represent a difficult group of patients to manage, both medically and surgically. Studies have revealed more vigorous inflammatory disease as well as poorer treatment outcomes compared to aspirin-tolerant patients [42]. Corticosteroids are often necessary in aspirin-sensitive patients for management of both sinonasal and pulmonary components of the disease. In addition to the multiple treatment options described previously in this chapter, aspirin-sensitive patients should also be considered for aspirin desensitization. Patients are treated with escalating doses of aspirin followed by daily maintenance therapy. Protocols for dose escalation vary widely and may be individualized. Outcome studies have revealed success of aspirin desensitization in reducing CRS exacerbations, hospitalizations for asthma, and use of systemic steroids [43].

Macrolide Therapy

Recent investigations have suggested that macrolide antibiotics may manifest anti-inflammatory effects beyond their antimicrobial properties. Excitement about long-term low-dose macrolide therapy began after Japanese reports of efficacy in treating patients with diffuse panbronchiolitis (a condition phenotypically similar to CF in which *Pseudomonas* and a variety of other bacteria may be involved) [44]. This therapy has also been evaluated in patients with CF in whom improved pulmonary function testing was demonstrated after 4 weeks of therapy [45].

Recent literature has suggested that this modality decreases symptoms of nasal obstruction and postnasal drip and reduces the quantity and viscosity of nasal secretions [46]. Authors have also reported decreased size of nasal polyps secondary to macrolide treatment [47]. Laboratory analysis has associated macrolides with reduction of proinflammatory cytokines (IL-1, IL-6, IL-8, leukotriene B4), neutrophil recruitment, and fibroblast proliferation [48,49]. In patients with panbronchiolitis or CF, it is possible that macrolides may retard biofilm formation by *Pseudomonas* and other organisms [50].

Although there is no standardized algorithm for macrolide administration, proposed dosing schemes for adults include clarithromycin 500 mg daily or azithromycin 500 mg every other day, and children may be treated with azithromycin 250 mg every other day [11,45]. Most experts agree that 4 weeks of therapy are necessary before symptomatic relief is realized, but selected patients with recalcitrant CRS may be able to achieve benefits only previously achieved with oral corticosteroids [11]. The practitioner must be familiar with the multiple drug interactions possible with macrolides that may lead to Q-T prolongation. The biochemical mechanism for the immunomodulatory effects of macrolides remains largely unknown.

Summary and Conclusions

CRS is a *chronic inflammatory* disease of multifactorial etiology. Medical treatment continues to evolve and, unfortunately, a standardized treatment algorithm has not been defined to date. It is likely that bacteria do play some role in the disease process, but not in the manner classically observed in acute infections. Thus, antibiotics are a significant component in the management. Patients should be treated with at least 3 weeks of a culture-directed or broad-spectrum oral antibiotic before consideration of surgery. In addition, antibiotic courses may be required postsurgically for acute exacerbations of CRS, where treatment duration is often longer than that required for isolated acute rhinosinusitis. Patients with CRS often benefit from saline nasal irrigation, particularly postsurgically. Furthermore, additional investigation is necessary to clarify the indications and pharmacokinetics of antibiotic-containing saline irrigations. Topical intranasal steroid sprays are considered a mainstay in the long-term management of CRS, but the role of oral steroids varies depending on the clinical scenario. Oral steroids are considered an important component in the management of patients with CRSwNP and, in particular, patients with AFS. Management of allergic rhinitis, which includes medical therapy, immunotherapy, and reduction of antigen exposure (via avoidance and nasal irrigation) can have a significant impact on patient symptoms and outcome. Ongoing research into the pathophysiology of CRS is necessary to develop more focused medical therapies.

References

1. Khalid AN, Hunt J, Perloff JR, Kennedy DW. The role of bone in chronic rhinosinusitis. Laryngoscope 2002;112:1951–1957.
2. Palmer J. Bacterial biofilms in chronic rhinosinusitis. Ann Otol Rhinol Laryngol Suppl 2006;196:35–39.
3. Bachert C, Gevaert P, Zhang N, et al. Role of staphylococcal superantigens in airway disease. Chem Immunol Allergy 2007;93:214–236.
4. Ramanathan M Jr, Lane AP. Innate immunity of the sinonasal cavity and its role in chronic rhinosinusitis. Otolaryngol Head Neck Surg 2007;136:348–356.
5. Benninger MS, Marple BF, Ferguson BJ, et al. Adult chronic rhinosinusitis: definitions, diagnosis, epidemiology, and pathophysiology. Otolaryngol Head Neck Surg Suppl 2003; 129:1–32.
6. Kingdom TT, Swain RE Jr. The microbiology and antimicrobial resistance patterns in chronic rhinosinusitis. Am J Otolaryngol 2004;25:323–328.
7. Brook I. Bacteriology of chronic sinusitis and acute exacerbation of chronic sinusitis. Arch Otolaryngol Head Neck Surg 2006;132:1099–1101.
8. Cincik H, Ferguson BJ. The impact of endoscopic cultures on care in rhinosinusitis. Laryngoscope 2006;116:1562–1568.
9. Tantilipikorn P, Fritz M, Tanabodee J, et al. A comparison of endoscopic culture techniques for chronic rhinosinusitis. Am J Rhinol 2002;16:255–260.
10. Dubin MG, Kuhn FA, Melroy CT. Radiographic resolution of chronic rhinosinusitis without polyposis after 6 weeks vs. 3 weeks of oral antibiotics. Ann Allergy Asthma Immunol 2007;98:32–35.
11. Vining EM. Evolution of medical management of chronic rhinosinusitis. Ann Otol Rhinol Laryngol Suppl 2006;196:54–60.
12. Conley DB, Tripathi A, Seiberling KA, et al. Superantigens and chronic rhinosinusitis: skewing of T-cell receptor V beta-distributions in polyp-derived CD4+ and CD8+ T cells. Am J Rhinol 2006;20:534–539.
13. Hwang PH, Woo RJ, Fong KJ. Intranasal deposition of nebulized saline: a radionuclide distribution study. Am J Rhinol 2006;20:255–261.
14. Vaughan WC, Carvalho G. Use of nebulized antibiotics for acute infections in chronic sinusitis. Otolaryngol Head Neck Surg 2002;127:558–568.
15. Desrosiers MY, Salas-Prato M. Treatment of chronic rhinosinusitis refractory to other treatments with topical antibiotic therapy delivered by means of a large-particle nebulizer: results of a controlled trial. Otolaryngol Head Neck Surg 2001;125:265–269.
16. Miller TR, Muntz HR, Gilbert ME, et al. Comparison of topical medication delivery systems after sinus surgery. Laryngoscope 2004;114:201–204.
17. Moss RB, King VV. Management of sinusitis in cystic fibrosis by endoscopic surgery and serial antimicrobial lavage. Reduction in recurrence requiring surgery. Arch Otolaryngol Head Neck Surg 1995;121:566–572.
18. Whatley WS, Chandra RK, MacDonald CB. Systemic absorption of gentamicin nasal irrigations. Am J Rhinol 2006;20:251–254.

19. Leonard DW, Bolger WE. Topical antibiotic therapy for recalcitrant sinusitis. Laryngoscope 1999;109:668–670.

20. Solares CA, Batra PS, Hall GS, et al. Treatment of chronic rhinosinusitis exacerbations due to methicillin-resistant *Staphylococcus aureus* with mupirocin irrigations. Am J Otolaryngol 2006;27:161–165.

21. Shin SH, Ponikau JU, Sherris DA, et al. Chronic rhinosinusitis: an enhanced immune response to ubiquitous airborne fungi. J Allergy Clin Immunol 2004;114:1369–1375.

22. Inoue Y MY, Shin SH, Ponikau JU, et al. Non pathogenic, environmental fungi induce activation and degranulation of human eosinophils. J Immunol 2005;175:5439–5447.

23. Ponikau JU, Sherris DA. The role of airborne mold in chronic rhinosinusitis. J Allergy Clin Immunol 2006;118:762–763.

24. Ponikau JU, Sherris DA, Weaver A, et al. Treatment of chronic rhinosinusitis with intranasal amphotericin B: a randomized, placebo-controlled, double-blind pilot trial. J Allergy Clin Immunol 2005;115:125–131.

25. Ebbens FA, Scadding GK, Badia L, et al. Amphotericin B nasal lavages: not a solution for patients with chronic rhinosinusitis. J Allergy Clin Immunol 2006;118:1149–1156.

26. Kennedy DW, Kuhn FA, Hamilos DL, et al. Treatment of chronic rhinosinusitis with high-dose oral terbinafine: a double-blind, placebo-controlled study. Laryngoscope 2005;115:1793–1799.

27. Rains BM III, Mineck CW. Treatment of allergic fungal sinusitis with high-dose itraconazole. Am J Rhinol 2003;17:1–8.

28. Allen DB. Systemic effects of intranasal steroids: an endocrinologist's perspective. J Allergy Clin Immunol Suppl 2000;106:179–190.

29. Allen DB. Do intranasal corticosteroids affect childhood growth? Allergy. 2000;55 (suppl 62):15–18.

30. Schleimer RP. Glucocorticoids: their mechanism of action and use in allergic diseases. In: Adkinson NF, Yunginger JW, Busse WW, et al, eds. Middleton's Allergy Principles and Practice. St. Louis: Mosby, 2003:912–914.

31. Pullerits T, Praks L, Ristioja V, et al. Comparison of a nasal glucocorticoid, antileukotriene, and a combination of antileukotriene and antihistamine in the treatment of seasonal allergic rhinitis. J Allergy Clin Immunol 2002;109:949–955.

32. Benninger MS, Hadley JA, Osguthorpe JD, et al. Techniques of intranasal steroid use. Otolaryngol Head Neck Surg 2004;130:5–24.

33. Kubba H, Spinou E, Robertson A. The effect of head position on the distribution of drops within the nose. Am J Rhinol 2000;14:83–86.

34. Lavigne F, Cameron L, Renzi PM, et al. Intrasinus administration of topical budesonide to allergic patients with chronic rhinosinusitis following surgery. Laryngoscope 2002;112:858–864.

35. Becker SS, Rasamny JK, Han JK, et al. Steroid injection for sinonasal polyps: the University of Virginia experience. Am J Rhinol 2007;21:64–69.

36. Landsberg R, Segev Y, DeRowe A, et al. Systemic corticosteroids for allergic fungal rhinosinusitis and chronic rhinosinusitis with nasal polyposis: a comparative study. Otolaryngol Head Neck Surg 2007;136:252–257.

37. Zieglmayer UP, Horak F, Toth J, et al. Efficacy and safety of an oral formulation of cetirizine and prolonged-release pseudoephedrine versus budesonide nasal spray in the management of nasal congestion in allergic rhinitis. Treat Respir Med 2005;4:2830–287.

38. McEvoy LK, Smith ME, Fordyce M, et al. Characterizing impaired functional alertness from diphenhydramine in the elderly with performance and neurophysiologic measures. Sleep 2006;29:957–966.

39. Nishioka GJ, Cook PR, Davis WE, et al. Immunotherapy in patients undergoing functional endoscopic sinus surgery. Otolaryngol Head Neck Surg 1994;110:406–412.

40. Grigoreas C, Vourdas D, Petalas K, et al. Nasal polyps in patients with rhinitis and asthma. Allergy Asthma Proc 2002;23:169–174.

41. Folker RJ, Marple BF, Mabry RL, et al. Treatment of allergic fungal sinusitis: a comparison trial of postoperative immunotherapy with specific fungal antigens. Laryngoscope 1998; 108:1623–1627.
42. Batra PS, Kern RC, Tripathi A, et al. Outcome analysis of endoscopic sinus surgery in patients with nasal polyps and asthma. Laryngoscope 2003;113:1703–1706.
43. Stevenson DD, Hankammer MA, Mathison DA, et al. Aspirin desensitization treatment of aspirin-sensitive patients with rhinosinusitis-asthma: long-term outcomes. J Allergy Clin Immunol 1996;98:751–758.
44. Kudoh S, Azuma A, Yamamoto M, et al. Improvement of survival in patients with diffuse panbronchiolitis treated with low-dose erythromycin. Am J Respir Crit Care Med 1998;157:1829–1832.
45. Saiman L, Marshall BC, Mayer-Hamblett N, et al. Macrolide Study Group. Azithromycin in patients with cystic fibrosis chronically infected with *Pseudomonas aeruginosa*: a randomized controlled trial. JAMA 2003;290:1749–1756.
46. Majima Y. Clinical implications of the immunomodulatory effects of macrolides on sinusitis. Am J Med Suppl 2004;117:20–25.
47. Gotfried MH. Macrolides for the treatment of chronic sinusitis, asthma, and COPD. Chest Suppl 2004;125:52–61.
48. Tamaoki J, Kadota J, Takizawa H. Clinical implications of the immunomodulatory effects of macrolides. Am J Med Suppl 2004;117:5–11.
49. Nonaka M, Pawankar R, Tomiyama S, et al. A macrolide antibiotic, roxithromycin, inhibits the growth of nasal polyp fibroblasts. Am J Rhinol 1999;13:267–272.
50. Gillis RJ, Iglewski BH. Azithromycin retards *Pseudomonas aeruginosa* biofilm formation. J Clin Microbiol 2004;42:5842–5845.

Chapter 7
Endoscopic Sinus Surgery

David W. Kennedy

Before 1985, sinus surgery was typically performed through open surgical approaches. At that time, the maxillary sinus was thought to be the most frequent site of sinus disease and the frontal sinus was considered to be the second most common site. When sinus disease within the maxillary sinus persisted despite medical therapy, one of the concepts was to provide dependent drainage to the sinus through an inferior meatal window, an opening created close to the floor of the sinus. If dependent drainage failed, the concept was then to strip the diseased mucosa from the sinus. Sinus surgery was frequently fraught with failure, and patients often ended up with increasing discomfort, persistent infection, and frequently repeated surgical interventions [1,2].

However, since that time, the results of surgical intervention have significantly improved, as has our understanding of sinusitis and its pathogenesis. In part, this occurred because as improved endoscopes were introduced, physicians both in Europe and in the United States began to use them more frequently for nasal endoscopy (Fig. 7.1). As we did so, we noted the frequency of involvement of the ethmoid sinuses and the adjacent middle meatus in both chronic and acute sinusitis and that, in many cases, this involvement occurred even before the maxillary sinus was affected. It also now became possible to identify endoscopically how inflammation in these areas appeared to affect the larger sinuses, causing obstruction and repeated infection (Figs. 7.2, 7.3) [3]. Around the same time, imaging—initially with polytomography and subsequently computed tomography (CT)—allowed improved radiographic visualization within the complex region of the ethmoid sinuses [4]. The ethmoid sinus area had previously been very poorly visualized on plain films because of the averaging created by the multiple ethmoid cells, cells that become superimposed upon each other and averaged in plain film imaging. CT confirmed what had been identified endoscopically: namely, that the ethmoid sinus was indeed the most frequently involved region in chronic sinusitis.

D.W. Kennedy
Department of Otorhinolaryngology – Head and Neck Surgery, University of Pennsylvania Medical Center, Philadelphia, PA, USA
e-mail: david.Kennedy@uphs.upenn.edu

E.R. Thaler, D.W. Kennedy (eds.), *Rhinosinusitis*, DOI: 10.1007/978-0-387-73062-2_7,
© Springer Science+Business Media, LLC 2008

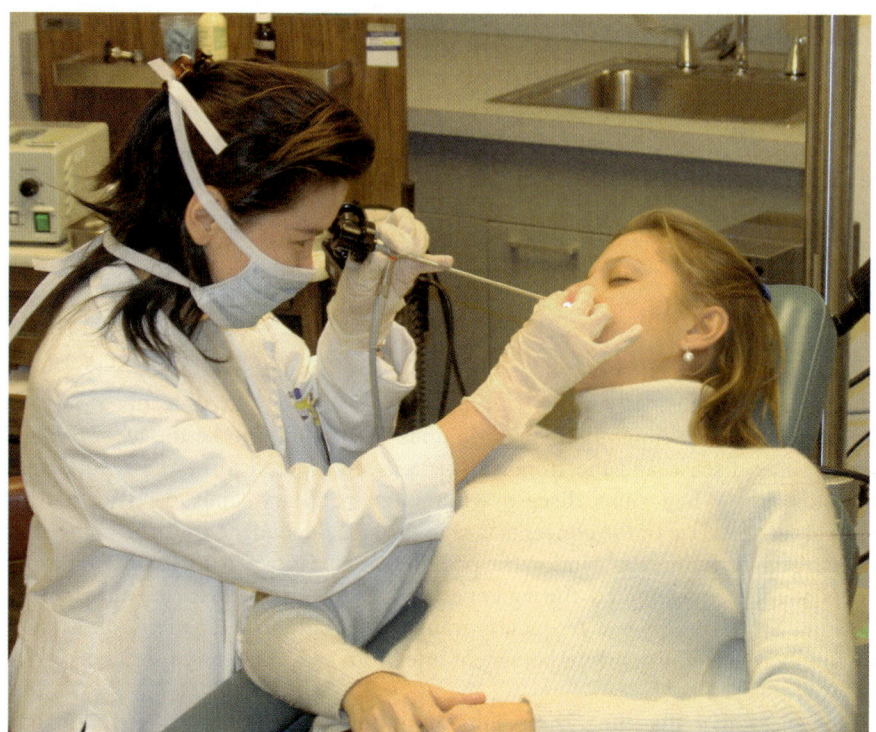

Fig. 7.1 Diagnostic nasal endoscopy under topical anesthesia with the rigid endoscope

We also began to better understand, at this time, the extent to which mucociliary clearance is a very active dynamic process, one that could be identified with microscopic and endoscopic visualization. Additionally, by reperforming experiments initially performed in the first half of the 20th century, we were able to

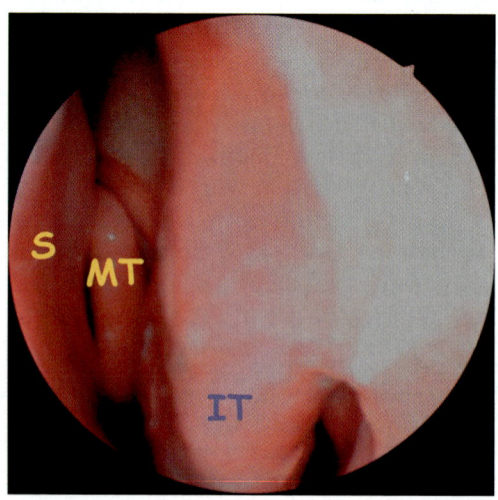

Fig. 7.2 Nasal endoscopy of nasal cavity demonstrating the normal anatomy. *IT*, inferior turbinate; *MT*, middle turbinate; *S*, nasal septum

Fig. 7.3 Nasal endoscopy of the left nasal cavity demonstrating the middle turbinate (*MT*) and nasal septum (*S*). The frontal sinus drainage pathway (*FS*) is obstructed by swelling in the region of the anterior ethmoid

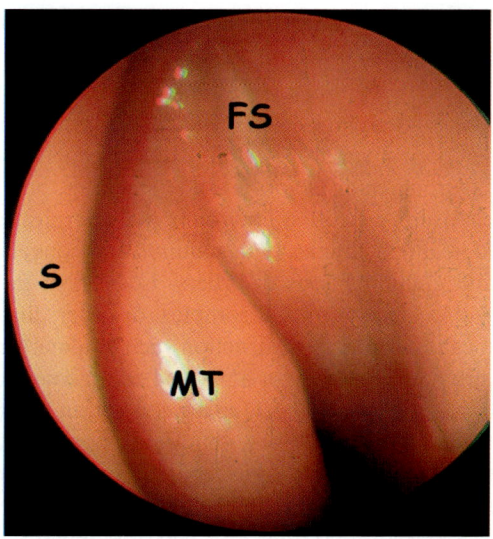

demonstrate conclusively that stripping mucosa was damaging to the sinuses in the long term and should be avoided whenever possible [5].

As a result of these observations and the advent of improved endoscopes, the concept of functional endoscopic sinus surgery (FESS) was born [3,6]. The keystones of this technique are accurate diagnosis of the underlying sites of persistent disease using both endoscopic visualization and CT imaging, the concept of a more limited surgical procedure performed endoscopically, as well as the preservation of mucosa with the goal of redeveloping mucociliary clearance. Since the introduction of FESS, the morbidity of surgical intervention has significantly decreased; and open surgical procedures are now rarely needed. By combining surgery with medical management and endoscopically directed postoperative care, we have demonstrated that it is possible to achieve a marked improvement in patient symptoms in more than 90% of patients with chronic rhinosinusitis and nasal polyposis. Moreover, we can maintain this improvement over at least an 8-year postoperative period [7]. In subsequent years, we have also developed some additional understanding of the causes of chronic rhinosinusitis, and of the application of surgery as an adjunct, rather than an alternative, to appropriate medical management.

In the early years of endoscopic sinus surgery—and to some extent still today—enthusiasm for the reduced morbidity, and the thought that perhaps many of these patients would be able to avoid continued medical therapy, led to overuse of endoscopic sinus surgery. As with other new surgical procedures the operation was not, and sometimes still is not today, always performed optimally and with the level of training that the techniques really require [8]. We now know that FESS requires meticulous attention to detail and mucosal preservation intraoperatively, as well as detailed postoperative follow-up, if the best possible results are to be achieved. The surgery should not be performed as an alternative to medical therapy, but rather to augment medical therapy, reduce recurrent infections, and improve overall quality of life.

The Role of Underlying Pathogenesis in Patient Selection for Surgery

The underlying causes of chronic rhinosinusitis are best divided into three categories: environmental factors, general host factors, and local host factors. Environmental factors include smoking, pollution, and viral, fungal, and bacterial exposure, as well as environmental allergies. General host factors include immunological deficiencies both acquired and congenital, ciliary dyskinesia, cystic fibrosis, and granulomatous disorders. Local host factors include persistent inflammation within the ostiomeatal complex, disorders that severely affect nasal airflow or cause local mucociliary obstruction such as a marked septal deformity, nasal polyps, prior turbinate resection, or a marked enlargement of some normal ethmoid cells such as a large concha bullosa (an air cell within the middle turbinate).

Patients who have continuing exposure to contributing environmental factors should either be removed from this environment or have the effects controlled before surgical intervention. If the sinuses are opened up, and areas of virgin mucosa are exposed to the presence of persistent environmental irritants or untreated allergies, it is likely that this healthier mucosa will also undergo chronic mucosal change and develop persistent inflammation over time. Indeed, a prior study that we performed looking at the causes of surgical failure over long-term follow-up demonstrated that one of the two most significant factors determining the need for revision surgical intervention was whether the patient continued to smoke, the other factor being the severity of preoperative disease [7]. In fact, so many of the patients who continued to smoke required revision surgical intervention over an 8-year follow-up period that we now recommend against surgical intervention in patients who have not yet quit smoking.

There is good evidence that patients with general host factors, which are clearly not modified by surgical intervention, do indeed benefit significantly from surgical intervention when carefully selected. However, patients with local host factors, such as localized mucosal and bone inflammation as major factors in their chronic rhinosinusitis, are most likely to have an excellent long-term favorable response to surgical intervention. The bacterial and fungal contamination associated with localized persistent inflammation acts as a reservoir for recurrent infection, but perhaps even more importantly, appears to significantly enhance the overall immunological reaction and mucosal reactivity [9,10].

The Role of Patient Symptoms in Selection for Surgery

Most adults get approximately four episodes of acute rhinosinusitis each year, although the frequency in children is higher. In some patients these acute infections linger longer than usual. However, if the infections resolve completely and only occur up to four times a year, this is rarely an indication for surgical intervention.

On the other hand, patients with persistent symptoms between acute episodes, or those who do not respond to medical treatment satisfactorily, are usually valid to consider for surgical intervention.

As noted previously, the sinuses most frequently involved in chronic rhinosinusitis are the ethmoid sinuses, and the most common symptoms of ethmoid sinusitis are nasal congestion and nasal obstruction. Another nonspecific symptom is nasal or postnasal discharge, but this is the symptom that typically responds least well to surgical intervention. Decreased sense of smell may occur from multiple etiologies, but the most common causes are viral infections, head trauma, or chronic rhinosinusitis. However, when hyposmia or anosmia comes on gradually, it is most commonly associated with chronic sinonasal disease and is generally a good predictor of chronic rhinosinusitis. Patients with chronic ethmoid sinusitis also sometimes complain of a feeling of facial pressure or discomfort, but true headache is an uncommon symptom of chronic rhinosinusitis, unless there is significant involvement of the frontal or sphenoid sinus. On the other hand, severe headache may certainly be seen with acute sinusitis. In general, chronic recurring headaches are much more likely to be associated with migraine than with chronic rhinosinusitis.

When the maxillary, frontal, or sphenoid sinuses become more involved the symptoms tend to become more localized. Chronic maxillary sinusitis may present as a feeling of pressure in the cheek or in the teeth. Chronic frontal sinusitis typically causes a feeling of pressure or discomfort on bending down, with the pressure localized in the forehead. Chronic sphenoid sinusitis may present as a feeling of pressure or discomfort on top of the head or behind the eyes.

Chronic rhinosinusitis is closely related to asthma. Indeed, it has sometimes been called asthma of the upper airways. Although there is no evidence that chronic rhinosinusitis is the cause of asthma, it is clear that severe sinusitis tends to exacerbate asthma and may lead to loss of asthma control [11]. There is now good evidence that in the presence of significant chronic rhinosinusitis on CT scan, successful surgical intervention in the sinuses results in significant long-term improvement of asthma, with decreased number of episodes, decreased medication usage, and improved quality of life [12,13].

Unilateral nasal congestion or nasal obstruction should give rise to consideration of a possible neoplasm. These patients should, therefore, typically undergo a CT scan and, when a unilateral area of opacification is observed, should be referred for nasal endoscopy and biopsy, and possibly for surgical intervention. A magnetic resonance imaging (MRI) scan will also help to differentiate tumor from retained secretion or mucocele.

The Role of Imaging and Endoscopy in Patient Selection for Surgery

Sinus CT scan demonstrates a snapshot of the sinuses out one point in time. Gwaltney et al. have demonstrated that the sinuses are involved in approximately

90% of patients who have an acute upper respiratory tract infection, however, these changes usually resolve approximately 2 weeks following the infection [14]. Additionally, approximately 30% of the asymptomatic population demonstrates areas of mucosal thickening on CT [15]. Following an acute bacterial sinusitis, resolution of the changes takes longer than with a viral infection, approximately 4 to 6 weeks.

In general, unless a complication is suspected, it is best to perform CT after an acute infection has been treated and the acute changes have resolved. The goal of CT scanning of the sinuses is usually to identify areas of persistent chronic inflammation that persist *between* episodes and may be a cause for recurrent acute infections. In general, CT is better than nasal endoscopy for demonstrating changes in the maxillary, frontal, or sphenoid sinuses. However, nasal endoscopy is more sensitive than CT for demonstrating changes within the ostiomeatal complex and middle meatus, not uncommonly demonstrating changes within these areas even when they are not visible on CT alone. Additionally, nasal endoscopy has the advantage that it can be repeated if necessary without exposing the patient to radiation. Nasal endoscopy, therefore, provides a way of monitoring patients over time and evaluating their response to medical therapy. Nasal endoscopy is also invaluable following surgical intervention, when patients frequently have persistent asymptomatic inflammation that needs to be treated and resolved if they are not to have further problems.

Allergic fungal sinusitis is less common than bacterial sinusitis and is much more frequently unilateral than chronic bacterial sinusitis. Patients with allergic fungal sinusitis typically demonstrate areas of increased opacification and inhomogeneity on CT because of the increased density of the fungus containing mucin [16]. Fungal balls within the sinuses frequently show areas of calcification. The diagnosis can be confirmed on MRI when the signal intensity from the mucin drops out on the T_2-weighted image.

Selecting Patients for Surgery

In general, the patient with chronic rhinosinusitis selected for surgery has persistent symptoms of chronic rhinosinusitis and significant CT changes or nasal endoscopic findings despite appropriate medical management. However, patients with worsening asthma should also be considered for surgical intervention if they have significant sinus involvement on CT scan. Nasal polyps, in contrast to polyps in the bowel, are not precancerous or potentially dangerous lesions. Rather, they are localized areas of mucosal edema that reflect the underlying inflammation. Accordingly, therefore, they do not need to be removed when asymptomatic, unless they are unilateral and a tumor is suspected (Fig. 7.4). Nasal polyps appear to regress late in life; however, at this point in time, patients with chronic rhinosinusitis may begin to have problems with recurrent chest infections and pneumonia. Intramucosal cysts are usually asymptomatic and rarely require surgical intervention, although occasionally they can give rise to local symptoms, or expand to where they extend out of the sinus. In the latter situation, the part of the cyst extending into the nose

Fig. 7.4 Coronal sinus computed tomography (CT) scan demonstrating a normal right anterior ethmoid and maxillary sinus. The left side of the nose, the ethmoid and maxillary sinuses, is totally opacified and obstructed, raising suspicion of a left-sided nasal tumor

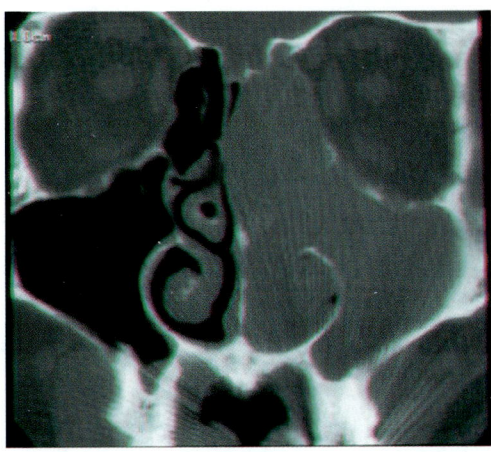

becomes polypoid, as with an antral-choanal or spheno-choanal polyp. Intramucosal cysts, which usually present as a rounded area of opacification within a sinus on CT and occur most frequently in the maxillary sinus, should be differentiated from mucoceles, which occur when a whole sinus is obstructed and the secretions fill and expand the sinus. Mucoceles occur most frequently in the frontal, sphenoid, or ethmoid sinuses and should be referred for surgical intervention as they can enlarge, sometimes quite rapidly, and begin to expand into the orbit or intracranial compartment. Sphenoid mucoceles may result in optic nerve compression and visual loss. Other indications for endoscopic surgery include intranasal and sinus tumors, cerebrospinal fluid (CSF) leaks, pituitary tumors, and skull base defects. Additionally, skull base tumors that have limited intracranial extension are increasingly being operated upon endoscopically (Table 7.1).

Patients with allergic fungal sinusitis should always be referred for surgical intervention. The thick mucus within the sinus in this situation contains the allergen (fungus) and must be drained if the sinuses are to be returned to health [17]. Fungal balls also require surgical removal and are frequently associated with surrounding bacterial inflammation. Invasive fungal sinusitis is usually seen in patients who are immunocompromised, and may be rapidly progressive (fulminant). It is an indication for urgent surgical intervention with, if possible, correction of the underlying

Table 7.1 Candidates for surgical intervention

- Mucoceles, tumors
- Acute sinusitis with threatened complications
- Nasal polyposis poorly responsive to medical therapy
- Chronic rhinosinusitis poorly responsive to medical therapy
- Recurrent acute sinusitis
  - More than four times per year (adults)
  - Persistent CT findings
- Patients with chronic sinusitis and worsening asthma

cause of immunocompromise, as well as immediate initiation of systemic antifungal therapy.

Patients with progressive unilateral symptoms or unilateral sinus disease on CT should be suspected of having a tumor or, possibly, fungal sinusitis until proven otherwise. At a minimum, these patients require nasal endoscopy and biopsy. However, in many cases surgical intervention is indicated. Many nasosinus tumors, particularly benign tumors, can now be removed endoscopically with minimal patient morbidity [18,19].

Selecting the Surgeon for Your Patients

As has been demonstrated with other types of surgery, the results of any surgical intervention are usually improved when the surgeon, and indeed the entire surgical team, perform a significant volume of the same type of surgical procedure. Although major surgical complications from the procedure are very rare, they can be devastating, and an excellent knowledge of the anatomy and instrumentation available is required if a complete surgical procedure is to be performed. On the other hand, the ideal surgeon should not perform an enormous number of these cases because, as you will see later in the chapter, each patient requires a significant amount of follow-up care after the procedure, and doing this correctly is very time consuming, requiring repeated in-office nasal endoscopy. Thus, it is impossible for a surgeon to do an extremely high volume of these cases and also take care of them ideally postoperatively. The ideal surgeon should also recognize that the surgery is really adjunctive to endoscopically directed medical therapy and that the latter is the real key to a long-term successful outcome. Although major complications are rare, minor complications are common and can severely affect a patient's subsequent quality of life [20]. As with other chronic diseases, the ideal surgeon should also be able to engage and motivate the patient in the long-term management of the disease.

Patient Preparation for Surgical Intervention

In addition to a general medical evaluation, it is important to try to minimize inflammation within the nose before surgical intervention. Bleeding is the enemy of the nasal endoscope, and the presence of inflammation will significantly increase intraoperative bleeding. Accordingly, patients should remain on the topical nasal steroids in the preoperative period and may be prescribed either a course of oral steroids and/or a course of antibiotics in the period immediately before the surgery [21]. The use of preoperative oral steroids becomes even more important in patients with asthma, where it is also critical to avoid bronchospasm, both intraoperatively and in the immediate postoperative period. As with inflammation, it is important that the patient's blood pressure is controlled so that bleeding can be minimized. The patient should, of course, be off aspirin for approximately 10 days and ibuprofen for at least

Table 7.2 Patient management before surgery

- Reduce inflammation
- Consider oral steroids (30 mg prednisone for 3–5 days)
- Off aspirin (10–14 days)
- Off ibuprufen and other NSAIDs (5 days)
- Off *Gingko biloba* and vitamin E
- Pulmonary function tests if asthmatic

5 days before the surgical procedure. Other therapies known to cause bleeding, such as *Ginkgo biloba* and vitamin E, should also be avoided (Table 7.2).

The patient should be aware that, in general, the surgery and the postoperative period are not painful, but that they will likely have a bloody nose following the surgery and that they will require prolonged endoscopic follow-up during the postoperative period (frequently weekly). The patient should also be aware of the need for significant medical therapy in the perioperative period and frequently for weeks or months following the surgical intervention. Surgical intervention is not an alternative to the use of topical nasal steroids or the avoidance of environmental irritants, and patients should be aware that they would need to be particularly careful in the postoperative period. In general, the nose is not packed following surgical intervention today, and patients are still able to breathe through the nose in the immediate postoperative period. Patients should also be aware that surgery is rarely a complete cure for chronic rhinosinusitis. Although it has markedly improved symptoms when combined with good medical therapy, it is not an alternative to appropriate medical therapy.

Major complications are extremely rare in the hands of skilled sinus surgeons. However, potential risks include major bleeding, CSF leak, or intraorbital damage, including diplopia or even loss of vision. However, because these major complications are so rare, the major decision-making factor in terms of having surgical intervention is not the potential for a major complication, but rather is centered around the amount of symptomatic improvement that is expected and whether this improvement is likely to be maintained long term. Long-term improvement is usually dependent on treatment of persistent and typically asymptomatic inflammation postoperatively and on long-term medical therapy, especially the use of long-term topical nasal steroids.

The Surgical Procedure

The majority of surgery today is performed endoscopically, working through the nose alongside the nasal endoscope. The surgery is typically performed under general anesthesia and takes 2 hours or more because meticulous care is required to avoid damage to, or stripping of, the surrounding mucosa. In general, the surgery begins with opening up the inflamed ethmoid sinuses and removal of all the bony partitions within the area of inflammation. Depending upon the extent of inflammation, the surgery is extended posteriorly into the posterior ethmoid sinuses and may involve opening up the maxillary, frontal, or even sphenoid sinuses. Because of the variability of sinus pneumatization, it is critical that the surgeon has a clear understanding of the anatomy and good three-dimensional conceptualization before the surgery is initiated. Increasingly, the surgery is performed with the aid of computer-assisted intraoperative surgical navigation. In this situation, the preoperative CT scan is downloaded into a computer in the operating room and this is then registered to the patient's head. Once the registration is complete, the movement of the instruments can be tracked on the CT image during the surgical procedure, providing the surgeon with additional anatomic information. However, the accuracy of these devices is still not sufficient that it can supplant an excellent knowledge and conceptualization of the anatomy. Although the use of laser was previously advocated for this type of surgery, the surgery is now typically performed with through-cutting forceps or a mechanical instrument called a microdebrider. The use of laser within the sinuses tends to cause collateral heat damage and is generally now considered best avoided. When the nasal septum is significantly deviated, this may need to be corrected so as to provide access before the sinus surgery is performed on the narrow side.

In some situations, standard endoscopic surgery may not be sufficient to create a long-term opening of the sinuses, and this is especially true in the case of severe chronic frontal sinusitis. In this situation, extended endoscopic approaches with more significant bone removal and, occasionally, removal of a portion of the nasal septum may be performed. However, these extended frontal sinus procedures should not be used for routine surgery in a previously unoperated patient because they involve a significant loss of mucosa and the potential for long-term scarring [22]. These extended surgical approaches may also allow access to remove tumors and other lesions from within the frontal sinus endoscopically.

Recently, the use of balloons to open the sinuses (balloon sinuplasty) has gained significant press, particularly in the form of publicity to the lay public. However, as the ethmoid sinuses are the most commonly involved sinuses and there is no balloon for opening this region, in the majority of cases, even if the balloon is used, it still has to be combined with standard surgical intervention. Additionally, the long-term results of balloon sinuplasty are not yet known; and the use of a balloon does not allow removal of the inflamed tissue, something that would appear to be a very significant limitation [23,24].

Although in most cases surgical intervention is performed endoscopically, there are still occasional cases in which open surgery is required. Most frequently this need occurs in extensive frontal sinus disease, where the anatomy is unfavorable for a wide opening through an endoscopic approach. In this situation, the sinus may need to be opened from above. This opening is performed through an incision, typically made behind the hairline, and the sinus is entered and opened to access the disease (osteoplastic flap). The sinus is then obliterated with fat taken from the abdomen before it is closed and the wound sutured. Such surgery, however, involves a significant degree of perioperative morbidity, and carries the added significant disadvantage that the ability to image the sinus with either CT or MRI is significantly impaired following the procedure. This limitation makes the interpretation of subsequent symptoms possibly related to frontal sinus disease, such as frontal headaches, difficult. Additionally, the failure rate of frontal sinus fat obliteration increases over time, approaching at least 25% as the years go by.

Postoperative Management

Patients are usually instructed not to blow the nose for several days following the surgery and to avoid any bending or heavy lifting. Most patients do not have any facial swelling or ecchymosis following endoscopic sinus surgery. Pain is typically minimal or absent, and the classical uncomfortable postoperative packing is essentially never used today. However, patients will usually have a bloody nasal discharge for several days to weeks and intermittent nasal congestion, which may also continue for a number of weeks. Many physicians will either place a sponge into the middle meatus, which is removed after the first or second postoperative day, or use an absorbable spacer in the middle meatus, which slowly dissolves in the first 2 to 3 weeks after the surgery. The advantage of using a sponge that can be removed is that it allows the surgeon to suction out blood and mucus from the sinuses in the early postoperative period. As we believe that bacteria and fungi exacerbate the inflammatory response, removal of the sponge and cleaning of the area would appear to be preferable.

The natural sequela, arising from the combination of surgical intervention and the presence of significant inflammation, is scarring. Furthermore, the chronic inflammation that leads to chronic rhinosinusitis does not resolve immediately following surgical intervention. Since the primary goal of the surgery is to create widely patent sinuses that can drain easily, and because inflammation and surgery cause scarring, it is clear that significant postoperative care is required if the primary goal of the surgery is to be achieved. This care entails treatment of the underlying inflammation with antibiotics and antiinflammatory medications, repeated nasal endoscopy, and, not infrequently, some minor removal of scar tissue until the sinus cavities have healed and the residual inflammation has resolved [25]. Saline nasal sprays instituted in the early postoperative period will reduce nasal crusting, and we usually recommend that patients use these every hour or so while awake in the early postoperative period. Patients may also be asked to perform more significant nasal lavage with saline, antibiotic, or steroid solutions [26]. Whenever possible, antibiotic therapy is directed based upon endoscopic culture, and antibiotics are usually prescribed for at least 2 weeks following the surgical intervention. When significant bone inflammation is present, antibiotics may be required for a significantly longer period of time. Oral steroids, when required to control either asthma or nasal mucosal inflammation, are usually slowly tapered in the postoperative period. However, in the presence of severe polyposis or allergic fungal sinusitis, prolonged oral steroid therapy may be required if a recurrence of disease is to be avoided. Fortunately, patients with nasal and sinus diseases usually respond to low doses of oral steroids. Avoidance of allergens and environmental irritants, and, especially, avoidance of exposure to smoke is critically important in the postoperative period (Table 7.3).

Table 7.3 Postoperative medical management

- Antibiotics (usually for 2 or more weeks)
- Nasal saline spray
- Long-term topical nasal steroids
- Possible slowly tapering oral steroids
- Possible antihistamines
- Possible antileukotrienes

Our postoperative regimen usually involves seeing the patient the day following the surgery and removing the middle meatal sponges and suctioning the nose under endoscopic visualization. The patient then returns weekly for 4 to 6 weeks, and less frequently thereafter until the cavity is fully healed and the residual inflammation has subsided. At each visit, a nasal endoscopy is performed under topical anesthesia and when the sinus cavities are raw. Particularly in the early postoperative period, an oral narcotic analgesic is beneficial before the visit because the cleanings are uncomfortable. When nasal endoscopy demonstrates a tendency to scarring, the immature scars are meticulously divided. Any residual areas of devitalized or inflamed bone are gently teased out, and careful attention is paid to ensure that the sinuses remain patent. Given the chronic and persistent nature of chronic rhinosinusitis and the tendency toward scarring in the postoperative period, it is particularly important that the patient returns for these postoperative visits until satisfactory healing is obtained. Convincing patients to return for these visits can be difficult because the patients are usually almost totally asymptomatic postoperatively, despite having ongoing persistent inflammation. Despite the relative lack of symptoms postoperatively, postoperative care, nasal endoscopy, and, when necessary, debridement are exceptionally important to the long-term outcome, and essential for most chronic disease if a late recurrence of chronic rhinosinusitis or nasal polyposis is to be avoided.

In the longer term, we regard these patients as "at-risk" patients for return of chronic sinusitis because the underlying factors associated with the onset of the disease probably have not been modified by the surgical intervention. Therefore, we recommend intermittent long-term nasal endoscopy and follow-up, until it is clear that the ethmoid cavity is stable and a recurrence of disease is unlikely. Early recurrent disease is usually asymptomatic, but it is important that it is identified at an early stage using nasal endoscopy if revision surgery is to be avoided [7]. Patients are usually recommended to use topical nasal steroids on a regular, ongoing, and long-term basis. The goal of the surgery should be to resolve the disease long term so as to avoid the necessity for subsequent surgical interventions, and not just reduce symptomatic relief, only to have the patient undergo revision surgery later.

Complications of Surgery

The most common complication of surgical intervention in the sinuses is persistence of inflammation, which may occur because of the underlying etiology of the disease, because of inadequate removal of the disease at the time of surgery, or because of limited postoperative care and postoperative medical therapy. Although major bleeding is uncommon with this type of surgery, postoperative bleeding is also always a potential risk. Spinal fluid leak can occur as a result of inadvertent intracranial entry, but typically this is identified and closed at the time of the surgical procedure. If a spinal fluid leak is suspected postoperatively, the patient is frequently asked to collect some fluid for a beta-2 transferrin test. Because tears may also contain glucose, the use of Dextrostix to identify a CSF leak is considered misleading and to have low specificity. Trauma to the extraocular muscles, resulting in diplopia or intraorbital hemorrhage resulting in visual loss, has also been reported. Minor complications are much more common, but can be extremely bothersome to the patient and occasionally become almost crippling. These problems include persistent or worsening of inflammation or significant alterations in airflow resulting from extensive turbinate resection, whether inadvertent or deliberate (empty nose syndrome). A nose with abnormally large air passages is extremely bothersome to the patient, because of increased nasal resistance as a result of the loss of laminar airflow and because of an increased tendency toward mucosal inflammation and crusting. There is some evidence that inferior turbinate resection may also increase the incidence of maxillary sinus infections.

Summary

The introduction of endoscopic sinus surgery has dramatically improved the results of surgical management of rhinosinusitis in terms of decreasing the associated morbidity. Superior results have also been demonstrated when compared to open surgical intervention. It has been shown that nasal-specific symptoms improve. Using the SF-36 overall health survey form, overall quality of life is significantly adversely affected by chronic rhinosinusitis, but it returns to normal, and medication usage is decreased compared to the preoperative status, by 7.8 years postoperatively. However, the surgery is not a panacea. Sinus surgery is technically challenging and is best thought of as adjunctive to an overall long-term medical therapy plan. It takes a significant period of time for the underlying chronic inflammation to settle down, and fairly intensive medical therapy and endoscopic follow-up are often required during that period.

References

1. Muntz HR, Lusk RP. Nasal antral windows in children: a retrospective study. Laryngoscope 1990;100:643–646.
2. Stefansson P, Andreasson L, Jannert M. Caldwell-Luc operation: long-term results and sequelaes. Acta Otolaryngol Suppl 1988;449:97–100.
3. Kennedy DW, Zinreich SJ, Rosenbaum AE, et al. Functional endoscopic sinus surgery. Theory and diagnostic evaluation. Arch Otolaryngol 1985;111:576–582.
4. Zinreich SJ, Kennedy DW, Rosenbaum AE, et al. CT of the paranasal sinuses: imaging requirement for endoscopic surgery. Radiology 1987;163:769–775.

5. Kennedy DW, Shaalan H. Reevaluation of maxillary sinus surgery: experimental study in rabbits. Ann Otol Rhinol Laryngol 1989;98(11):901–906.
6. Kennedy DW. Functional endoscopic sinus surgery. Technique. Arch Otolaryngol 1985;111:643–649.
7. Senior BA, Kennedy DW, Tanabodee J, et al. Long-term results of functional endoscopic sinus surgery. Laryngoscope 1998;108(2):151–157.
8. Stankiewicz JA. Complications of endoscopic nasal surgery: occurrence and treatment. Am J Rhinol 1987;1:45–49.
9. Conley DB, Tripathi A, Ditto AM, et al. Chronic sinusitis with nasal polyps: staphylococcal exotoxin immunoglobulin E and cellular inflammation. Am J Rhinol 2004;18(5):273–278.
10. Bernstein JM, Ballow M, Schlievert PM, et al. A superantigen hypothesis for the pathogenesis of chronic hyperplastic sinusitis with massive nasal polyposis. [Erratum appears in Am J Rhinol 2004;18(1):62.] Am J Rhinol 2003;17(6):321–326.
11. Slavin RG. Sinusitis in adults and its relation to allergic rhinitis, asthma, and nasal polyps. J Allergy Clin Immunol 1988;82:950–956.
12. Senior BA, Kennedy DW, Tanabodee J, et al. Long-term impact of functional endoscopic sinus surgery on asthma. Otolaryngol Head Neck Surg 1999;121:66–68.
13. Park AH, Lau J, Stankiewicz J, et al. The role of functional endoscopic sinus surgery in asthmatic patients. J Otolaryngol 1998;27(5):275–280.
14. Gwaltney JM Jr, Phillips CD, Miller RD, et al. Computed tomographic study of the common cold [see comments]. N Engl J Med 1994;330:25–30.
15. Havas TE, Motbey JA, Gullane PJ. Prevalence of incidental abnormalities on computed tomographic scans of the paranasal sinuses. Arch Otolaryngol 1988;114:856–859.
16. Zinreich SJ, Kennedy DW. Fungal sinusitis: diagnosis with CT and MR imaging. Radiology 1988;169:439-444.
17. Marple BF, Mabry RL. Allergic fungal sinusitis: learning from our failures. Am J Rhinol 2000;14(4):223–226.
18. Woodworth BA, Bhargave GA, Palmer JN, et al. Clinical outcomes of endoscopic and endoscopic-assisted resection of inverted papillomas: a 15-year experience. Am J Rhinol 2007;21(5):591–600.
19. Wolfe SG, Schlosser RJ, Bolger WE, et al. Endoscopic and endoscope-assisted resections of inverted sinonasal papillomas. Otolaryngol Head Neck Surg 2004;131(3):174–179.
20. Kennedy DW, Shaman P, Han W, et al. Complications of ethmoidectomy: a survey of fellows of the American Academy of Otolaryngology-Head and Neck Surgery. Otolaryngol Head Neck Surg 1994;111(5):589–599.
21. Wright ED, Agrawal S, Wright ED, et al. Impact of perioperative systemic steroids on surgical outcomes in patients with chronic rhinosinusitis with polyposis: evaluation with the novel Perioperative Sinus Endoscopy (POSE) scoring system. Laryngoscope 2007;117(11 pt 2 suppl 115):1–28.
22. Gross WE, Gross CW, Becker D, et al. Modified transnasal endoscopic Lothrop procedure as an alternative to frontal sinus obliteration. Otolaryngol Head Neck Surg 1995;113:427–434.
23. Brown CL, Bolger WE, Brown CL, et al. Safety and feasibility of balloon catheter dilation of paranasal sinus ostia: a preliminary investigation. [see comment]. Ann Otol Rhinol Laryngol 2006;115(4):293–299.
24. Bolger WE, Brown CL, Church CA, et al. Safety and outcomes of balloon catheter sinusotomy: a multicenter 24-week analysis in 115 patients. Otolaryngology - Head Neck Surg 2007;137(1):10–20.
25. Bugten V, Nordgard S, Steinsvag S, et al. The effects of debridement after endoscopic sinus surgery. Laryngoscope 2006;116(11):2037–2043.
26. Bachmann G, Hommel G, Michel O. Effect of irrigation of the nose with isotonic salt solution on adult patients with chronic paranasal sinus disease. Eur Arch Oto-Rhino-Laryngol 2000;257(10):537–541.

Chapter 8
Allergy and Rhinosinusitis

John H. Krouse

Clinicians have observed a relationship between allergy and acute and chronic rhinosinusitis (RS) for many years. This association appears to be common, and has been described by a number of authors over the past several decades [1]. As both RS and allergy reflect inflammatory disorders of the upper respiratory system, it is compelling to speculate that these two illnesses share common pathophysiological mechanisms and that treatment of nasal allergies would have an important benefit in the management of patients with RS. The science supporting this relationship, however, is largely anecdotal and epidemiologic, and mechanisms through which allergy predisposes a patient to RS are currently speculative.

This chapter discusses the relationship between nasal allergies and RS. The epidemiology and pathophysiology of nasal allergy are first reviewed, followed by a clinical overview of allergic rhinitis. Diagnostic methods used to evaluate the patient suspected of nasal allergy are outlined, and treatment methods to address allergy among patients with RS are discussed. It is important for physicians treating patients with RS to understand the role of allergy in the expression of symptoms among these individuals and to initiate relevant therapeutic options to decrease morbidity and improve quality of life.

Epidemiology and Burden of Nasal Allergy

Nasal allergies are common and are experienced by patients of all ages. The term that is used to describe a nasal disorder caused by allergic hypersensitivity is *allergic rhinitis* (AR). AR implies that nasal inflammation is triggered in an individual by hyperactive immune responses to known sensitizing agents. Epidemiologic studies have consistently positioned AR among the most common chronic illnesses in the United States (Fig. 8.1). In one recent study, it was estimated that more than 58 million Americans, or about 20% of the population, are bothered by symptoms

J.H. Krouse
Department of Otolaryngology, Wayne State University, Detroit, MI, USA
e-mail: jKrouse@med.wayne.edu

E.R. Thaler, D.W. Kennedy (eds.), *Rhinosinusitis*, DOI: 10.1007/978-0-387-73062-2_8,   107
© Springer Science+Business Media, LLC 2008

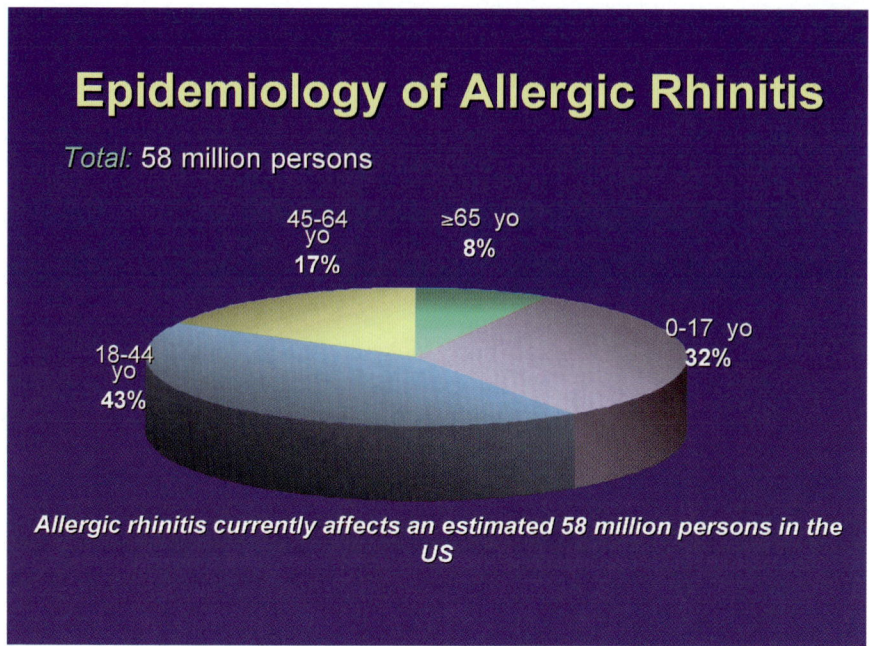

Fig. 8.1 Proportion of U.S. patients with allergic rhinitis by age. *yo*, years old

of AR [2]. It is also important to recognize that among patients with AR, many individuals also have symptoms that are worsened by nonallergic triggers, such as cigarette smoke, newsprint, and strong odors [3].

Although AR can affect individuals of any age, it is most commonly a disease of later childhood, adolescence, and young adulthood. Symptoms tend to be expressed most vigorously between the ages of 10 and 40 years [4], while the diagnosis of AR is usually made before the age of 10 [5]. In fact, there is strong evidence that the prevalence of AR among children has more than doubled since 1990 [6]. It is likely that the increasing prevalence of AR among children that has been noted will result in a greater number of adults with AR over the next several decades.

Because of the prevalence and symptomatic morbidity of AR, treatment of nasal allergies carries a significant economic cost. The financial burden of the direct treatment of AR has been estimated to range up to $9 billion (U.S.) [7], with up to $6 billion attributable to medication costs alone [8]. Since AR frequently coexists among patients with RS, treatment of AR among these individuals will add to the significant baseline costs associated with the diagnosis and treatment of RS.

Pathophysiology of Allergy

The allergic response involves a specific immune-mediated hypersensitivity to a generally innocuous substance in an individual who is genetically capable of generating such a response. This genetic predisposition to develop allergic diseases is known as *atopy*. Not all individuals have inherited this predisposition to respond in this manner, and these individuals will not develop allergic hypersensitivities with exposure. A review of the immunology relevant to the allergic response will be useful. In addition, a list of terms commonly used in allergy diagnosis and treatment is presented in Table 8.1.

The term *immunity* is based on a Latin word meaning exemption. It refers to the processes through which the immune system is able to protect the individual from invasion by foreign substances that could be injurious. In carrying out this process, the immune system must be able to identify and neutralize substances that are potentially dangerous, yet *exempt* host tissues from injury. As such, the immune system is a primary line of defense through which the body is able to protect itself from pathogenic substances and organisms.

The immune system carries out its function through the coordinated response of a variety of humoral and cellular mediators. These components of the immune system must interact in a controlled and balanced manner to process foreign substances, identify host cells, and neutralize potentially harmful materials before they cause serious injury to the body. Cellular mediators involved in this system include director cells, such as macrophages and lymphocytes, and effector cells such as neutrophils, mast cells, and eosinophils. Lymphocytes are centrally involved in immune function and are divided into several subclasses, including B lymphocytes, T lymphocytes, and NK (natural killer) cells. B and T lymphocytes are both critical in the development and activation of the allergic response. In addition, eosinophils and mast cells are important leukocytes involved in the allergic response.

Humoral mediators include various cytokines, which are polypeptide messengers involved in coordination of the immune response, as well as immunoglobulins, which are antibodies involved in the binding of antigens and the stimulation of innate defense mechanisms. The primary immunoglobulin involved in the allergic response is immunoglobulin E (IgE), which is produced in very small amounts by B lymphocytes and plasma cells. IgE is developed in response to antigen exposure in an atopic individual and is bound to the surface of mast cells. These mast cells are present in both the nasal and sinus mucosa, as well as in other mucosal tissues and in the systemic circulation.

Table 8.1 Definitions of terms used in allergy

Atopy	The genetic predisposition to develop allergic sensitization
Antigen	Any substance capable of generating an immune response
Allergen	An antigen that is capable of generating an allergic response
Allergy	Type-1 hypersensitivity response, primarily mediated by IgE
Histamine	Primary mediator of the immediate hypersensitivity response
Immunotherapy	Desensitization therapy for allergic disease
In vitro tests	Allergy testing through serum sampling for immunoglobulins
In vivo tests	Allergy testing through patient exposure to suspected antigens
Lymphocytes	Director cells of the immune system
RAST testing	Type of in vitro test for allergic sensitivity
Rhinitis	Inflammatory condition affecting the nasal mucosa

Although the normally functioning immune system protects host tissues from injury and avoids exaggerated responses to innocuous substances, in some circumstances the immune system reacts inappropriately, resulting in the identification of nonthreatening substances as dangerous or in the destruction of normal tissues. These processes are broadly referred to as *hypersensitivity reactions* and are classified into several types. The allergic response is classified as a type I hypersensitivity response and is mediated by sensitization to innocuous substances in atopic individuals, production of IgE antibodies, and histamine-mediated production of symptoms on exposure. The type I hypersensitivity response is seen in a variety of conditions, including allergic rhinitis, allergic conjunctivitis, urticaria, and asthma, and in its most pronounced form is expressed with *anaphylaxis*. In anaphylaxis, exposure to a sensitized antigen results in prompt and overwhelming release of histamine into the systemic circulation, resulting in wheezing, bronchoconstriction, hypotension, and potentially death. For purposes of this chapter, discussion of hypersensitivity responses is limited to those seen in allergic rhinitis.

As noted earlier, AR is an immune-mediated nasal disorder that involves an inflammatory response of the nasal and sinus mucosa (Fig. 8.2). While it is primarily mediated by IgE, some evidence exists that may implicate other types of immune mechanisms [9]. When atopic individuals are exposed to antigens, they can become sensitized to those antigens. Antigen-presenting cells (APC), such as macrophages, capture these antigens and process them for presentation to T-helper lymphocytes. This APC–antigen complex binds to the T lymphocyte through a specific receptor and triggers activation of the T cell. Cytokines communicate with other cells of the immune system, including B lymphocytes, and stimulate amplification of the allergic response after sensitization. B lymphocytes are critical in the allergic response as they synthesize IgE antibodies specific for the sensitized antigen. These

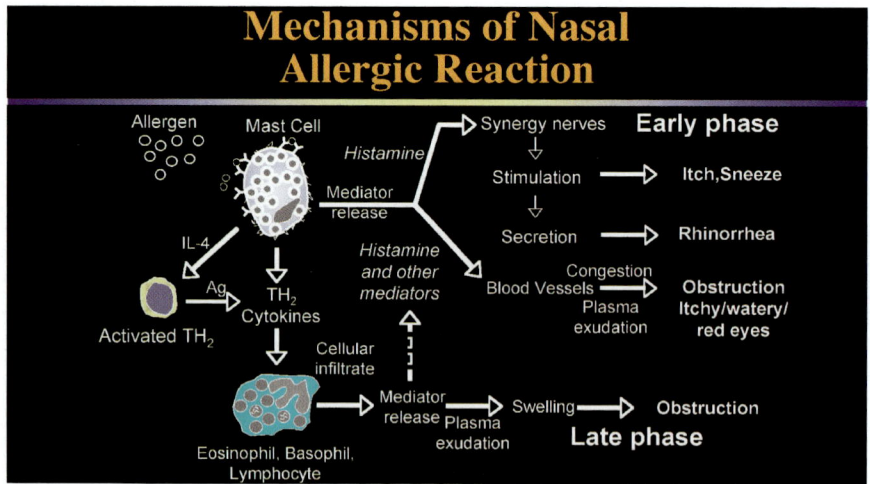

Fig. 8.2 Early- and late-phase allergic response: mediators and symptoms

IgE antibodies bind to the surface of mast cells and basophils and maintain memory for specific antigens that allows recognition of the antigen on future exposure.

On subsequent exposure, this antigen will cross-link adjacent IgE molecules bound to the surface of mast cells in the nasal mucosa, activating the mast cell through a calcium-dependent process, and allowing both release of preformed inflammatory mediators, such as *histamine,* and the synthesis of newly formed mediators, such as *leukotrienes.* Histamine provokes immediate nasal symptoms through prompt binding to histamine-1 (H1) receptors on cells of the nasal mucosa. Within 5 to 10 min after exposure, patients will complain of the four classic symptoms of AR: sneezing, itching, rhinorrhea (nasal discharge), and nasal congestion. While the effects of histamine decline within minutes after release, symptoms of AR are maintained and often worsened by prolonged mediators of inflammation such as the cysteinyl leukotrienes.

The nasal symptoms of AR are often accompanied by nonnasal symptoms as well. Ocular symptoms are common in patients with AR, as are symptoms such as palatal itching and ear fullness. In addition, patients with AR have a higher prevalence of lower respiratory inflammation and asthma than do nonallergic individuals. Nasal symptoms are also frequently exacerbated in patients with concurrent AR and RS.

Allergic Rhinitis: Overview

The term *rhinitis* refers to an inflammatory disorder of the nasal mucosa. The inflammation that is present in rhinitis can be caused by many different mechanisms, some of them allergic and many of them nonallergic. Nonallergic rhinitis can be stimulated by a variety of triggers, such as respiratory irritants, viral and bacterial infections, medications, and hormonal variations. The mucosal inflammation caused by rhinitis can be mild to severe; severe inflammation can be critical in contributing to the pathogenesis of RS by impairing ventilation and drainage through the sinus ostia.

AR is usually classified in the United States on the basis of its correspondence with well-defined geographic seasons. If AR shows a strong seasonal variability, it is referred to as *seasonal allergic rhinitis* (SAR), which is attributable to pollens and seasonal variations in mold spores. If AR is present throughout most or all of the year, it is referred to as *perennial allergic rhinitis* (PAR), which is generally attributable to animal dander, dust mites, other arthropods such as cockroaches, and indoor molds. Many patients have elements of both SAR and PAR, and complain of year-round symptoms with seasonal exacerbations. While this system can often be useful in classifying AR, especially in more temperate climates, it does not explain the nature of symptoms in climates with more frequent or prolonged periods of pollination, such as Southern California.

In patients with SAR, there is a clear association between the pollen counts in a specific region and the development and expression of symptoms. As pollen counts rise seasonally, inflammatory mediators in both the nasal mucosa and the serum begin to rise. The presence of increased antigen loads causes mast cells to release histamine and other mediators, and proinflammatory cytokines increase cellular influx into the nasal tissues. Eosinophils are drawn into the nasal mucosa in AR as in chronic RS and cause tissue inflammation and local injury. As pollen counts decline at the end of the season, inflammation also begins to wane and symptoms become less prominent.

In contrast, among patients with PAR, while there can be fluctuations in symptoms with variations in antigen load throughout the year, symptoms are present at some level on an almost constant basis. Because the antigens are constantly present, wide fluctuations in symptoms are less common with PAR than with SAR. In addition, symptoms such as nasal congestion and postnasal drainage appear to be more common in PAR. Since PAR symptoms overlap with symptoms frequently expressed in chronic RS, diagnostic confusion can often be present. It is important to evaluate if PAR is a comorbidity of chronic RS in a particular individual, and to determine whether symptoms expressed by the patient are caused by allergy alone or by inflammatory changes related to RS.

A separate system that has come into common use outside the United States is a classification model for AR known as *ARIA* (allergic rhinitis and its impact on asthma). The ARIA guidelines present a system for categorizing AR that is similar conceptually to that used widely for the classification of asthma [10]. In the ARIA guidelines, AR is classified according to the severity of the patient's symptoms and the time pattern over which they occur. Symptoms that occur throughout the majority of the year on essentially a daily basis are referred to as *persistent*, while symptoms that occur only a few days a week or only for a few weeks of the year are termed *intermittent*. Severity of symptoms is classified in the ARIA guidelines by the degree to which they effect the patient's quality of life, sleep, and daytime function. If the patient's symptoms are bothersome but do not interrupt sleep or interfere with daytime activities, the severity of AR is considered *mild*. On the other hand, if the patient's symptoms cause significant difficulties with sleep, adversely affect daytime function, or bring about impairment in quality of life, the severity of AR is considered *moderate-severe*. ARIA allows for a consideration of the patient's AR along four dimensions combining chronicity and severity, with the four classifications being (1) mild intermittent, (2) mild persistent, (3) moderate-severe intermittent, and (4) moderate-severe persistent. These categories are familiar to clinicians who are used to treating patients with asthma, and allow for treatment guidelines based upon an objective analysis of the patient's symptoms.

Diagnosis of Allergic Rhinitis

History

The most important element of the diagnostic process among patients suspected of having AR is the history. The history will assist in the assessment of whether the patient's symptoms are truly allergic in their pathophysiology or whether other mechanisms may be involved (e.g., nonallergic rhinitis). Since AR is usually first seen in childhood, it is important in all individuals suspected of having AR to determine the age at which they first had symptoms. As AR is frequently not the initial allergic illness experienced by patients, it is also important to inquire whether individuals had any episodes of other atopic illnesses in childhood, such as perioral or perianal eczema, atopic dermatitis, or asthma. In addition, atopic children may also have experienced frequent episodes of otitis media or RS, which may help with determining the likelihood of an individual having an allergic component to their present symptoms.

Since AR has a genetic predisposition, family history is also relevant in assessing the patient. If one or both parents of the patient have AR, the likelihood of the patient having AR increases significantly. The absence of a family history, however, does not preclude the diagnosis of AR.

Assessment of seasonality is an important component of the patient history because many patients with AR have a strong seasonal pattern to the onset and resolution of their symptoms. In patients with SAR, symptoms will closely track pollen counts for relevant antigens, and the presence of clear seasonal relationships strongly suggests a diagnosis of SAR. The absence of seasonal variation does not exclude the presence of AR, however, as patients with PAR often have relatively consistent symptoms throughout the year. Seasonal variability in patients with PAR is also common, as many patients with PAR also have concurrent SAR.

In addition to seasonal variability, patients are often able to describe discrete triggers that will bring about the rapid development of symptoms. It is important, therefore, to inquire about specific triggers of which the patient is aware. Patients often notice symptoms worsening with marked exposure to antigens, as is often seen with allergy to cat dander, dust mites, and ragweed or grass pollen. The absence of patient awareness of discrete triggers does not exclude allergic sensitivities to those antigens, however, as patients often accommodate to the presence of antigens within their environments.

Physical Examination

It is important to examine not only the nose among patients with AR but to evaluate the head and neck for comorbid signs as well. An inspection of the face often suggests signs of AR among both children and adults. Patients with AR often have puffiness of the eyelids or the cheeks, as well as darkening of the skin under the eyes, referred to as "allergic shiners." These findings are seen secondary to nasal congestion and inflammation. Fine lines may be noted in the lids, referred to as "Dennie's lines," which are secondary to spasms of the eyelid musculature. In addition, injection or redness of the conjunctivae may also be seen.

In patients with AR, the nasal examination often shows signs of acute or chronic inflammation. The mucosa in the nose of a patient with AR is often pale, gray to bluish-white, and is frequently boggy and edematous. In contrast, patients with nonallergic or infectious rhinitis often have an inflamed, hyperemic, and angry-appearing nasal mucosa. The inferior turbinates are often swollen in the patient with AR, and this edema will usually decrease rapidly with administration of a vasoconstricting drug such as oxymetazoline. The nose should also be examined for other signs of nasal pathology, including purulent discharge, which would be common in acute and chronic RS, and nasal polyps, which are commonly seen in patients with chronic RS. Examination of the nose can be conducted using an otoscope, but more thorough examination of the posterior portion of the nasal cavity often requires an endoscopic examination.

In addition, patients with AR often have changes in their pharyngeal mucosa secondary to the increased immune responsiveness of the mucosa. It is common to see "cobblestoning" in the posterior pharyngeal wall among patients with AR. This smoothly irregular surface seen in the posterior oropharynx is caused by the presence of numerous lymphoid follicles in the pharyngeal submucosa. Examination of the skin for signs of atopic dermatitis or eczema can also confirm the presence of allergic findings that often accompany AR. In addition, auscultation of the lungs is important as many patients with AR have concurrent asthma as part of their spectrum of disease.

Allergy Testing

When a patient with symptoms of rhinitis is suspected of being allergic, and when the clinician wishes to confirm a diagnosis of allergy, testing can be conducted using one of several methods (Table 8.2). Because allergy is an important contributor to the expression of symptoms in patients with RS, it is reasonable to consider allergy testing in all patients with recurrent episodes of acute RS and in many, if not all, patients with chronic RS. Confirmation of the presence of allergies in these populations can significantly alter treatment and testing should be utilized as a component of the diagnostic process in patients with problematic RS.

Screening Tests

Screening tests can be used as an initial approach to detect the presence of allergic hypersensitivity. The results should be interpreted as suggestive of the presence of

Table 8.2 Common tests used for diagnosis of allergy

Screening Tests	Specific Tests
Total IgE level	In Vivo (Skin) Tests
Nasal cytology	Prick testing
	Intradermal testing
	Modified quantitative testing
	Intradermal dilutional testing
	In Vitro Tests
	RAST testing
	ELISA testing

allergy rather than conclusive [11]. Screens can be useful, however, since they can often be done quickly using routine methods available to both primary care physicians and specialists.

One commonly used screening test is *total IgE*. Through venipuncture, a blood sample can be collected for global assessment of IgE in the patient's serum. When the concentration of total IgE is elevated (usually above 100 μg/mL), this finding is considered suggestive of the presence of allergy. Significant elevations usually correlate with clinically relevant allergy, while total IgE levels within the normal range do not rule out the presence of allergic disease or elevated levels specific to individual antigens. Total IgE levels should therefore be considered suggestive rather than diagnostic of the presence of allergy [12].

Another commonly used screening method is *nasal cytology*. As eosinophils are frequently present in significant quantity in the mucus of allergic individuals, a sample of the nasal mucus can be gathered using a small swab or nasal spoon and examined microscopically for the presence of eosinophils. Abundant numbers of eosinophils would be suggestive of allergy, although nasal eosinophils are also elevated among patients with chronic RS as well. The presence of increased eosinophils may therefore be more important in patients with recurrent acute RS than in individuals with chronic RS; elevations in the acute RS population would suggest the presence of allergy as a potential cofactor in the recurrence of the patient's disease. Results of nasal cytology, however, can be unreliable and should be judged with caution when evaluating the presence of nasal allergy [13].

Confirmatory Tests

In contrast to the use of screening tests, assessment techniques are available to accurately confirm the presence of allergic hypersensitivity and to quantify or estimate the degree of that hypersensitivity. Confirmatory testing for allergy can be conducted using two methods: (1) *in vivo testing*, in which assessment is conducted through introducing suspected antigens directly into the skin; and (2) *in vitro testing*, in which serum sampling is done to assess the presence of, and to quantify the amount of, specific IgE antibodies in the systemic circulation.

In vivo testing, also known as *skin testing*, is the most commonly used method of allergy testing both in the United States and internationally. In all types of skin testing, a small amount of a suspected antigen is introduced into the skin using one of several well-accepted methods. Patients allergic to that antigen will have IgE specific to the antigen bound to the surface of mast cells through prior exposure and sensitization. When the antigen is reintroduced into the skin, it will bind to these IgE antibodies, resulting in cross-linking of adjacent IgE molecules, degranulation of preformed histamine-containing cytoplasmic granules, and release of histamine into the skin. Histamine will bind to cellular receptors in the skin, resulting in localized tissue inflammation. Local inflammation is expressed through a reaction known as *wheal and flare*, in which transudation and release of plasma into the tissues cause a discrete area of swelling (wheal) and tissue irritation results in local erythema of the skin (flare). This response is very rapid, and is usually noted within 5 to

10 min after introduction of the antigen. The absence of response suggests that the patient does not have IgE specific to that antigen, so long as the ability of the skin to react to challenge has been established using appropriate control tests. The size and dimensions of the wheal and flare are loosely correlated with the degree of skin reactivity.

One common skin testing method uses a technique known as *prick testing* (also known as prick/puncture testing). In prick testing, a small amount of an antigen is placed into the superficial dermis using either a small introducer or lancet. Multiple-pronged testing devices are also available that allow the concurrent evaluation of several suspected antigens (Fig. 8.3). Prick testing has been conducted for more than 100 years with a high degree of safety, accuracy, and utility.

Another common method of skin testing involves a technique known as *intra-dermal testing* (ID testing). In contrast to prick testing, ID tests introduce a discrete amount of a dilute antigen into the skin using a syringe and a fine-gauge needle, raising a wheal of reproducible dimension (Fig. 8.4). This technique is similar to the method used with Mantoux testing for tuberculosis. ID testing introduces antigen at a slightly deeper level into the skin than prick testing. In ID testing, the change in the size of the wheal over a 10-min period is assessed; accepted systems are used for measuring and quantifying the degree of response. Initial ID testing using antigens of a single concentration is rarely done because there can be an increased risk of systemic reaction using this technique. For that reason, ID testing is conducted

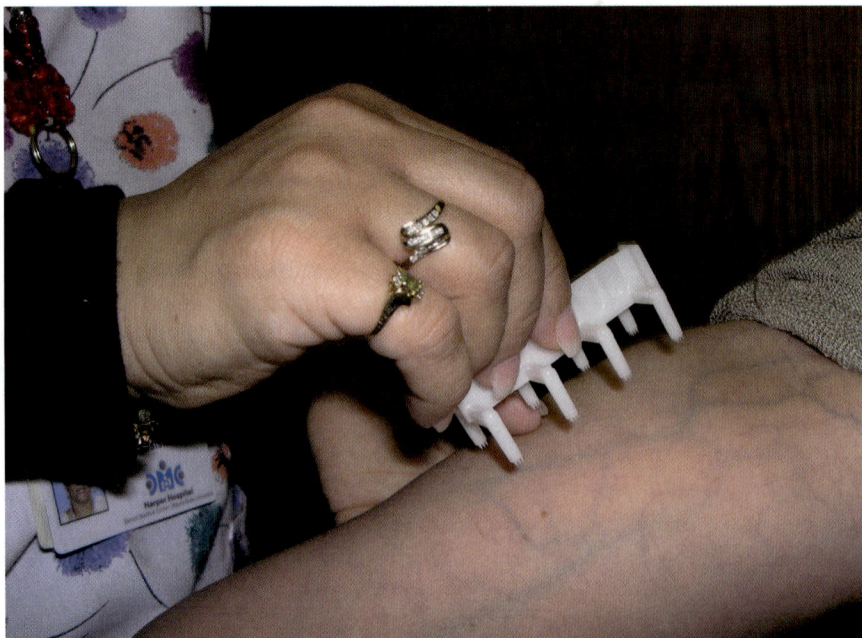

Fig. 8.3 Skin testing for allergic rhinitis using the multiple-prick method

Fig. 8.4 Skin testing for allergic rhinitis using the intradermal method

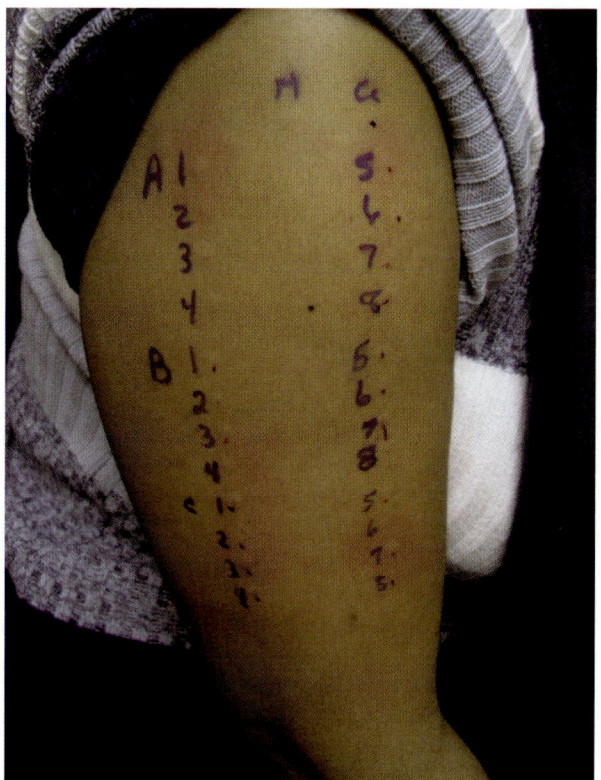

following the prior use of prick testing or in a sequential manner using multiple ID tests starting at very dilute concentrations and progressing to more concentrated antigens. The serial use of multiple antigens of increasing concentration is well established and is referred to either as *serial endpoint titration* (SET) or as *intradermal dilutional testing* (IDT). Blended testing methods using a combination of prick and ID tests have also been used for many years, and current systems allow more accurate quantification of allergic sensitivity with these techniques with approaches such as *modified quantitative testing* (MQT) [14].

Because skin testing carries the risk of large local reactions and, rarely, of severe systemic reactions, anaphylaxis, and death, skin testing should be conducted only by clinicians who are trained and experienced in its use. When properly done, however, it is safe and well tolerated.

In vitro allergy testing involves the use of clinical laboratory analysis for the presence of specific IgE antibodies. In this assay, serum drawn from a patient suspected of allergy is evaluated using one of several methods in which both the presence and the amount of specific IgE are assessed to one or more suspected allergens. Serum is incubated with anti-IgE antibodies and complexes are formed with patient IgE antibodies for specific allergens if they are present in the serum. Using a tagged radioactive or immunoreactive label, these complexes can be quantified and the presence and severity of allergy to each individual antigen can be assessed. Accuracy of results from in vitro testing compare favorably with those obtained through skin testing. The advantage of in vitro testing is that it is simple, rapid, safe, and can be conducted even when patients are on medications that may interfere with skin testing results (e.g., antihistamines). Disadvantages of in vitro testing include higher costs and slightly decreased sensitivity when compared with skin testing [15].

The Association of Allergy and Rhinosinusitis

The majority of information supporting a comorbid link between AR and RS has been gathered from epidemiologic studies conducted over the past 20 years. These data suggest a relationship in the development and expression of symptoms among patients with RS, although a true pathogenetic link has been difficult to establish.

In one classic study, a group of 224 young adults with acute maxillary RS were matched with a group of 103 young adults without RS and evaluated with skin testing for the presence of allergy. Results demonstrated that patients with RS had a numerically higher prevalence of skin-test positivity than did healthy control subjects (45% vs. 33%). These findings suggest that AR may play a role in the development of RS, at least in a subset of sensitive individuals [16].

In another important study, 40 subjects with perennial AR were compared with 30 nonallergic subjects to assess the relative presence of physical and radiologic signs of RS. All subjects had computed tomography (CT) scans of their sinuses to evaluate the presence of findings consistent with RS. Results demonstrated a higher prevalence of RS among patients with perennial AR than among their nonallergic counterparts. These findings again suggest that AR may contribute to the development or persistence of RS in some individuals [17].

While it may be difficult to describe a causal relationship between AR and RS, several research studies suggest that the presence of AR may affect the severity of symptoms among individuals with RS, as well as impact resistance to medical therapy. Among a sample of 200 consecutive patients who underwent sinus surgery and also had in vitro testing for routine allergens, 80% of individuals demonstrated significantly elevated levels of specific IgE for one or more antigens. As the prevalence of allergy in the general population is estimated at 25% to 30%, this observation would suggest that the presence of allergy may contribute to the development of chronic RS, or at least affect its severity and response to medical therapy [18].

In another study, 50 consecutive patients who underwent sinus surgery had skin testing for inhalant allergy, received CT scans to assess the severity of chronic RS, and completed quality-of-life instruments to evaluate the perceived impact of their disease. Patients with RS reported significant adverse impact on their quality of life. In addition, the presence and severity of allergy on skin testing was significantly associated with decrements in perceived quality of life. Changes on CT scan, however, did not appear to be associated with quality of life [19]. These findings were confirmed in a similar study, in which allergy was judged to be an independent predictor of the severity of RS and its response to surgical treatment [20].

Other studies have suggested that the severity of disease among patients with chronic RS is associated with the presence of allergy. In one such study, 104 patients undergoing sinus surgery had preoperative and intraoperative assessments that included CT scans, in vitro allergy tests, sinus cultures, tissue and serum eosinophilias, and quality-of-life measurements. Among patients who underwent surgery, the extent of disease on CT scan and the presence of eosinophils in the sinus tissue were associated with elevations of specific IgE on in vitro allergy testing. The authors suggested that this relationship might be more vigorous among patients with extensive disease. They further suggested that both chronic RS and AR appeared to share similar immune mechanisms [21]. Other authors have reported similar relationships between the presence of allergy and the severity of RS [22–24].

Despite epidemiologic evidence linking AR and RS, convincing mechanisms that would account for the observed association between these two diseases have not been developed. It does appear that instillation of an antigen into the nose among allergic patients known to be sensitive to that antigen will reproduce symptoms consistent with RS. In one such study, 37 patients with known chronic RS and AR were challenged with installation of antigen directly into the nose [25]. Among this group of patients, 29 individuals complained of upper respiratory symptoms in the sinuses and ears. Changes were also noted on sinus radiographs among these individuals. The authors of this study argued that antigen exposure in sensitized individuals causes significant changes in the sinonasal mucosa, resulting in localized edema, mucociliary dysfunction, and increased mucous production. While this model could account for symptom exacerbations among allergic individuals with chronic RS, it is unable to explain the initial development of RS among atopic patients.

In a similar study, nasal antigen challenge among a group of patients with known AR demonstrated changes in the sinuses related to the presence of the antigen. In this study, sensitive patients had antigen instilled into one side of the nose, and eosinophils were harvested from both maxillary sinuses. An increase in eosinophils collected by sinus lavage was noted bilaterally. The authors of this study suggested that a direct neurogenic reflex was responsible for these changes within the sinuses, and that inflammation could be found in the sinuses simply by installation of antigen into the nose [26].

This series of studies suggests that the presence of AR appears to be involved as a cofactor in the disease expression of patients with both acute and chronic RS. Although a direct pathogenic relationship may be difficult to establish, evidence demonstrates that patients with both AR and RS appear to have increased symptoms secondary to their RS, can have their symptoms exacerbated by exposure to antigens, and can be more resistant to treatment, both surgical and medical. For that reason, it is important to recognize the presence of allergies among patients with RS and to assure that management strategies are implemented that address the allergic component of these patients' symptoms.

Treatment of Allergic Rhinitis in the Patient with Rhinosinusitis

Management of the patient with AR involves a coordinated strategy designed to both modify the burden of disease and decrease its symptomatic expression. Optimal management often utilizes a multifaceted approach to therapy and may involve input from several disciplines to maximize outcome. The treatment of AR has generally been conceptualized to include one or more of three important strategies: (1) allergen avoidance, (2) pharmacotherapy, and (3) antigen-specific immunotherapy (Table 8.3).

Avoidance

Since AR is a disease that is triggered by exposure to antigens to which an individual has been previously sensitized, it is logical to attempt to control the contact that a patient may have with relevant antigen triggers. The ability to exert effective environmental controls in patients with AR is an important therapeutic adjunct that allows specific treatment interventions to be more successful [27].

To allow effective allergen avoidance, it is first important to identify those allergens that are relevant in the expression of the patient's symptoms. The most valuable element of the diagnostic workup of the patient with AR is therefore the allergy history, as important triggers to the development of symptoms can often be readily identified. For example, among patients who are allergic to cat dander, it is quite common for them to realize that they become much more symptomatic when in the presence of cats than when away from them. This simple observation can lead to a treatment strategy of cat avoidance that can decrease the burden of exposure and improve patient symptoms. Clinicians should therefore be diligent in conducting a complete allergy history.

Table 8.3 Management options for treatment of allergic rhinitis

Environmental control procedures
    Antigen avoidance
Pharmacotherapy
    Antihistamines
        Oral
        Topical
    Decongestants
        Oral
        Topical
    Corticosteroids
        Oral/parenteral
        Topical
    Leukotriene modifiers
    Mast cell stabilizers
    Anticholinergics
Immunotherapy
    Subcutaneous
    Sublingual

In addition to exploring the patient's allergy history, other triggers to the exacerbation of symptoms should also be established. Many patients with AR also have nonallergic triggers—such as cigarette smoke and strong odors—and exposure to these triggers can worsen their allergic disease. Decreasing exposure to nonallergic triggers among patients with AR can limit the expression of their disease and their symptoms of AR and RS.

Three basic strategies should be employed in practicing good environmental controls in allergen avoidance:

1. Remove the source of the antigen (if possible)
2. Remove accumulated antigen
3. Prevent the return of the antigen

As it is not equally plausible to effectively reduce exposure to all relevant antigens, selective implementation of these three strategies can result in optimal management.

For example, it may not be possible to remove the source of outdoor pollens such as grass or ragweed antigens during their season. It is often possible, however, to decrease exposure to the outdoor environment and to prevent the accumulation of grass or ragweed pollen inside the home. Keeping windows closed during pollen seasons, using air conditioning to ventilate and cool the air, and employing whole-house or room filtration devices can modify the inside environment sufficiently to decrease patient exposure and lessen symptoms. In another example, if a patient is allergic to cat dander, it is possible to remove cats from the home, or to at least limit their presence throughout the house. It may take several months to clear cat dander from the home after removal of the animal, but the decline in the burden of antigen in the environment will improve patient symptoms and lessen nasal inflammation.

While effects of managing allergen exposure have not been directly assessed in the treatment of acute and chronic RS, it would be logical to limit contact with sensitized antigens to decrease local inflammation in the nasal and sinus mucosa. As has been demonstrated in experimental models, nasal inhalation of antigens in sensitive individuals will increase sinus mucosal thickening and the presence of eosinophils. Since these processes are relevant in the development of symptoms among patients with RS, it is reasonable to decrease exposure to known allergens. Simple strategies to limit allergen burden can be safely and easily applied.

Pharmacotherapy

The mainstay of therapy for the treatment of AR is the use of medications designed to decrease allergic symptoms, downregulate inflammatory processes in the nose, and improve patient quality of life. Many classes of medications have been used in the treatment of patients with AR, and their efficacy has been well established (for a listing of these medication classes, see Table 8.4). The utility of these agents

Table 8.4 Medications for allergic rhinitis (AR): effects on symptoms

Agent	Sneezing	Itching	Congestion	Rhinorrhea	Eye Symptoms
Oral antihistamines	+++	+++	+/–	++	+++
Nasal antihistamines	++	++	++	+	–
Intranasal corticosteroids	++	++	+++	++	+
Leukotriene modifiers	+	+	+	+	+
Oral decongestants	–	–	+++	–	–
Nasal decongestants	–	–	+++	–	–
Nasal mast cell stabilizers	+	+	+/–	+	–
Topical anticholinergics	–	–	–	+++	–

+++, marked benefit; ++, substantial benefit; +, some benefit; +/–, questionable benefit; –, no benefit.

in treating concurrent RS has only been established in a smaller subset of these medications. This section reviews the medical management of AR, and special note is made of evidence that directly impacts the treatment of patients with RS.

Antihistamines

The most frequently prescribed class of medications for the management of AR is the antihistamines. These products have been widely used in the treatment of patients with AR since the 1950s, and their use continues to be common today. Antihistamines were developed in the 1940s and came into widespread use shortly thereafter. Antihistamines work primarily as selective antagonists to the histamine-1 (H1) receptor, in which they bind to these surface receptors on target cells, change the confirmation of these receptors, and occupy and deactivate the response of the receptor to the binding of histamine. Antihistamines have a wide range of clinical efficacy, as well as marked variability in their adverse event profile.

The earliest antihistamines in general use included medications such as diphenhydramine, chlorpheniramine, and hydroxyzine. In general, these agents were poorly selective H1 antagonists that exerted relatively poor binding at the H1 receptor and therefore required significant doses to exhibit a clinical effect. While they could demonstrate clinical efficacy at sufficient dose levels, these agents were also highly lipophilic and readily crossed the blood–brain barrier. When bound to central H1 receptors, these earlier (or *first-generation*) antihistamines uniformly caused significant central nervous system effects, including sedation, somnolence, drowsiness, and cognitive and psychomotor impairment. In addition, because these agents were relatively nonselective, their use was also accompanied by anticholinergic side effects such as blurred vision, dry mouth, and urinary retention. They are also frequently associated with increased mucous tenacity, which can be problematic in a patient with RS in whom mucociliary clearance is an essential goal of therapy.

Newer, or *second-generation*, antihistamines demonstrate significantly greater receptor selectivity than their older counterparts. As a result, they are usually effective at significantly lower doses and are not associated with the range and severity of adverse effects noted with first-generation agents. The first group of these newer antihistamines was introduced in the 1980s and included medications such as terfenadine, astemizole, and loratadine. These agents demonstrated good binding affinity at the H1 receptor and exerted significant clinical antihistaminic effect. Cardiac toxicity and impaired liver clearance caused both terfenadine and astemizole to be removed from the market in the 1990s. Loratadine continues to be available in the United States as an over-the-counter (OTC) preparation. Newer second-generations antihistamines available for clinical use in the United States include fexofenadine, cetirizine, desloratadine, and levocetirizine. Topical agents available for use in the eye and nose include azelastine, olapatadine, and epinastine.

These newer antihistamines have been shown to be equally effective as older medications without the significant adverse effects noted with agents such as diphenhydramine. As oral agents, loratadine, fexofenadine, and desloratadine are classified as "nonsedating," meaning that they do not exert significant sedation at recommended doses. Both cetirizine and levocetirizine are mildly sedating at recommended doses. Sensitive individuals can complain of sedation with these agents, and antihistamines should be evaluated for their sedating effects on an individual basis.

While no antihistamine is indicated for the primary or adjuvant treatment of RS, it is reasonable to treat patients who have concurrent AR and RS with appropriate allergy medications, including antihistamines. Two studies suggest that the use of antihistamines can be of benefit in treating patients with AR and RS. One study demonstrated that the addition of loratadine to the antibiotic treatment of patients with acute RS decreased patient symptoms when compared with the addition of a placebo [28]. In addition, in an animal model, the use of desloratadine was shown to inhibit allergic symptoms and reduce sinonasal infection among sensitized mice [29]. Aside from these studies, the treatment of AR among patients with RS has not been directly examined.

Despite the lack of research in this area, from the standpoint of relevant comorbidities, it would appear to be beneficial in treating patients with AR and RS with concurrent antibiotic and antihistamine therapy. First-generation antihistamines with anticholinergic side effects should be avoided because of their effects on mucous clearance, as well as their sedation and impairment effects. Additional research is indicated in this area.

Decongestants

A common symptom noted by patients with both acute and chronic RS is nasal congestion. Patients with RS frequently complain of facial pressure, nasal blockage, and sinonasal obstruction. For this reason, decongestant medications are often recommended as adjuvant treatment for RS, especially in the early treatment of patients with acute RS. Decongestants can be administered by either the topical or oral route and work through alpha-receptors in the nasal mucosa to stimulate vasoconstriction and decrease nasal obstruction. Decongestants are nonselective alpha-agonists and affect receptors not only in the nose but also in the brain, cardiovascular system, and prostate. Common agents used as decongestants include topical oxymetazoline and phenylephrine, and oral pseudoephedrine and phenylephrine.

Decongestants are widely used for nasal obstruction and show significant and rapid benefit when used either orally or topically. Although nasally applied agents are more efficacious and work more quickly, they are also accompanied by the rapid development of tachyphylaxis and tolerance. Rebound congestion can occur within days, and prolonged use can result in significant nasal inflammation through a syndrome known as rhinitis medicamentosa. This dependency seen with topical decongestants, and to a lesser extent oral decongestants, limits the use of this class of medications.

The side effect profile of decongestant medications reflects the nonselective alpha-agonistic activity of the class. Central nervous system effects such as anxiety, tremulousness, insomnia, and irritability are very common and are dose-related. Cardiovascular effects are common, and include hypertension, cardiac irritability, tachycardia, and arrhythmia. In addition, decongestants cause prostatic hypertrophy by their alpha-agonistic effects on the prostate, resulting in urinary retention in older men. These side effects can be quite bothersome, and, in extreme cases, dangerous for patients at risk.

Despite the potential beneficial impact of treating nasal congestion in patients with RS, there is little evidence supporting the use of oral or topical decongestants among these patients. No studies support the use of oral agents such as pseudoephedrine, despite their frequent use. Topical treatment with oxymetazoline has been shown to be of benefit in only a few small studies. In one investigation, the use of topical oxymetazoline was shown to not only improve nasal airflow but to modulate proinflammatory cytokines among patients with acute RS [30]. This benefit was supported in another small-scale study [31]. In contrast, two studies suggest that the use of topical oxymetazoline in patients with RS may inhibit bacterial clearance and natural defense mechanisms in acute bacterial RS [32,33]. For this reason, the use of topical decongestants in patients with acute RS should be applied with caution. There is no benefit of these agents for patients with chronic RS.

Corticosteroids

Corticosteroid medications are widely used in both the treatment of AR and RS. Corticosteroids are available in both topical and systemic forms. Systemic formulations can be administered both orally and parenterally. While injectable "depot" formulations of corticosteroids have been widely used in practice, current guidelines in the treatment of AR recommend against their use for safety reasons [34]. Oral corticosteroids are used short term in the treatment of AR but are often used over longer periods in the management of patients with chronic RS.

The use of oral steroids in the treatment of chronic RS is widespread and well established by expert opinion. Several papers suggest that in patients with chronic

RS oral corticosteroids should be considered a component of their maximal medical therapy [35,36]. The use of oral steroids is limited by the well-known side effect profile of this class of drugs, including elevations in intraocular pressure, cataract formation, musculoskeletal and joint effects, and mental status aberrations. When used in the treatment of acute or chronic RS, oral steroids should be limited to the shortest period that is feasible to bring about therapeutic benefit.

During the past two decades, topical intranasal corticosteroids (INCS) have become widely used in the primary management of patients with AR. They have been shown to be safe and effective for use in children as young as 2 years of age, and newer agents such as fluticasone propionate and mometasone furoate are free from growth suppression and significant systemic effects. Their benefit in the treatment of AR is well established; and INCS have been shown consistently to be the most efficacious agents in the management of patients with AR. Currently available INCS include flunisolide, beclomethasone dipropionate, triamcinolone acetonide, budesonide, fluticasone propionate, mometasone furoate, and fluticasone furoate.

INCS have also been extensively studied for the treatment of patients with acute and chronic RS. A series of studies describes the benefit of INCS in the management of patients with acute RS, both as monotherapy and as an adjunct to the use of antibiotics. A recent Cochrane review of INCS in the treatment of the symptoms of acute RS concludes that there is significant benefit in using INCS along with antibiotic therapy [37]. INCS have been shown to contribute to a more rapid and complete reduction of symptoms than when antibiotics are used without INCS. Support for the adjuvant use of INCS [38–41], as well as for the use of INCS alone in the treatment of acute RS [42], is widely noted in the literature. The use of INCS as an adjunct to antibiotics in patients with acute RS brings about a more rapid resolution of symptoms such as headache, facial pressure, and nasal congestion. Evidence supports the use of INCS in the adjuvant treatment of patients with acute RS.

INCS have been studied less extensively in the treatment of chronic RS. The use of INCS appears to decrease the bacterial burden among this group of patients. In one study, preoperative use of INCS resulted in the decreased recovery of pathogenic bacteria at the time of surgery in a group of patients undergoing sinus surgery for chronic RS [43]. In another study, 167 patients with chronic RS were randomized to receive either budesonide nasal spray or placebo over a 20-week period. Allergic patients on budesonide demonstrated decreased nasal congestion and nasal discharge and improved sense of smell when compared with patients treated with placebo. Nonallergic patients with chronic RS did not demonstrate these effects. Both allergic and nonallergic patients in this study demonstrated improved nasal airflow [44]. Similar findings were noted with beclomethasone dipropionate [45].

Treatment of patients with chronic RS with nasal polyps using INCS has also been shown to be effective. Several studies have confirmed the efficacy of mometasone furoate in the treatment of nasal polyps [46,47]. This treatment appears to be effective in both allergic and nonallergic patients, and demonstrates both reduction in nasal congestion as well as improvement in the endoscopically assessed volume of polypoid tissue present in the nasal cavity. Similar findings have been noted with fluticasone propionate [48,49], beclomethasone dipropionate [48,49], and budes-onide [50].

Research with INCS strongly supports the use of these agents in the treatment of acute RS, chronic RS without nasal polyps, and chronic RS with nasal polyps. These agents appear to be safe and well tolerated. Adverse event profiles with these medications are favorable. INCS treatment appears to have benefit in patients with both allergic and nonallergic RS, although some evidence suggests an enhanced benefit in patients with AR. INCS should be used as adjuvant treatment in the management of both acute and chronic RS.

Leukotriene Modifiers

Another class of medications that shows benefit in the treatment of AR is the leukotriene modifiers. Leukotrienes are arachidonic acid metabolites that are potent proinflammatory agents in the nasal and sinus mucosa. They have been shown to be involved in chronic inflammatory respiratory diseases such as AR and asthma and are implicated in sinonasal diseases such as chronic RS with and without nasal polyps. Medications that are available to treat asthma include montelukast, zafir-lukast, and zileuton, although montelukast is the only one of these three agents to be approved for the treatment of AR. Both montelukast and zafirlukast are leukotriene receptor antagonists, and zileuton is an inhibitor of the 5-OH-lipoxygenase enzyme, involved in the conversion of arachidonic acid to the leukotrienes.

Montelukast has been used extensively in the treatment of AR. It is shown to have benefits in both seasonal and perennial AR and has efficacy relative to that seen with loratadine in several clinical trials. More recently, the use of montelukast in patients with RS has been reviewed. A retrospective review of the use of montelukast in chronic RS with polyposis suggested that this medication could show significant efficacy in this subset of patients [51]. Efficacy supporting the use of montelukast was also seen in 10 patients with chronic RS. The addition of montelukast to their routine medical therapy brought about incremental improve-ment in symptom control among this sample. Although objective measures did not demonstrate improvement in nasal airflow, patient-reported symptoms did improve, suggesting that there may be adjuvant benefit in adding montelukast in this group [52]. While these data should be considered preliminary, there may be benefit to adding montelukast to the regimen of allergic patients with RS, especially in the group that has chronic RS with nasal polyps. Additional research is warranted.

Immunotherapy

The third treatment principle that is used in the management of patients with AR is antigen-specific immunotherapy. Immunotherapy involves the administration of small but increasing amounts of antigen to which a patient has been shown to be sensitive, usually through the subcutaneous route. In the past several years in the

United States, immunotherapy has also been administered sublingually, or under the tongue, in an attempt to decrease side effects and improve patient adherence. Sublingual immunotherapy is currently the primary treatment for the immune management of allergies across Europe and the United Kingdom.

Immunotherapy is generally used among patients with AR who are poorly responsive to medical therapy. It can be used as the sole treatment method for these patients, or more frequently in combination with pharmacotherapy and allergen avoidance. The benefit of immunotherapy is that over time it can modulate the allergic response among patients with AR, reducing the effect of proinflammatory mediators of allergic inflammation and decreasing patient hypersensitivity and symptoms. It is therefore used as a method of desensitization to allergens to which the patient is known to be allergic. Immunotherapy has been a common treatment for AR for at least a century.

Efficacy of immunotherapy in the treatment of AR has been well established. Large-scale meta-analytic reviews completed by the Cochrane group have demonstrated that both subcutaneous [53] and sublingual [54] immunotherapy show significant benefit in the treatment of AR when compared with placebo treatments. These findings strongly support the role of antigen-specific immunotherapy in the treatment of patients with AR.

Among patients with concomitant AR and RS, the use of immunotherapy has not been well established. Since studies suggest that both allergic rhinitis and chronic RS may have similar immune mechanisms, some authors have argued that immunotherapy should be employed in the treatment of allergic patients with chronic RS [55]. Immunotherapy has been commonly used as part of the treatment for patients with allergic fungal sinusitis and has shown good efficacy in one series of patients [56]. In addition, in one series, immunotherapy has been shown to be an effective adjuvant therapy following sinus surgery in both allergic and nonallergic patients for symptom control [57]. Unfortunately, little additional evidence exists to support the use of immunotherapy in this population.

As with other methods of treatment for patients with AR, it would be prudent to optimally manage allergic disease in patients with both AR and RS to decrease the contribution of inflammation secondary to allergy. Despite the absence of supporting data, antigen-specific immunotherapy should be considered as part of the comprehensive treatment of patients with both recurrent acute RS and chronic RS.

Framework for Managing Concurrent Allergic Rhinitis and Rhinosinusitis

Present models consider RS to be an inflammatory disease that has many interacting elements and potential pathophysiological triggers. While acute RS may most commonly involve an infectious pathology, recurrent acute RS and chronic RS likely have several mechanisms that contribute to their pathogenesis and symptom expression. The role of inflammatory processes, such as allergic disease in RS, must be evaluated and managed to optimize patient outcome and control recurrent and chronic symptoms.

Much is understood about how adequate ventilation and drainage of the sinuses contribute to normal functioning and freedom from disease. In large part, ventilation and drainage of the sinuses relies on a normal anatomic framework of the sinuses and functional, patent openings between the sinuses and the nose. In addition, an increasing body of evidence supports the role of various types of inflammatory processes in RS, including the role of allergy and concurrent AR. With worsening mucosal inflammation, the sinuses become less able to remain healthy and patients develop increasing symptoms. In managing the patient with RS, therefore, it is valuable to consider the relative input of both these broad areas in developing the most effective treatment strategy.

RS can therefore be modeled as a disease that involves the interaction between two areas: structural and physiological. The clinician should attempt to assess the relative contributions of these two factors in approaching patients with chronic and recurrent sinus disease. Structural issues concern the anatomy of the nose and facial framework. Any significant anatomic abnormalities, such as a badly deviated nasal septum or abnormally pneumatized sinus cells, can contribute to anatomic dysfunction. In addition, the clinician must evaluate any underlying acute or chronic physiological issues, such as allergy and other inflammatory diseases. Through understanding the relative input of these two potential contributors, the clinician can best assess the factors affecting the individual patient's symptoms and can prescribe appropriate therapeutic strategies to maximize treatment and improve patient outcomes (Table 8.5).

In patients with recurrent acute RS and with chronic RS, it is therefore important to understand the role of allergy in contributing to their disease. As noted earlier, an allergy workup in this setting would involve a thorough patient history, a focused physical examination, and the possible use of skin or in vitro allergy tests to confirm the presence of an inhalant allergy. In the case of significant allergic disease, it would be reasonable to manage the patient's AR using appropriate methods of allergen avoidance, pharmacotherapy, and immunotherapy as indicated. If the patient fails appropriate medical management, and if allergy appears to be a significant component of the patient's disease, then evaluation by an otolaryngologist with special training in allergy would be appropriate both to confirm the presence of allergy and to offer specific treatment for allergic disease such as immunotherapy.

Table 8.5 Framework for managing allergic rhinitis and rhinosinusitis

Structural issues	Physiological issues
Deviated nasal septum	Allergic rhinitis
Concha bullosa	Persistent infection
Haller cells	Immunodeficiency
Polypoid obstruction	Polypoid obstruction
Stenotic ostia	Samter's triad
Foreign body	
CONSIDER SURGERY	CONSIDER MEDICAL MANAGEMENT

Conclusion

Allergic rhinitis and rhinosinusitis are comorbid conditions that share elements of pathogenesis and symptom expression. Among patients with RS, allergic factors appear to be of importance and can make treatment of RS more challenging and less successful. A thorough evaluation of the potential role for allergy in each individual patient with RS will allow clinicians to institute specific therapy for AR that will decrease the patient's symptoms and improve quality of life. The clinician should, therefore, be vigilant to the presence of allergy among patients with RS—especially those who have recurrent or chronic symptoms—and should consider aggressive management of allergy among these patients to decrease morbidity and to potentially improve control of their RS.

References

1. Sanders SH. Allergic rhinitis and sinusitis. Otolaryngol Clin N Am 1971;4:565–578.
2. Settipane RA. Demographics and epidemiology of allergic and nonallergic rhinitis. Allergy Asthma Proc 2001;22:185–189.
3. Stankiewicz J, Osguthorpe JD. Medical treatment of sinusitis. Otolaryngol Head Neck Surg 1994;110:361–362.
4. Naclerio R, Solomon W. Rhinitis and inhalant allergens. JAMA 1997;278:1842–1848.
5. Settipane GA. Allergic rhinitis: update. Otolaryngol Head Neck Surg 1986;94:470–474.
6. Nimmagadda SR, Evans R III. Allergy: etiology and epidemiology. Pediatr Rev 1999;20: 111–115.
7. Reed SD, Lee TA, McCrory DC. The economic burden of allergic rhinitis: a critical evaluation of the literature. Pharmacoeconomics 2004;22:345–361.
8. Stempel DA, Woolf R. The cost of treating allergic rhinitis. Curr Allergy Asthma Rep 2002;2:223–230.
9. Wang DY, Gordon BR, Chan YH, et al. Potential non-IgE mediated food allergies: comparison of open challenge and DBPCFC. Otolaryngol Head Neck Surg (in press).
10. Bousquet J, Van Cauwenberge P, Khaltaev N; ARIA Workshop Group; World Health Organization. Allergic rhinitis and its impact on asthma. J Allergy Clin Immunol 2001;108: S147–S334.
11. Krouse JH, Stachler RJ, Shah A. Current in vivo and in vitro screens for inhalant allergy. Otolaryngol Clin N Am 2003;36:855–868.
12. Salkie ML. Role of clinical laboratory in allergy testing. Clin Biochem 1994;27:343–355.
13. Mullarkey MF, Hill JS, Webb DR. Allergic and non-allergic rhinitis: their characterization with attention to the meaning of nasal eosinophilia. J Allergy Clin Immunol 1980;65:122–126.
14. Krouse JH, Mabry RL. Skin testing for inhalant allergies 2003: current strategies. Otolaryngol Head Neck Surg 2003;129:S33–S49.
15. Poon AW, Goodman CS, Rubin RJ. In vitro and skin testing for allergy: comparable clinical utility and costs. Am J Manag Care 1998;4:969–985.
16. Savolainen S. Allergy in patients with acute maxillary sinusitis. Allergy 1989;44:116–122.
17. Berrettinin S, Carabelli A, Sellari-Franceschini S, et al. Perennial allergic rhinitis and chronic sinusitis: correlation with rhinologic risk factors. Allergy 1999;54:242–248.
18. Emanuel IA, Shah SB. Chronic rhinosinusitis: allergy and sinus computed tomography relationships. Otolaryngol Head Neck Surg 2000;123:687–691.
19. Krouse JH. Computed tomography stage, allergy testing, and quality of life in patients with sinusitis. Otolaryngol Head Neck Surg 2000;123:389–392.
20. Stewart MG, Donovan DT, Parke RM Jr, et al. Does the severity of sinus tomography findings predict outcome in chronic sinusitis? Otolaryngol Head Neck Surg 2000;123:81–84.

21. Newman LJ, Platts-Mills TA, Phillips CD, et al. Chronic sinusitis: relationship of computed tomographic findings to allergy, asthma, and eosinophilia. JAMA 1994;271:363–367.
22. Ramadan HH, Fornelli R, Ortiz AO, et al. Correlation of allergy and severity of sinus disease. Am J Rhinol 1999;13:345–347.
23. Lane AP, Pine HS, Pillsbury HC. Allergy testing and immunotherapy in an academic otolaryngology practice. Otolaryngol Head Neck Surg 2001;124:9–15.
24. Yariktas M, Doner F, Demirci M. Rhinosinusitis among the patients with perennial or seasonal allergic rhinitis. Asian Pac J Allergy Immunol 2003;21:75–78.
25. Pelikan Z, Pelikan-Filipak M. Role of nasal allergy in chronic maxillary sinusitis—diagnostic value of nasal challenge with antigen. J Allergy Clin Immunol 1990;86:484–491.
26. Baroody FM, Saengpanich S, deTineo M, et al. Nasal allergy challenge leads to bilateral maxillary sinus eosinophil influx [abstract]. J Allergy Clin Immunol 2002;109:S216.
27. Ferguson BJ. Environmental controls in allergy. Curr Opin Otolaryngol 1995;3:44–49.
28. Braun JJ, Alabert JP, Michel FB, et al. Adjunct effect of loratadine in the treatment of acute sinusitis in patients with allergic rhinitis. Allergy 1997;52:650–655.
29. Kirtsreesakul V, Blair C, Yu X, et al. Desloratadine partially inhibits the augmented bacterial responses in the sinuses of allergic and infected mice. Clin Exp Allergy 2004;34: 1649–1654.
30. Tuettenberg A, Koelsch S, Knop J, et al. Oxymetazoline modulates proinflammatory cytokines and the T-cell stimulatory capacity of dendritic cells. Exp Dermatol 2007;16:171–178.
31. Inanli S, Ozturk O, Korkmaz M, et al. The effects of topical agents of fluticasone propionate, oxymetazoline, and 3% and 0.9% sodium chloride solutions on mucociliary clearance in the therapy of acute bacterial rhinosinusitis in vivo. Laryngoscope 2002;112:320–325.
32. Bende M, Fukami M, Arfors KE, et al. Effect of oxymetazoline nose drops on acute sinusitis in the rabbit. Ann Otol Rhinol Laryngol 1996;105:222–225.
33. Min YG, Kim HS, Suh SH, et al. Paranasal sinusitis after long-term use of topical nasal decongestants. Acta Otolaryngol 1996;116:465–471.
34. Dykewicz MS, Fineman S, Skoner DP, et al. Diagnosis and management of rhinitis. Complete guidelines of the Joint Task Force on Practice Parameters in Allergy, Asthma and Immunology. American Academy of Allergy, Asthma and Immunology. Ann Allergy Asthma Immunol 1998;81:478–518.
35. Gillespie MB, Osguthorpe JD. Pharmacologic management of chronic rhinosinusitis, alone or with nasal polyposis. Curr Allergy Asthma Rep 2004;4:478–485.
36. Lund VJ. Maximal medical therapy for chronic rhinosinusitis. Otolaryngol Clin N Am 2005;38:1301–1310.
37. Zalmanovici A, Yaphe J. Cochrane Database Syst Rev 2007; 2:CD005149.
38. Nayak AS, Settipane GA, Pedinoff A, et al. Effective dose range of mometasone furoate in the treatment of acute rhinosinusitis. Ann Allergy Asthma Immunol 2002;89: 271–278.
39. Meltzer EO, Charous BL, Busse WW, et al. Added relief in the treatment of acute recurrent sinusitis with adjunctive mometasone furoate nasal spray. The Nasonex Sinusitis Group. J Allergy Clin Immunol 2000;106:630–637.
40. Yilmaz G, Varan B, Yilmaz T, et al. Intranasal budesonide spray as an adjunct to oral antibiotic therapy for acute sinusitis in children. Eur Arch Otorhinolaryngol 2000;257:256–259.
41. Dolor RJ, Witsell DL, Hellkamp AS, et al. Comparison of cefuroxime with or without intranasal fluticasone for the treatment of rhinosinusitis. The CAFFS Trial: a randomized controlled trial. JAMA 2001;286:3097–3105.
42. Meltzer EO, Bachert C, Staudinger H. Treating acute rhinosinusitis: comparing safety and efficacy of mometasone furoate nasal spray, amoxicillin, and placebo. J Allergy Clin Immunol 2005;116:1289–1295.
43. Desrosiers M, Hussain A, Frenkiel S, et al. Intranasal corticosteroid use is associated with lower rates of bacterial recovery in chronic rhinosinusitis. Otolaryngol Head Neck Surg 2007;136:235–239.

44. Lund VJ, Black JH, Szabo LZ, et al. Efficacy and tolerability of budesonide aqueous nasal spray in chronic rhinosinusitis patients. Rhinology 2004;42:57–62.
45. Giger R, Pasche P, Cheseaux C, et al. Comparison of once- versus twice-daily use of beclomethasone dipropionate aqueous nasal spray in the treatment of allergic and non-allergic chronic rhinosinusitis. Eur Arch Otorhinolaryngol 2003;260:135–140.
46. Stjarne P, Mosges R, Jorissen M, et al. A randomized controlled trial of mometasone furoate nasal spray for the treatment of nasal polyposis. Arch Otolaryngol Head Neck Surg 2006;132:179–185.
47. Small CB, Hernandez J, Reyes A, et al. Efficacy and safety of mometasone furoate in nasal polyposis. J Allergy Clin Immunol 2005;116:1275–1281.
48. Lund VJ, Flood J, Sykes AP, et al. Effect of fluticasone in severe polyposis. Arch Otolaryngol Head Neck Surg 1998;124:513–518.
49. Holmberg K, Juliusson S, Balder B, et al. Fluticasone propionate aqueous nasal spray in the treatment of nasal polyposis. Ann Allergy Asthma Immunol 1997;78:270–276.
50. Jankowski R, Schrewelius C, Bonfils P, et al. Efficacy and tolerability of budesonide aqueous nasal spray treatment in patients with nasal polyps. Arch Otolaryngol Head Neck Surg 2001;127:447–452.
51. Parnes SM. The role of leukotriene inhibitors in patients with paranasal sinus disease. Curr Opin Otolaryngol Head Neck Surg 2003;11:184–191.
52. Wilson AM, White PS, Gardiner Q, et al. Effects of leukotriene antagonist therapy in patients with chronic rhinosinusitis in a real life rhinology clinic setting. Rhinology 2001;39:142–146.
53. Calderon MA, Alves B, Jacobson M, et al. Allergen injection immunotherapy for seasonal allergic rhinitis. Cochrane Database Syst Rev 2007;1:CD001936.
54. Wilson DR, Torres LI, Durham SR. Sublingual immunotherapy for allergic rhinitis: systematic review and meta-analysis. Cochrane Database Syst Rev 2003;2:CD002893.
55. Nguyen LH, Fakhri S, Frenkiel S, et al. Molecular immunology and immunotherapy for chronic sinusitis. Curr Allergy Asthma Rep 2003;3:505–512.
56. Mabry RL, Mabry CS. Allergic fungal sinusitis: the role of immunotherapy. Otolaryngol Clin N Am 2000;33:433–440.
57. Nishioka GJ, Cook PR, Davis WE, et al. Immunotherapy in patients undergoing functional endoscopic sinus surgery. Otolaryngol Head Neck Surg 1994;110:406–412.

Chapter 9
Complementary and Alternative Medicine in Rhinology

Marcelo B. Antunes, Edwin Tamashiro, and Noam A. Cohen

Complementary and alternative medicine encompasses a wide range of practices. Eisenberg et al. defined this practice as "medical interventions not taught widely at U.S. medical schools or generally available at U.S. hospitals" [1]. Recently, a great interest has developed for the practice of complementary and alternative medicine (CAM), as evidenced by the number of publications on this subject. In 1999, the National Institutes of Health (NIH) established the National Center for Complementary and Alternative Medicine (NCCAM), which is funding research in this area. This is a further indication that "Western Medicine" is embracing certain aspects of the alternative practices and attempting to glean knowledge from these long-practiced remedies. Unfortunately, for practitioners in the U.S. many of the studies evaluating the efficacy of CAM have been published in languages other than English.

In 1990, a survey reported that one third of the population of the United States used some form of CAM, and of those, nearly three-quarters did not inform their physicians of such practice [1]. In a subsequent study focusing on the changes in patients' practices between 1990 and 1997, the authors demonstrated that the use of CAM increased from 33.8% to 42.1%. Expenditure on CAM and CAM-related products was estimated to be $13.7 billion in 1990 and increased to approximately $21.2 billion in 1997 [2]. Moreover, this study estimated that the number of visits to practitioners of complementary medicine exceeded that of the number of visits to primary care physicians.

The use of CAM in otorhinolaryngology permeates all the discipline's subspecialties, and thus the American Academy of Otolaryngology – Head and Neck Surgery (AAO-HNS) has established a Committee on Alternative Medicine to serve as a resource for information on this practice. The most common forms of CAM employed are herbal medicines, acupuncture, homeopathy, massage, mind–body medicine, and chiropractic manipulation [3]. In most of these arenas there is no evidence of safety or efficacy. In rhinology, there are several conditions for which

N.A. Cohen
Department of Otorhinolaryngology – Head and Neck Surgery, University of Pennsylvania, Philadelphia, PA, USA
e-mail: Cohenn@uphs.upenn.edu

E.R. Thaler, D.W. Kennedy (eds.), *Rhinosinusitis*, DOI: 10.1007/978-0-387-73062-2_9,   133
© Springer Science+Business Media, LLC 2008

CAM has been widely used, including the common cold/upper respiratory infections, allergic rhinitis, acute rhinosinusitis (ARS), and chronic rhinosinusitis (CRS). In 2001, a survey of 175 patients with rhinosinusitis in Northern California reported that 43% of patients used some form of CAM to alleviate their symptoms, with herbal medicine being utilized by 26% of subjects [4]. Krouse et al. in 1999 reported on the use of CAM by 120 patients and found that 35% of the cohort underwent chiropractic treatment, 29% herbal medicines, and 19% acupuncture for the treatment of their sinus conditions [5]. Thus, clinicians must be aware of these practices and actively query their patients on the use of CAM, not only for their potential benefits, but because they may have potential adverse effects, interact with traditional therapies, or complicate surgical intervention.

Herbal Medicines

Herbal medicines are the most common form of CAM used by rhinology patients for several different disease entities [4]. The most commonly used herbs for rhinologic symptoms are *Echinacea*, Sinupret® (a combination of five herbs), bromelain (an extract of pineapple), and a myriad of Chinese herbs and extracts. Less commonly used herbs are Bi Yuan Shu, Esberitox, Myrtol, cineole, and *Ecballium elaterium*. The compositions of these herbal medicines are summarized in Table 9.1.

Echinacea is one of the best-studied herbs. Although there are multiple species of the plant, *Echinacea pallida* and *Echinacea purpurea* are most commonly used in CAM [6]. The therapeutic effects of echinacea have long been debated, with some authors suggesting that this herb may have an immunomodulatory effect on lymphocytes [7,8]. Scientific evidence demonstrating beneficial clinical effects for the common cold is conflicted, with several studies demonstrating symptomatic improvement [9,10] and others demonstrating no benefit [11,12]. However, a recent meta-analysis of three studies that assessed the efficacy of echinacea in the prevention of symptomatic experimental rhinovirus infection demonstrated that the

Table 9.1 Summary of herbal medicines

Herbal medicine	Herbal components
Echinacea	*Echinacea pallida* and *Echinacea purpurea*
Sinupret	*Gentiana lutea, Primula veris, Rumex* sp., *Sambucus nigra, Verbana officinalis*
Bromelain	*Ananas comosus,* extract from pineapple
Esberitox	*Thuja ocidentalis, Echinacea angustifolia, Baptista tinctoria*
Myrtol	Alpha-pinene, D-limonene, and 1,8-cineole, extracted from pine, lime, and *Eucalyptus globulus*
Cineole	Essential oil extracted from *Eucalyptus globulus*
Bi Yuan Shu	Chinese herb mixture that contains a number of different herbs including *Magnolia lilifora, Xanthium strumairium, Astragalus membranaceus, Angelica dahurica,* and *Scutellaria baicalensis*
Ecballium elaterium	Herb extracted from cucumber, used mostly in Turkey
Shea butter	*Butyrospermum parkii*
Butterbur	*Petasites hybridus*

likelihood of experiencing the common cold was significantly higher with placebo than with the herb [13]. The Cochrane collaboration reviewed several studies on echinacea and its effects on the common cold, and the concluding recommendations were that clinicians should be aware that the majority of the echinacea products have not been tested. Nevertheless, the herb may be beneficial for common cold symptoms in adults if started early [14].

Sinupret® is a trademarked preparation developed in Germany composed of a blend of five herbs: European elder, common sorrel, cowslip, European vervain, and gentian. Three trials investigated the effect of this preparation as an adjunct treatment for acute rhinosinusitis (ARS) in patients being treated with antibiotics [15]. In two of the trials, a statistically significant improvement was demonstrated with the addition of the herbal preparation in the therapeutic regimen, while the third study demonstrated a trend toward improvement but did not reach significance. One trial evaluated the effect of Sinupret in chronic rhinosinusitis (CRS) and reported both clinical and radiologic improvement following 7 days of oral administration three times per day [16].

Bromelain is a pineapple extract with antiinflammatory, antithrombotic, and fibrinolytic properties. Proteolytic activity of the substance modifies tissue permeability, with resultant reduction of edema [17]. The modulation of tissue permeability and fibrinolysis promotes the resorption of the edema and enhances tissue permeability for some antibiotics. Additionally, bromelain modulates function of adhesion molecules and immune cells, including their cytokine production. In vitro, bromelain stimulates production of tumor necrosis factor (TNF)-α, interleukin (IL)-1β, and IL-6 [18,19]. Three double-blind, placebo-controlled studies have demonstrated a significant improvement in sinusitis symptoms with the use of bromelain [20–22]. In all these trials, the patients were using antibiotics with adjuvant bromelain or placebo. These studies were predominated by patients with ARS. The significance of beneficial effects varied among the studies as to outcomes of symptoms, including nasal obstruction, headache, nasal discharge, and nasal mucosal inflammation.

The Chinese herb Bi Yuan Shu has been evaluated in CRS with and without nasal polyps following functional endoscopic sinus surgery (FESS). Three hundred forty patients were randomized to receive the herb in addition to the standard treatment of antibiotic and topical steroids. Quality-of-life outcomes were determined on days 7, 14, 30, and 60. The patients who received Bi Yuan Shu demonstrated significant improvement when questioned about pain, breathing difficulty, purulent discharge, and hyposmia, but not cough [15]. The utilization of the Chinese herbal extracts in the management of allergic rhinitis also appears to have some efficacy. Xue et al. demonstrated that a mixture of 18 different herb extracts resulted in improvement in symptoms when compared to placebo, as measured by quality-of-life questionnaires [23]. Furthermore, in conjunction with acupuncture, Chinese herbs have been demonstrated to have a significant improvement in quality of life compared to sham acupuncture and nonspecific herbs [24]. Yang et al. used a mixed formula of Chinese herbs to treat perennial allergic rhinitis for 3 months and found that patients with high titers of IgE had significant improvement in a symptom score. Moreover, the levels of IgE decreased after treatment. The authors also compared cytokine production by mononuclear cells and COX-2 mRNA expression before and after therapy and found that the formula enhanced IL-10, but decreased IL-5, interferon (INF)-γ production, and COX-2 expression after 3 months of treatment [25].

Several other herbal extract combinations including Esberitox, Myrtol, and cineole have been demonstrated to be effective in reducing the symptoms of acute rhinosinusitis with short-term (<14 days) use [15,26]. *Isodon Japonicus* has been used in Korea as an antiinflammatory medicine. An experimental study in an allergic mouse model demonstrated that this herb inhibited mast cell-derived, immediate-type allergic reactions and decreased production of TNF-α [27].

Ecballium elaterium is the only herb that has been tested in an animal model of sinusitis [28]. The authors used a well-established rabbit model for sinusitis and treated the animals with an aqueous solution of *Ecballium elaterium* or normal saline irrigation. The endpoint of the study was evaluation of inflammatory mediators in the tissue, specifically nitric oxide (NO) metabolites. Evidence suggesting antiinflammatory activity of the herb was demonstrated by significant higher levels of NO metabolites in the control group. However, upper aerodigestive tract edema resulting from *Ecballium elaterium* therapy in patients with atopy has been reported [29].

Butterbur (*Petasites hybridus*) is a shrub-like plant native to Europe. Extracts of the root have been used to treat allergies and asthma. Three clinical trials have been conducted to study the effect of this herb on rhinitis. One compared the herb with cetirizine and found that both treatments are equally effective in terms of quality-of-life endpoints [30]. A second trial demonstrated that butterbur was equivalent to fexofenadine [31]. However, a recent randomized placebo-controlled trial failed to detect any significant effect on symptoms or inspiratory peak flow [32]. Last, shea butter (from *Butyrospermum parkii*) placed on the upper lip was found to be more effective as a nasal decongestant[33] than oxymetazoline drops.

It is not surprising that herbal medicines have measurable clinical effect considering the amount of active pharmacologic components they have. However, one must keep in mind that despite the general belief that herbal therapies are safe, they are not completely devoid of side effects and pharmacologic interactions (see Table 9.2) [34].

Table 9.2 Side effects of herbal therapies [34]

Herb	Adverse effects
Echinacea	Liver toxicity
	Short-term use: immunostimulant
	Long-term use: immunosuppressive
Garlic	Inhibits platelet aggregation
Ginkgo	Inhibits platelet-activating factor
Ginger	Increased bleeding time
St. John's wort	Central serotonin, noradrenaline and dopamain antagonist
	Induction of cytochrome p450
Valerian	Potentiation of GABA

Acupuncture

Acupuncture is probably the form of CAM that has the widest acceptance in the medical community. In 1997, an NIH consensus statement [35] concluded that there was enough evidence of the value of acupuncture to encourage further studies of its physiology and clinical value. The theoretical function of acupuncture is to restore the balance of "vital flows" by inserting needles into specific points where the "meridians" for vital flow lie. When investigating the scientific merit of the technique, sham acupuncture is performed as a control.

Recently, a survey of acupuncturists in Northern California was performed assessing their management of sinus and nasal symptoms [36]. With a 22% response rate they reported that the overall efficacy of their treatment was 4.2 on a five-point scale (1 = not effective and 5 = very effective). The improvement was generally in subjective symptoms such as facial pain, headache, pressure, and congestion. The most common acupuncture points to treat nasal and sinus problems were LI4, located on the back side of the hand between the thumb and first finger, and LI20, located in the nasolabial groove, at the midpoint of the lateral border of the ala nasi (Fig. 9.1). However, most of the practitioners reported using the types of herbal medicines discussed previously as adjuvant therapy.

The majority of the studies with acupuncture and rhinitis are not randomized nor controlled. A pilot study to evaluate the effect of acupuncture in allergic rhinitis demonstrated an improvement in airway resistance; however, the effect did not reach significance [37]. A case series studied the radiologic outcome pre- and postacupuncture and found no difference in CT scan scores [36]. Additionally, two randomized placebo-controlled trials failed to demonstrate a benefit in rhinitis symptoms [38,39]. Attempting to address the mechanism of action of acupuncture, Petti et al. compared levels of IL-2, IL-6, and IL-10 in allergic patients before and after acupuncture and demonstrated that only levels of IL-10 had a significant reduction in symptoms compared to the sham or no treatment groups [40]. A direct comparison of acupuncture with conventional medical therapy for chronic rhinosinusitis—consisting of 2 to 4 weeks of antibiotics, steroids, and nasal irrigation—demonstrated statistically significant improvement in radiographic scoring and quality-of-life measures with conventional therapy, while traditional acupuncture demonstrated a nonsignificant improvement in symptom scores [41].

Homeopathy

Homeopathy was founded in the beginning of the 1800s and is based on the principle that disease can be cured by application of the inciting substance in ultra-diluted formulations. Remedies are selected according to the patient's symptoms and are prepared with special techniques. The use of homeopathy in rhinitis has been investigated by several studies. A meta-analysis of seven studies that evaluated the efficacy of homeopathic medicine revealed that this practice probably reduces the duration of influenza [42]. Three double-blinded, placebo-controlled

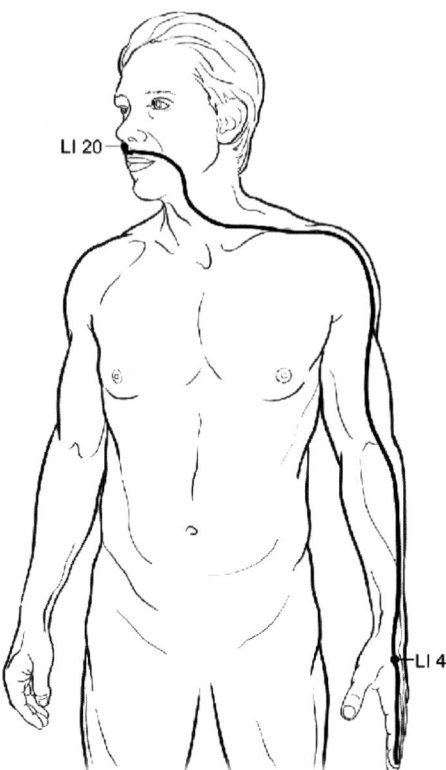

Fig. 9.1 Illustration of LI4 and LI20, the most common meridians used by acupuncturists to treat rhinitis and rhinosinusitis. LI4 or Large Intestine 4 is called "He Gu," which is the command Point of the Face and Mouth. It is located on the dorsum of the hand, approximately at the midpoint of the second metacarpal bone, in the belly of the first interosseus dorsalis muscle. LI20 or Large Intestine 20 is called "Ying Xiang," which is the Meeting Point on the Large Intestine Channel with the Stomach Channel. It is located in the nasolabial groove, 0.5 cm lateral to the nostril. (Illustration by Alice Y. Chen.)

trials have investigated the effectiveness of homeopathy in rhinitis. Using a visual analogue symptom scale, Reilly et al. and Kim et al. reported significant differences favoring the homeopathy treatment groups for allergic diseases compared to placebo [43,44], while a direct comparison of homeopathy with cromolyn for exacerbations of hay fever found that both therapies were equally effective [45]. Evaluation of the homeopathic remedy Betula 30c in double-blinded, placebo-controlled studies for management of allergic rhinitis symptoms [46], or as a prophylaxis for allergic rhinitis [47], demonstrated no benefit from the intervention. Last, two meta-analyses directed at evaluating the efficacy of homeopathic intervention compared to placebo in various diseases concluded that the effects of homeopathy cannot be completely due to placebo effect, but that insufficient evidence exists to conclude whether the practice is efficacious [48,49]. This result was largely caused by the poor methodological quality of the trials.

Other Complementary and Alternative Therapies

Vitamin C

Vitamin C (ascorbic acid) has long been part of folkloric medicine as a preventative and treatment for the common cold. A meta-analysis of 30 trials evaluating the efficacy of vitamin C in preventing or reducing the duration of the common cold concluded that there is no evidence demonstrating the utility of vitamin C in prevention and only a very modest benefit in reducing the duration of symptoms [50]. However, a prospective study analyzing serum antioxidant levels (including vitamin C) demonstrated significantly lower serum levels in children with chronic rhinosinusitis than age- and gender-matched healthy children [51]. Last, a study using intranasal vitamin C solution to treat allergic rhinitis demonstrated that, after 2 weeks of therapy, 74% of treated patients exhibited a decrease in nasal blockage, secretion, and edema, while in the placebo group only 24% of the patients had improvement in their symptoms [52].

Urtica dioca

Although *Urtica dioca* (stinging nettle) has been commonly used to treat allergies, the antiinflammatory mechanism is not entirely clear. The extract of the plant's hairs contains both serotonin and histamine [53] and, although counterintuitive, histamine has been demonstrated to downregulate polymorphonuclear leukocytes and reduce the production of leukotrienes [54]. There is no evidence of its efficacy in the management of rhinosinusitis, but a trial in patients with allergic rhinitis demonstrated benefits in global assessments [55].

Nasal Irrigation

Nasal irrigation and inhalation of vaporized water is often recommended as a home remedy for various sinonasal conditions. One study in patients with allergic rhinitis revealed that normal saline irrigation significantly reduced levels of histamine and leukotriene C4 in nasal washings [56]. A randomized clinical trial with hypertonic saline nasal irrigation in patients with acute or chronic rhinosinusitis demonstrated that the scores on the Rhinosinusitis Disability Index (RSDI) and Sino-nasal Outcomes Test (SNOT-20) significantly improved after an average of 2.4 irrigations per week [57]. Another study also demonstrated that nasal irrigations for 2 weeks and reflexology massage improve symptoms in chronic rhinosinusitis [58]. Recently, Chiu et al. demonstrated that 1% baby shampoo irrigations in normal saline, twice a day for 1 month, improved symptom scores of patients with recurrent sinusitis following functional endoscopic sinus surgery [59].

Humming

Humming increases the production of nitric oxide (NO) by healthy sinuses and increases the gas exchange between the sinus cavity and the nasal cavity [60]. A study conducted on patients with allergic rhinitis evaluated NO level changes produced by humming after quiet exhalation. It found that in those patients for whom the NO levels did not increase (non-hummers), compared with those whose levels increased (hummers), there was significantly worse sinus ostium obstruction detected by nasal endoscopy [61]. Last, a case report stated that strong humming for 1 h daily lessened symptoms of chronic rhinosinusitis and accelerated recovery [62].

Phototherapy

Phototherapy has an immunosuppressive effect and is able to inhibit allergic reactions in the skin. A randomized double-bind study evaluated the effect of a mixture of UV-A (25%), UV-B (5%), and visible light (70%) applied intranasally (rhinophototherapy) three times weekly for three weeks on allergic rhinitis induced by ragweed. This treatment demonstrated a significant improvement in symptoms (sneezing, rhinorrhea, nasal itching), as well as a reduction of the number of eosinophils and the levels of eosinophil cationic protein and IL-5 in nasal secretions [63]. This finding confirmed a prior randomized double-blind study, using low-energy narrow-band red light phototherapy, which demonstrated significant improvement in symptoms and endoscopic scores of patients with allergic rhinitis [64].

Conclusions

Over the centuries, many remedies have been concocted and practiced to treat the symptoms of allergic rhinitis and rhinosinusitis. Although anecdotal evidence supports these practices, few corroborative clinical trials have been performed. The brevity of this chapter illustrates the paucity of evidence available to support or refute some of these practices.

References

1. Eisenberg DM, Kessler RC, Foster C, et al. Unconventional medicine in the United States. Prevalence, costs, and patterns of use. N Engl J Med 1993;328:246–252.
2. Eisenberg DM, Davis RB, Ettner SL, et al. Trends in alternative medicine use in the United States, 1990–1997: results of a follow-up national survey. JAMA 1998;280:1569–1575.
3. Ernst E, Fugh-Berman A. Complementary and alternative medicine: what is it all about? Occup Environ Med 2002;59:140–144; quiz 144, 184.

4. Blanc PD, Trupin L, Earnest G, et al. Alternative therapies among adults with a reported diagnosis of asthma or rhinosinusitis : data from a population-based survey. Chest 2001;120: 1461–1467.

5. Krouse JH, Krouse HJ. Patient use of traditional and complementary therapies in treating rhinosinusitis before consulting an otolaryngologist. Laryngoscope 1999;109:1223–1227.

6. Asher BF, Seidman M, Snyderman C. Complementary and alternative medicine in otolaryngology. Laryngoscope 2001;111:1383–1389.

7. Melchart D, Linde K, Worku F, et al. Results of five randomized studies on the immunomodulatory activity of preparations of Echinacea. J Altern Complement Med 1995;1:145–160.

8. Sun LZ, Currier NL, Miller SC. The American coneflower: a prophylactic role involving nonspecific immunity. J Altern Complement Med 1999;5:437–446.

9. Percival SS. Use of echinacea in medicine. Biochem Pharmacol 2000;60:155–158.

10. Barrett B, Vohmann M, Calabrese C. Echinacea for upper respiratory infection. J Fam Pract 1999;48:628–635.

11. Barrett BP, Brown RL, Locken K, et al. Treatment of the common cold with unrefined echinacea. A randomized, double-blind, placebo-controlled trial. Ann Intern Med 2002;137: 939–946.

12. Melchart D, Linde K, Fischer P, et al. Echinacea for preventing and treating the common cold. Cochrane Database Syst Rev 2000;CD000530.

13. Schoop R, Klein P, Suter A, et al. Echinacea in the prevention of induced rhinovirus colds: a meta-analysis. Clin Ther 2006;28:174–183.

14. Linde K, Barrett B, Wolkart K, et al. Echinacea for preventing and treating the common cold. Cochrane Database Syst Rev 2006;CD000530.

15. Guo R, Canter PH, Ernst E. Herbal medicines for the treatment of rhinosinusitis: a systematic review. Otolaryngol Head Neck Surg 2006;135:496–506.

16. Richstein A, Mann W. Treatment of chronic sinusitis with Sinupret. Ther Ggw 1980;119: 1055–1060.

17. Maurer HR. Bromelain: biochemistry, pharmacology and medical use. Cell Mol Life Sci 2001;58:1234–1245.

18. Desser L, Rehberger A. Induction of tumor necrosis factor in human peripheral-blood mononuclear cells by proteolytic enzymes. Oncology 1990;47:475–477.

19. Desser L, Rehberger A, Paukovits W. Proteolytic enzymes and amylase induce cytokine production in human peripheral blood mononuclear cells in vitro. Cancer Biother 1994;9: 253–263.

20. Ryan RE. A double-blind clinical evaluation of bromelains in the treatment of acute sinusitis. Headache 1967;7:13–17.

21. Seltzer AP. Adjunctive use of bromelains in sinusitis: a controlled study. Eye Ear Nose Throat Mon 1967;46:1281–1288.

22. Taub SJ. The use of bromelains in sinusitis: a double-blind clinical evaluation. Eye Ear Nose Throat Mon 1967;46:361–362.

23. Xue CC, Thien FC, Zhang JJ, et al. Treatment for seasonal allergic rhinitis by Chinese herbal medicine: a randomized placebo controlled trial. Altern Ther Health Med 2003;9:80–87.

24. Brinkhaus B, Hummelsberger J, Kohnen R, et al. Acupuncture and Chinese herbal medicine in the treatment of patients with seasonal allergic rhinitis: a randomized-controlled clinical trial. Allergy 2004;59:953–960.

25. Yang SH, Hong CY, Yu CL. Decreased serum IgE level, decreased IFN-gamma and IL-5 but increased IL-10 production, and suppressed cyclooxygenase 2 mRNA expression in patients with perennial allergic rhinitis after treatment with a new mixed formula of Chinese herbs. Int Immunopharmacol 2001;1:1173–1182.

26. Federspil P, Wulkow R, Zimmermann T. Effects of standardized Myrtol in therapy of acute sinusitis: results of a double-blind, randomized multicenter study compared with placebo. Laryngorhinootologie 1997;76:23–27.

27. Shin TY, Kim SH, Choi CH, et al. *Isodon japonicus* decreases immediate-type allergic reaction and tumor necrosis factor-alpha production. Int Arch Allergy Immunol 2004;135:17–23.

28. Uslu C, Karasen RM, Sahin F, et al. Effect of aqueous extracts of *Ecballium elaterium* Rich, in the rabbit model of rhinosinusitis. Int J Pediatr Otorhinolaryngol 2006;70:515–518.
29. Kloutsos G, Balatsouras DG, Kaberos AC, et al. Upper airway edema resulting from use of *Ecballium elaterium*. Laryngoscope 2001;111:1652–1655.
30. Schapowal A. Randomised controlled trial of butterbur and cetirizine for treating seasonal allergic rhinitis. BMJ 2002;324:144–146.
31. Lee DK, Gray RD, Robb FM, et al. A placebo-controlled evaluation of butterbur and fexofenadine on objective and subjective outcomes in perennial allergic rhinitis. Clin Exp Allergy 2004;34:646–649.
32. Gray RD, Haggart K, Lee DK, et al. Effects of butterbur treatment in intermittent allergic rhinitis: a placebo-controlled evaluation. Ann Allergy Asthma Immunol 2004;93:56–60.
33. Tella A. Preliminary studies on nasal decongestant activity from the seed of the shea butter tree, *Butyrospermum parkii*. Br J Clin Pharmacol 1979;7:495–497.
34. Skinner CM, Rangasami J. Preoperative use of herbal medicines: a patient survey. Br J Anaesth 2002;89(5):792–795.
35. Acupuncture. NIH Consensus Statement 1997; 15: 1–34.
36. Pletcher SD, Goldberg AN, Lee J, et al. Use of acupuncture in the treatment of sinus and nasal symptoms: results of a practitioner survey. Am J Rhinol 2006;20:235–237.
37. Davies A, Lewith G, Goddard J, et al. The effect of acupuncture on nonallergic rhinitis: a controlled pilot study. Altern Ther Health Med 1998;4:70–74.
38. Passalacqua G, Bousquet PJ, Carlsen KH, et al. ARIA update: I. Systematic review of complementary and alternative medicine for rhinitis and asthma. J Allergy Clin Immunol 2006;117:1054–1062.
39. Magnusson AL, Svensson RE, Leirvik C, et al. The effect of acupuncture on allergic rhinitis: a randomized controlled clinical trial. Am J Chin Med 2004;32:105–115.
40. Petti FB, Liguori A, Ippoliti F. Study on cytokines IL-2, IL-6, IL-10 in patients of chronic allergic rhinitis treated with acupuncture. J Tradit Chin Med 2002;22:104–111.
41. Rossberg E, Larsson PG, Birkeflet O, et al. Comparison of traditional Chinese acupuncture, minimal acupuncture at non-acupoints and conventional treatment for chronic sinusitis. Complement Ther Med 2005;13:4–10.
42. Vickers AJ, Smith C. Homoeopathic Oscillococcinum for preventing and treating influenza and influenza-like syndromes. Cochrane Database Syst Rev 2000;CD001957.
43. Reilly D, Taylor MA, Beattie NG, et al. Is evidence for homoeopathy reproducible? Lancet 1994;344:1601–1606.
44. Kim LS, Riedlinger JE, Baldwin CM, et al. Treatment of seasonal allergic rhinitis using homeopathic preparation of common allergens in the southwest region of the US: a randomized, controlled clinical trial. Ann Pharmacother 2005;39:617–624.
45. Weiser M, Gegenheimer LH, Klein P. A randomized equivalence trial comparing the efficacy and safety of Luffa comp.-Heel nasal spray with cromolyn sodium spray in the treatment of seasonal allergic rhinitis. Forsch Komplementarmed 1999;6:142–148.
46. Aabel S, Laerum E, Dolvik S, et al. Is homeopathic "immunotherapy" effective? A double-blind, placebo-controlled trial with the isopathic remedy Betula 30c for patients with birch pollen allergy. Br Homeopath J 2000;89:161–168.
47. Aabel S. No beneficial effect of isopathic prophylactic treatment for birch pollen allergy during a low-pollen season: a double-blind, placebo-controlled clinical trial of homeopathic Betula 30c. Br Homeopath J 2000;89:169–173.
48. Linde K, Clausius N, Ramirez G, et al. Are the clinical effects of homeopathy placebo effects? A meta-analysis of placebo-controlled trials. Lancet 1997;350:834–843.
49. Cucherat M, Haugh MC, Gooch M, et al. Evidence of clinical efficacy of homeopathy. A meta-analysis of clinical trials. HMRAG. Homeopathic Medicines Research Advisory Group. Eur J Clin Pharmacol 2000;56:27–33.
50. Douglas RM, Chalker EB, Treacy B. Vitamin C for preventing and treating the common cold. Cochrane Database Syst Rev 2000;CD000980.

51. Unal M, Tamer L, Pata YS, et al. Serum levels of antioxidant vitamins, copper, zinc and magnesium in children with chronic rhinosinusitis. J Trace Elem Med Biol 2004;18:189–192.
52. Podoshin L, Gertner R, Fradis M. Treatment of perennial allergic rhinitis with ascorbic acid solution. Ear Nose Throat J 1991;70:54–55.
53. Oliver F, Amon EU, Breathnach A, et al. Contact urticaria due to the common stinging nettle (*Urtica dioica*): histological, ultrastructural and pharmacological studies. Clin Exp Dermatol 1991;16:1–7.
54. Flamand N, Plante H, Picard S, et al. Histamine-induced inhibition of leukotriene biosynthesis in human neutrophils: involvement of the H2 receptor and cAMP. Br J Pharmacol 2004;141:552–561.
55. Mittman P. Randomized, double-blind study of freeze-dried *Urtica dioica* in the treatment of allergic rhinitis. Planta Med 1990;56:44–47.
56. Georgitis JW. Nasal hyperthermia and simple irrigation for perennial rhinitis. Changes in inflammatory mediators. Chest 1994;106:1487–1492.
57. Rabago D, Pasic T, Zgierska A, et al. The efficacy of hypertonic saline nasal irrigation for chronic sinonasal symptoms. Otolaryngol Head Neck Surg 2005;133:3–8.
58. Heatley DG, McConnell KE, Kille TL, et al. Nasal irrigation for the alleviation of sinonasal symptoms. Otolaryngol Head Neck Surg 2001;125:44–48.
59. Chiu AG, Palmer JN, Woodworth BA, et al. Baby shampoo nasal irrigations for the symptomatic post-FESS patient. Am J Rhinol 2007;(in press).
60. Weitzberg E, Lundberg JO. Humming greatly increases nasal nitric oxide. Am J Respir Crit Care Med 2002;166:144–145.
61. Maniscalco M, Sofia M, Weitzberg E, et al. Humming-induced release of nasal nitric oxide for assessment of sinus obstruction in allergic rhinitis: pilot study. Eur J Clin Invest 2004;34: 555–560.
62. Eby GA. Strong humming for one hour daily to terminate chronic rhinosinusitis in four days: a case report and hypothesis for action by stimulation of endogenous nasal nitric oxide production. Med Hypotheses 2006;66:851–854.
63. Koreck AI, Csoma Z, Bodai L, et al. Rhinophototherapy: a new therapeutic tool for the management of allergic rhinitis. J Allergy Clin Immunol 2005;115:541–547.
64. Neuman I, Finkelstein Y. Narrow-band red light phototherapy in perennial allergic rhinitis and nasal polyposis. Ann Allergy Asthma Immunol 1997;78:399–406.

Chapter 10
Radiology: Its Diagnostic Usefulness in Rhinosinusitis

Laurie A. Loevner

This chapter addresses imaging modalities available to assess disease processes of the sinonasal cavity and provides some direction on when and how to use them. To understand the pathogenesis and imaging appearances of rhinosinusitis and other pathological processes that may affect the paranasal sinuses, a brief review of sinus development and anatomy as it pertains to mucociliary clearance is essential. Subsequently, focused imaging assessment of disease processes, including rhinosinusitis and neoplasms, is covered.

Development

The maxillary sinuses are the first of the paranasal sinuses to develop, beginning in the first trimester of gestation and usually completed by adolescence [1]. The ethmoid air cells arise from numerous evaginations from the nasal cavity, beginning with the anterior air cells, and progressing to the posterior air cells. The ethmoid air cells start to develop between the end of the first trimester and the mid-second trimester of gestation, and their final adult proportions are usually attained during puberty. The sphenoid sinus is present by the second trimester of pregnancy, and usually finishes its growth by the time a child reaches 10 years of age. The frontal sinuses are the only sinuses that are consistently absent at birth. Their development is variable, beginning during the first few years of life, and is completed in early adolescence [1].

Anatomy

To understand the disease processes that may affect the paranasal sinuses and the nasal cavity, it is important to understand the anatomy as well as the normal drainage patterns of the sinonasal cavity [1,2]. The paranasal sinuses and nasal

L.A. Loevner
Department of Otorhinolaryngology – Head and Neck Surgery, University of Pennsylvania, Philadelphia, PA, USA
e-mail: laurie.loevner@uphs.upenn.edu

E.R. Thaler, D.W. Kennedy (eds.), *Rhinosinusitis*, DOI: 10.1007/978-0-387-73062-2_10,   145
© Springer Science+Business Media, LLC 2008

cavity are lined by ciliated columnar epithelium, which contains both mucinous and serous glands. The common drainage pathway for the frontal sinuses, maxillary sinuses, and anterior ethmoid air cells is through the ostiomeatal complex [2]. The ostiomeatal unit comprises a drainage pathway that consists of the maxillary sinus ostium, the infundibulum, the hiatus semilunaris, and the middle meatus (Fig. 10.1a,b). This drainage conduit is centered about the uncinate process (an osseous extension of the lateral nasal wall). Secretions that accumulate within the maxillary sinuses circulate toward the maxillary sinus ostium propelled by cilia within this sinus. From the maxillary ostium, mucus circulates through the infundibulum located lateral to the uncinate process. Secretions progress through the hiatus semilunaris, an air-filled channel above the tip of the uncinate process and anterior and inferior to the ethmoidal bulla (the largest ethmoid air cell), and then pass into the middle meatus, the nasal cavity, and ultimately into the nasopharynx. They are then swallowed.

The frontal sinuses drain inferiorly via the frontal ethmoidal recess/nasofrontal duct into the middle meatus, the common drainage site also for the anterior ethmoid air cells, which have ostia in contact with the infundibulum of the ostiomeatal complex. The nasofrontal duct is the channel between the inferomedial frontal sinus and the anterior part of the middle meatus. The anteriormost ethmoid air cells, the agger nasi cells, are located in front of the middle turbinates, which are in turn located anterior, lateral, and inferior to the frontal ethmoidal recess. Inconstant ethmoid air cells located along the anterosuperior maxillary surface just inferior to the orbital floor, referred to as maxilloethmoidal or Haller cells, are present in less than one-half of imaged patients. These cells are important because if they are opacified they may obstruct the infundibulum of the ostiomeatal unit.

The posterior ethmoid air cells are located behind the middle turbinate and secretions drain through the superior meatus, the supreme meatus, and/or other tiny ostia under the superior turbinate into the sphenoethmoidal recess, the nasal cavity, and finally into the nasopharynx (Fig. 10.1c,d). Cilia are necessary for the drainage of the sphenoid sinuses as secretions must be propelled to the ostia that is located above the sinus floor.

The three sets of turbinates in the nasal cavity include the superior, middle, and inferior turbinates. Occasionally, there may be a supreme turbinate located above the superior turbinate. When the middle turbinate is aerated, it is termed a concha bullosa, present in up to 30% to 50% of patients. Large or opacified concha bullosa may obstruct the ostiomeatal complex, the common drainage passageway of the frontal sinus, maxillary sinus, and anterior ethmoid air cells.

The nasal septum separates the right and left nasal turbinates, dividing the nasal cavity in half. The anterior and inferior nasal septum is made up of cartilage. The posterior portion of the nasal septum is osseous. The superior posterior osseous portion is the perpendicular plate of the ethmoid bone, and the inferoposterior osseous portion is the vomer. The septum within the nasal cavity is lined by squamous epithelium; e remainder of the nasal cavity and the paranasal sinuses are lined by columnar epithelium.

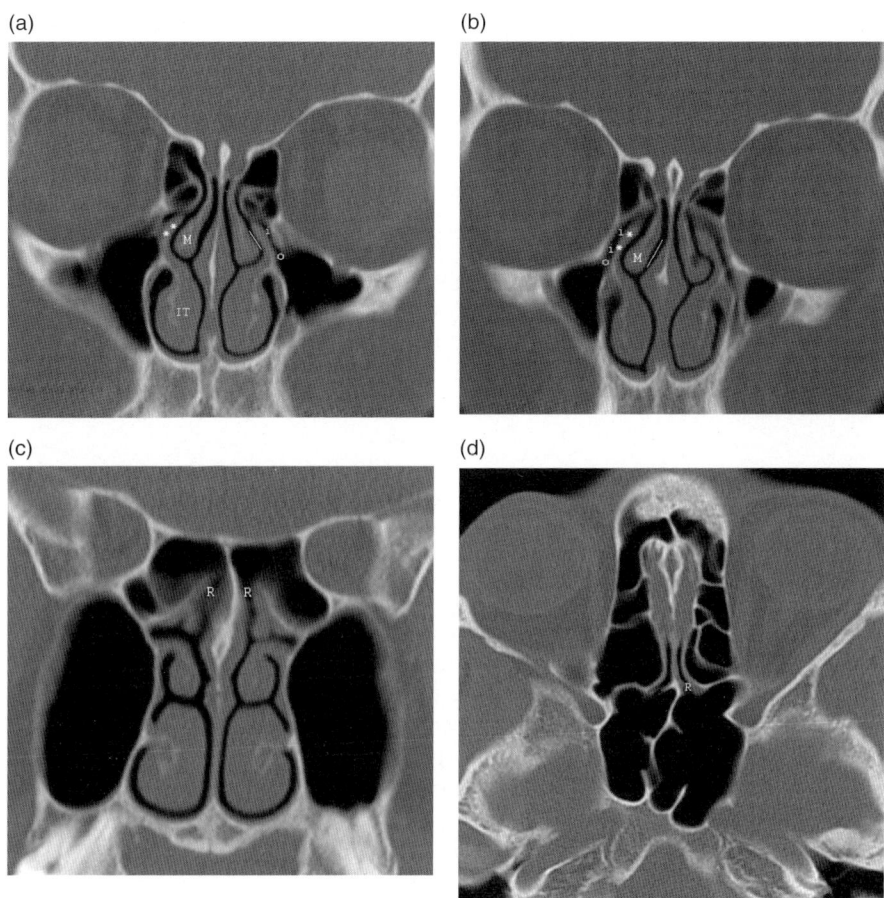

Fig. 10.1 Normal anatomy of the mucociliary drainage of the paranasal sinuses. (**a, b**) Coronal computed tomography (CT) images in bone algorithm show the normal drainage pathway of the maxillary sinus, anterior ethmoid air cells, and frontal sinus via the ostiomeatal complex (*OMC*). *, uncinate process; *O*, maxillary sinus ostium; *i*, infundibulum; *white line*, middle meatus; *m*, middle turbinate; *IT*, inferior turbinate. Coronal (**c**) and axial (**d**) CT images in bone algorithm show the normal drainage of the posterior ethmoid air cells and the sphenoid sinus via the sphenoethmoidal recess into the nasal cavity (*R*)

The nasolacrimal duct runs from the lacrimal sac at the medial canthus, along the anterior and lateral nasal wall, and drains into the inferior meatus. There is normal cyclical passive congestion and decongestion of each side of the nasal cavity and ethmoid air cells, which includes temporary mucosal thickening in these structures.

Blood supply to the sinonasal structures comes from the internal and external carotid arteries. The arterial supply to the frontal sinuses is from supraorbital and supratrochlear branches of the ophthalmic artery, while venous drainage is through the superior ophthalmic veins. The ethmoid air cells and sphenoid sinus also receive blood supply from branches of the sphenopalatine artery (arising from the external carotid circulation) as well as ethmoidal branches of the ophthalmic artery (arising from the internal carotid circulation). Venous drainage is via nasal veins into the nasal cavity, and/or ethmoidal veins that drain into the ophthalmic veins, which then subsequently drain into the cavernous sinus. Branches of the maxillary artery that arise from the external carotid circulation supply the maxillary sinuses predominantly. These sinuses drain through facial and maxillary veins, the latter communicating with the pterygoid venous plexus. The venous drainage pattern of the paranasal sinuses (ultimately communicating with the cavernous sinus and pterygoid venous plexus) is responsible for the potential intracranial complications of rhinosinusitis including meningitis, subdural empyema, and venous thrombosis.

Imaging Sinonasal Disease: The Radiologist's Arsenal

Plain Film Radiographs

Several years ago, computed tomography (CT) replaced plain film radiographs as the mainstay in evaluating sinonasal disease. In the 1980s, functional endoscopic sinonasal surgery (FESS) supplanted external procedures such as the Caldwell-Luc and maxillary antrostomy for the treatment of rhinosinusitis, which has required much greater anatomic precision than is provided by plain film radiographs. Overlapping structures on plain film radiographs limit evaluation of the ostiomeatal complex, as well as the individual paranasal sinuses. There is also insufficient detail regarding the osseous confines of the sinonasal cavity.

Plain film radiographs are sometimes obtained in intensive care unit settings when rhinosinusitis is suspected or needs to be excluded in fevers of unknown origin and the patient is too sick to come to the radiology department for CT imaging. However, portable CT units are rapidly multiplying, making access to portable CT scans in hospitalized patients the new reality.

Computed Tomography

As functional endoscopic sinonasal surgery (FESS) has replaced external surgical procedures for treating rhinosinusitis, CT imaging has become necessary to provide the surgeon with precise anatomic information. Functional endoscopic sinonasal surgery is performed through an intranasal endoscope, and CT provides the precise anatomic information as seen by the endoscopist. Surgery is directed toward removing blockages to mucociliary clearance at the ostiomeatal complex. For the surgeon performing FESS, coronal CT is ideal as it simulates the appearance of the sinonasal cavity from an endoscopic view.

Direct coronal thin section imaging (1.5 to 3 mm) is frequently obtained through the paranasal sinuses. Using the newer helical CT scanners, high-quality axial reformatted images may be created from these coronal images. Alternatively, direct axial CT imaging is performed with subsequent creation of coronal reformatted images. Many computer software programs allow instant three-plane reconstructions (for instance, coronal and sagittal reconstructions from axial images). Intravenous contrast material is usually not necessary in sinonasal CT imaging for inflammatory disease. If CT imaging shows findings like bone destruction or extension of disease outside the sinonasal cavity concerning a more aggressive process such as a neoplasm or invasive rhinosinusitis [3,4], magnetic resonance (MR) imaging should be obtained without and with intravenous contrast administration, which is a more sensitive study. If the patient has a contraindication to MR imaging (i.e., pacemaker) and an enhanced study is indicated, then contrast-enhanced CT is the appropriate alternative study.

Magnetic Resonance Imaging

Because of its excellent soft tissue resolution and multiplanar capabilities, MR imaging has become an increasingly important technology in assessing patients with both benign and malignant neoplasms of the sinonasal cavity, as well as meningoencephaloceles and aggressive infections such as invasive fungal rhinosinusitis. A combination of sagittal, axial, and coronal imaging provides excellent anatomic information regarding the extent of sinonasal tumors. Multiple different image acquisitions (sequences) are obtained, including T_1-weighted and T_2-weighted as well as contrast-enhanced multiplanar imaging. In most instances, excellent anatomic resolution may be acquired from an MR examination performed in a standard head coil. On occasion, imaging of the sinonasal cavity may be performed with a surface coil positioned over the face (the sinus of interest). Imaging of sinonasal malignancies and aggressive infections must include high-resolution views not only of the sinonasal cavity but also of the orbits, skull base, and the intracranial compartment. Magnetic resonance imaging allows discrimination of inflammation and inspissated secretions from neoplasm and other nonneoplastic masses (i.e., encephalocele) and is valuable in assessing for extension of disease (neoplasms and aggressive infections such as invasive fungus) outside the sinonasal cavity into the intracranial compartment, the eye, and the base of skull [3].

Sinonasal secretions have variable signal intensity patterns on MR related to multiple factors including the protein concentration relative to mobile water protons, viscosity, and cross-linking of glycoproteins [5]. As the protein concentration in secretions increases relative to free water, the signal intensity on T_1-weighted imaging changes from hypointense (dark) to hyperintense (bright) to hypointense again. On T_2-weighted images, secretions with low protein content are initially bright; however, as the protein content and viscosity increase, the signal intensity decreases.

Imaging Disease Processes of the Paranasal Sinuses

Inflammatory Disease/Rhinosinusitis

Most cases of acute rhinosinusitis are related to an antecedent viral upper respiratory tract infection. The resultant swelling causes apposition of the mucosal surfaces within the paranasal sinuses, leading to obstruction of the normal drainage pathways. Inadequate drainage of secretions results in bacterial overgrowth and sinus infection. In patients with suspected acute rhinosinusitis, unenhanced coronal CT imaging may be obtained to assess for radiologic findings (air-fluid levels, mucoid material, mucosal disease, and/or blockage of the drainage passageways) to support this clinically suspected diagnosis (Fig. 10.2a,b) [4]. In some instances (usually at the clinician's discretion), the patient may be managed expectantly for rhinosinusitis without imaging, with imaging reserved for those patients refractory to medications and antibiotics. If imaging is contemplated to follow up a patient treated for rhinosinusitis, it is best to obtain imaging 4 to 6 weeks following therapy as the radiologic findings may lag behind the clinical response.

In patients being assessed with CT imaging for chronic rhinosinusitis, it is important for the radiologist to report the areas of mucosal thickening in the paranasal sinuses as well as the drainage passageways of the ostiomeatal complex and sphenoethmoidal recess (Fig. 10.3a,b) [4]. The location of rhinosinusitis is as important as the extent of disease in producing symptoms. Evaluation of the nasal cavity and of the walls of the sinuses (medial orbital walls, cribriform plate, sphenoid sinus roof) and identification of anatomic variants are also essential. The presence of air-fluid

(a)   (b)

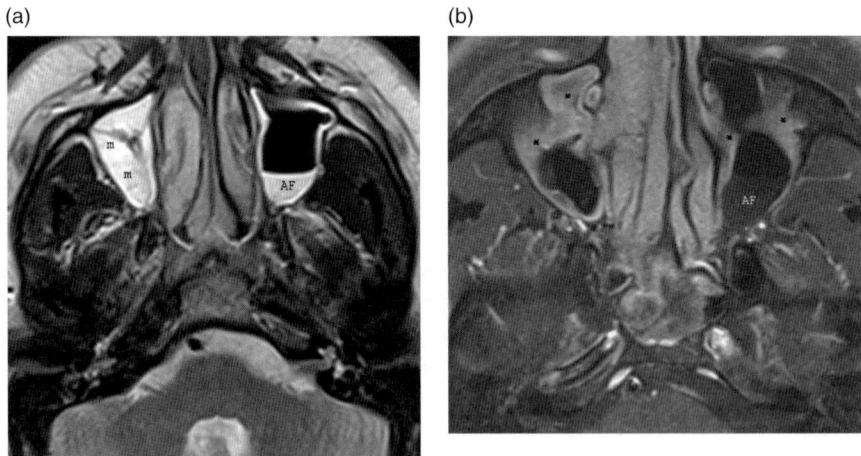

Fig. 10.2 Acute rhinosinusitis in a patient with left facial pain and nasal congestion. (**a**) Axial T_2-weighted and (**b**) contrast-enhanced T_1-weighted magnetic resonance (MR) images show mucosal disease in the bilateral maxillary sinuses (*), and an air-fluid (*AF*) level in the left maxillary sinus. *m*, middle turbinate

(a)   (b)

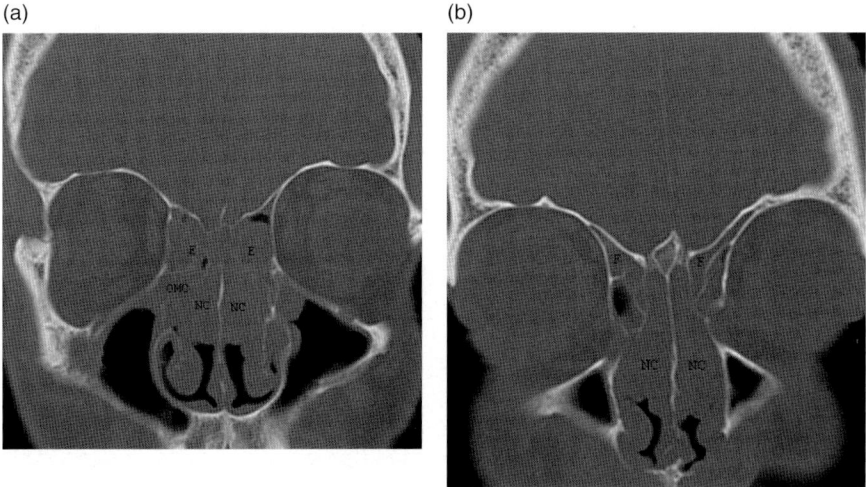

Fig. 10.3 CT imaging of chronic rhinosinusitis before functional endoscopic sinonasal surgery (FESS). (**a**) Coronal images [note: (**b**) is anterior to (**a**)] show mucosal disease in the bilateral maxillary sinuses, opacification of the ethmoid air cells (*E*), opacification of the nasal cavity (*NC*), and opacification of the frontal sinuses (*F*). The ostiomeatal complexes (*OMC*) are obstructed

levels should be noted. Hyperdense sinus contents on CT may reflect the presence of inspissated secretions, fungal elements, or hemorrhage in the setting of trauma or instrumentation.

When evaluating patients for chronic rhinosinusitis and potential functional endoscopic sinus surgery (FESS), it is important to evaluate certain anatomical landmarks on high quality, thin section unenhanced CT images of the sinonasal cavity. Direct coronal images may be obtained, or direct thin section axial images may be obtained and coronal reformations created from these. The medial orbital walls, cribriform plate, and the roof and lateral walls of the sphenoid sinus should be evaluated for osseous defects or deficiencies. A defect in the lamina papyracea may result in orbital penetration and subsequent hematoma formation, whereas a dehiscence in the cribriform plate or sphenoid sinus could result in a cerebrospinal fluid (CSF) leak, intracranial complications (meningitis, encephalocele), or carotid artery complications (perforation with acute subarachnoid hemorrhage; pseudoaneurysm formation). The radiologist and clinician must also assess for anatomic variants or secondary changes of the drainage passageways that may impact on surgery. For instance, is there an atelectatic infundibulum/ostiomeatal complex (OMC) in which the uncinate process or middle turbinate is opposed to the orbital floor (Fig. 10.4a,b)? If so, and the endoscopist is unaware, vigorous removal may result in orbital penetration (Fig. 10.5).

Post-FESS scanning is not accurate in distinguishing inflammation, granulation, and fibrous tissue. The absence of disease on a postoperative study is reliable, but the converse is not true. False-positive studies are common. In cases of suspected

(a)   (b)

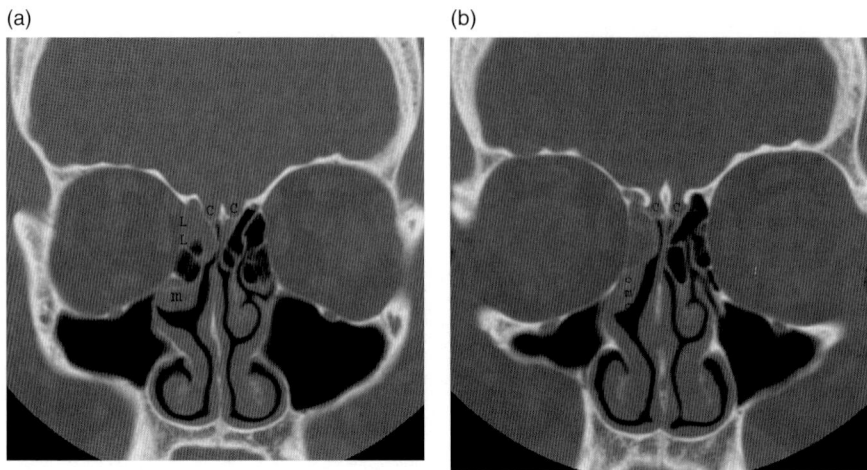

Fig. 10.4 Atelectatic right uncinate process/OMC identified in a patient before FESS for chronic rhinosinusitis. (**a, b**) Contiguous direct coronal CT images show the right *OMC* (uncinate process and middle turbinate) are apposed to the orbital wall. The cribriform plate (*C*) and lamina papyracea (*L*) are intact. The right ethmoid air cells are opacified. *m*, middle turbinate

Fig. 10.5 Defect in the orbital floor following FESS. The * shows a defect in the floor of the right orbit with herniation of orbital fat into the defect. The patient had intermittent diplopia

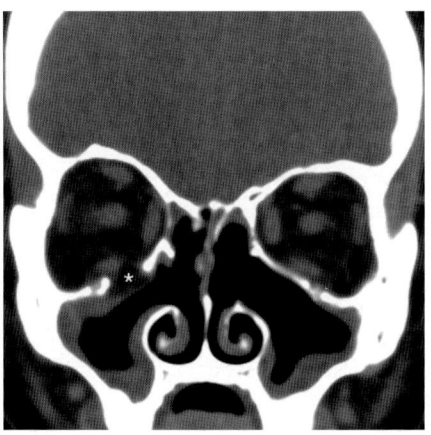

complications following FESS, CT scan is the study of choice. Many of these complications are evident within 24 to 48 h following instrumentation. Computed tomography is accurate in identifying orbital hematomas and optic nerve injury in the orbit, as well as other orbital injuries (medial rectus contusion). A CSF leak caused by inadvertent injury to the cribriform plate or overly vigorous removal of the attachment of the middle turbinate to the fovea ethmoidalis may be immediately evident in the operating room, or it may present days to weeks after surgery with nasal drainage (CSF leak) or symptoms of meningitis (Fig. 10.6a,b).

Complications of acute rhinosinusitis include periorbital cellulitis and abscess formation (Fig. 10.7a,b), meningitis, thrombophlebitis (including cavernous sinus

(a)   (b)

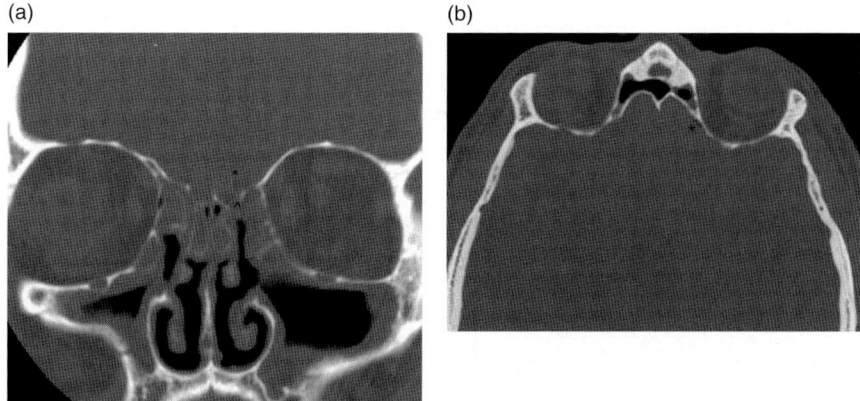

Fig. 10.6 Cerebrospinal fluid (CSF) leak and meningitis presenting approximately 2 weeks following FESS. Coronal (**a**) and axial (**b**) CT scans show intracranial air (*), seen as hypodense or dark areas. There is a surgically created defect in the left fovea ethmoidalis (^)

(a)   (b)

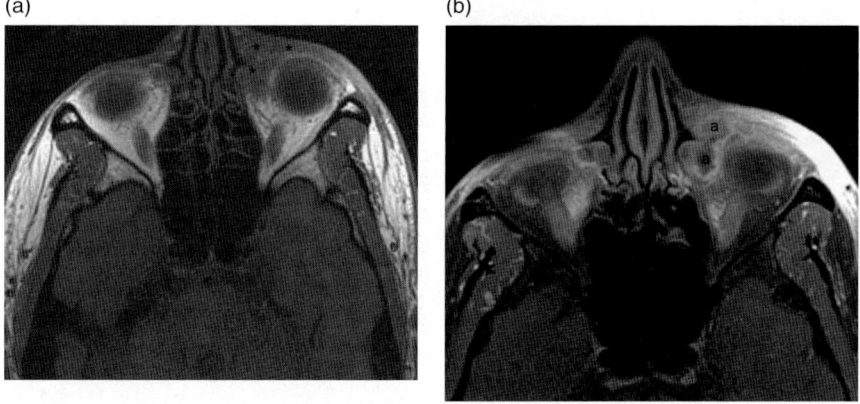

Fig. 10.7 Periorbital cellulitis and abscess formation complicating acute rhinosinusitis. (**a**) Unenhanced axial T_1-weighted MR image shows periorbital soft tissue (*) in the left eyelid and preseptal tissues. (**b**) Enhanced axial T_1-weighted MR image at the same level as (**a**) shows areas of fluid with rim enhancement consistent with abscess formation (*a*)

thrombosis), subdural empyema, brain abscess, and perineural and perivascular spread of infection (especially in invasive fungal disease). These acute complications are most accurately assessed with combined brain and orbital MR imaging including contrast-enhanced imaging; however, contrast enhanced CT is reliable in assessing orbital and periorbital infection so long as there is not concern for extension to the orbital apex or intracranial compartment (in which case MR should be obtained).

Mucoceles may complicate chronic rhinosinusitis (Fig. 10.8a,b,c,d), facial trauma (Fig. 10.9a,b,c), or sinus surgical instrumentation. Mucoceles develop from obstruction of sinus ostia or septated compartments of a sinus and represent mucoid secretions encased by mucus-secreting epithelium (the sinus mucosa). In more than 90%

(a)   (b)

(c)   (d)

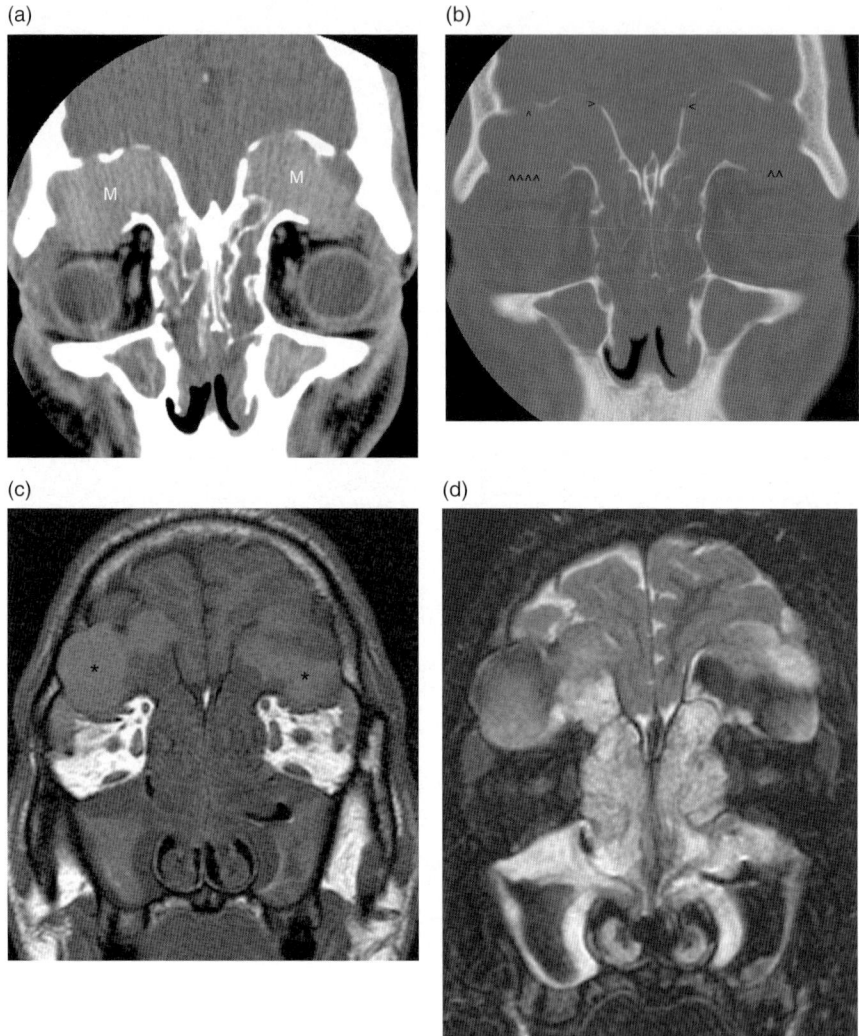

Fig. 10.8 Bilateral frontal sinus mucoceles complicating chronic rhinosinusitis. This case shows multiple, expansile slow-growing mucoceles (*M*) in the bilateral frontal sinuses (the remainder of the paranasal sinuses are opacified from chronic sinus infections). (**a**) The material within the mucoceles is hyperdense on unenhanced CT (consistent with mucoid material). (**b**) Note the multiple areas of osseous expansion and bone thinning (^ and >). Corresponding MR images show the material to be hyperintense (**c**) on T1W images (very common) and heterogeneous (**d**) on T2W images. Also note the very proteinaceous inspissated secretions in the bilateral maxillary sinuses (**c**), bright on T_1-weighted imaging, and (**d**) simulating air on T_2-weighted imaging

(a)   (b)

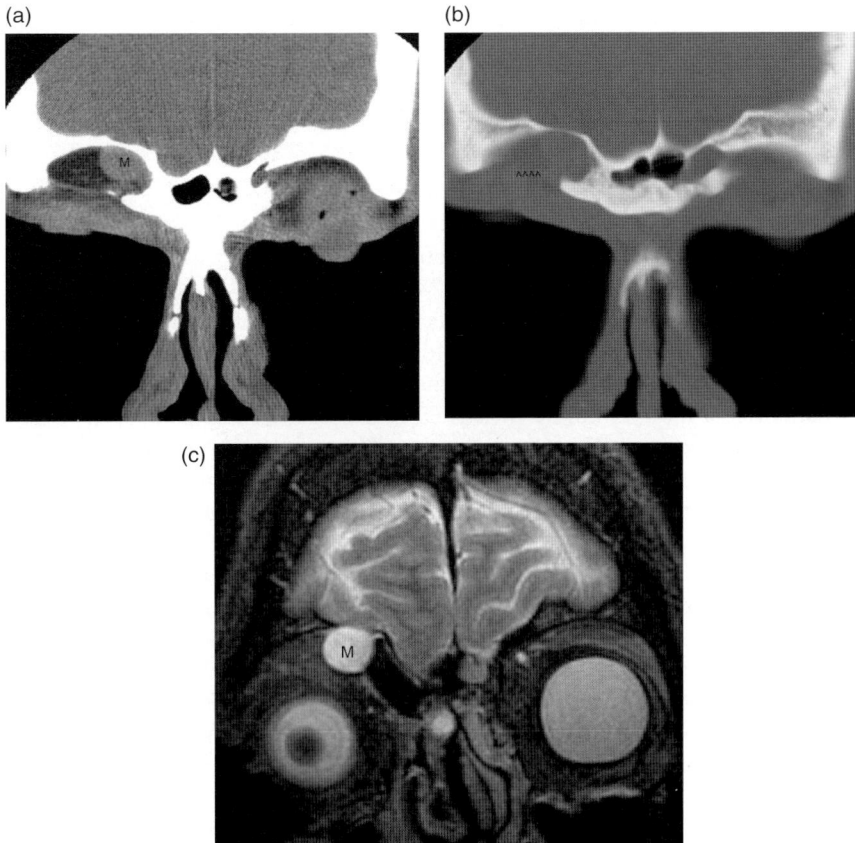

(c)

Fig. 10.9 Right orbital mucocele complicating remote trauma. (**a**) Coronal CT image in soft tissue detail shows the hyperdense mucocele (*M*) in the right frontal sinus. (**b**) Corresponding coronal CT image in bone algorithm shows the osseous expansion associated with the mucocele, as well as the deficient bone at the floor of the sinus (^^). (**c**) Coronal T_2-weighted MR image shows to best advantage the relationship of the mucocele (*M*) to the frontal sinus and adjacent orbit

of cases, mucoceles occur in the frontal sinuses or the ethmoid air cells. When symptomatic, mucoceles present with signs and symptoms related to mass effect including frontal swelling, headache, or orbital pain. Orbital extension may result in proptosis and diplopia. Secondary infection (mucopyocele) or direct extension into the anterior cranial fossa is not infrequent. Advances in endoscopic sinus surgery have led to an acceptance of simple drainage procedures, even for some seemingly very complicated mucoceles.

In the radiologic evaluation of mucoceles, CT best demonstrates the osseous changes of the sinus walls, which may be remodeled and expanded, thinned, and, with large mucoceles, partially dehiscent (see Figs. 10.8a–d, 10.9a–c). However, MR imaging best detects its interface with the intraorbital and intracranial structures (Fig. 10.8a–d). When necessary, enhanced MR imaging is useful in distinguishing a mucocele (which demonstrates peripheral enhancement) from a neoplasm (which typically demonstrates solid enhancement) [6,7]. Mucoceles may show a spectrum of signal characteristics on MR imaging (see Fig. 10.8a–d) that are dependent on their protein content, and usually they demonstrate rim enhancement (compared to tumors, which typically show more solid enhancement) [5–8].

Congenital Lesions

Meningo(encephalo)cele refers to herniation of the meninges, CSF, and/or brain through an osseous defect in the cranium. Meningoencephaloceles are more common than meningoceles. Congenital encephaloceles are caused by an abnormality in the process of invagination of the neural plate [9,10]. During embryogenesis, the dura around the brain contacts the dermis in the facial/nasion region as the neural plate regresses. When there is failure of dermal regression, an encephalocele, dermoid cyst, sinus tract, or nasal glioma may develop. The term nasal glioma is a misnomer as it is not a true neoplasm. With nasal gliomas, there is a fibrous connection with the intracranial compartment. Dermoid sinus tracts may have an intracranial connection in up to 25% of cases and may be complicated by infection (osteomyelitis, meningitis, and abscesses). Nasofrontal and sphenoethmoidal encephaloceles are frequently clinically occult, and the differential diagnosis is broad when seen through the endoscope on office examination. Anterior basal encephaloceles have an association with other developmental anomalies (Fig. 10.10a,b,c), including migrational abnormalities, agenesis of the corpus callosum, and cleft lip and palate [10].

In the setting of trauma or surgery, most meningoencephaloceles involve the nasal cavity and paranasal sinuses or the temporal bone. Patients may present with rhinorrhea.

A combination of imaging modalities, including nuclear scintigraphy, CT, and/or MR imaging, can be used to assess CSF leaks and meningoencephaloceles. It is important to determine whether the CSF leak is caused by a dural laceration or a meningo(encephalo)cele. Following the placement of pledgets in the nares, intrathecal instillation of indium-diethylenetriaminepentaacetic acid (DTPA) may be used to confirm and localize the CSF leak. Once a leak is established, coronal CT may be performed for anatomic localization. In the hands of skilled ENT surgeons and radiologists, iodinated contrast CT cisternography is rarely necessary. If an encephalocele is suspected, MR imaging in the sagittal and coronal planes is most useful in establishing this diagnosis by showing direct continuity of the tissue in the sinonasal cavity with the intracranial brain (see Fig. 10.10a–c). Although imaging may be useful in detecting CSF leaks, fluorescein injected intrathecally followed by endoscopic evaluation may allow direct visualization of an active leak.

Neoplasms

Computed tomography and MR imaging play complementary roles in evaluating tumors of the sinonasal cavity, and frequently both are obtained in the assessment of patients with newly diagnosed sinonasal masses. Computed tomography provides

(a)   (b)

(c)

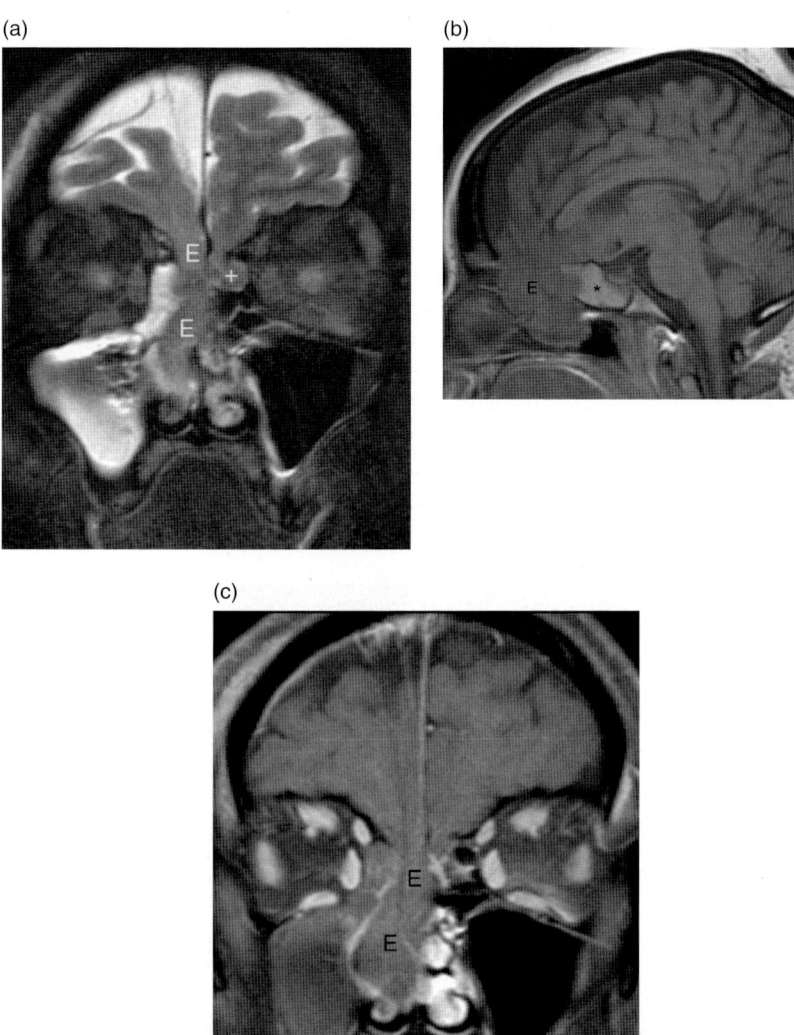

Fig. 10.10 Large congenital basal encephalocele associated with bilateral frontal lobe cortical dysplasia. (**a**) Coronal T-weighted MR image shows tissue similar in signal characteristics to brain and contiguous with the brain extending into the right sinonasal cavity through a defect in the cribriform plate consistent with an encephalocele (*E*). Note the small left encephalocele (+). (**b**) Sagittal T_1-weighted MR image shows the encephalocele (*E*). Also note the T_1 bright proteinaceous inspissated secretions in the sphenoid sinus (*). (**c**) Coronal contrast enhanced T_1-weighted MR image shows the absence of solid enhancement in the encephalocele (*E*)

bone detail, while MR provides superior soft tissue resolution as well as multiplanar capabilities. Magnetic resonance is also better in evaluating the intraorbital and intracranial extension of neoplastic processes. Imaging findings on CT scans that should raise one's index of suspicion for something other than inflammatory disease include unilateral nasal mass/tissue, unilateral opacification of the olfactory strut, bone destruction, and extension outside the sinuses. In these cases, MR imaging may provide important additional information. Unilateral opacification of the olfactory strut usually represents a CSF leak (Fig. 10.11a,b,c), meningoencephalocele, or a neoplasm such as an esthesioneuroblastoma (Fig. 10.12a,b).

Typically, benign neoplasms when large enough expand the paranasal sinus that they affect and secondarily remodel the adjacent bone; however, osseous destruction from benign lesions is less common than with malignancies. It should be noted that in the paranasal sinuses, it is not unusual for contained malignant tumors to have benign features, and that benign tumors may be relatively aggressive in appearance. Caution is always required when evaluating masses within the sinuses. Fibroosseous lesions that may involve the paranasal sinuses include osteomas, fibrous dysplasia,

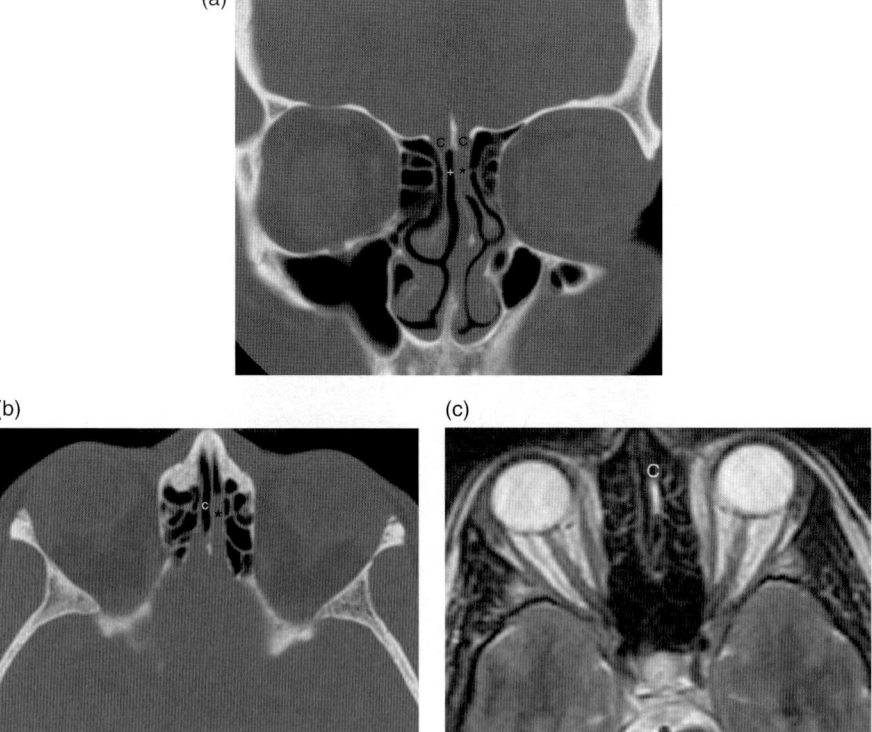

Fig. 10.11 Unilateral opacification of the left olfactory strut representing a CSF leak (*). Coronal (**a**) and axial (**b**) CT images show opacification of the left olfactory strut (*). (**c**) Axial T$_2$-weighted MR image shows that the material in the left olfactory strut (*) is similar to CSF (similar to the vitreous in the orbital globes). *C*, cribriform plate; +, clear olfactory strut

(a) (b)

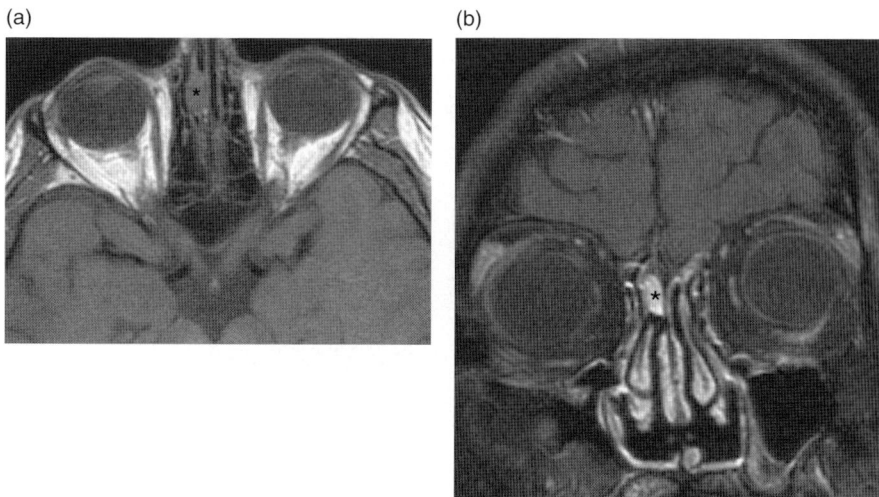

Fig. 10.12 Esthesioneuroblastoma. (**a**) Axial unenhanced T_1-weighted image shows a small expansile mass in the right olfactory strut (*). (**b**) Coronal fat-suppressed enhanced T_1-weighted image shows solid enhancement of the mass consistent with tumor (*)

ossifying or nonossifying fibromas, and chondromas or other chondroid lesions. These lesions frequently have radiologically characteristic appearances.

Papillomas

Papillomas arise from the columnar epithelium and include the following subtypes: inverted, cylindrical, and fungiform. In general, papillomas occur unilaterally in the sinonasal cavity [11]. The most common papilloma is the inverted papilloma, which is more common in men in the fourth through sixth decades of life. This is a benign neoplasm; however, squamous cell carcinoma may be present within these in up to 15% of cases [11,12]. Inverted papillomas may show a rather aggressive appearance with bony destruction. This neoplasm typically arises from the lateral nasal wall at the level of the middle turbinate, or less commonly, within the maxillary sinus itself (Fig. 10.13a,b,c). Although no imaging features characteristically suggest the diagnosis of an inverting papilloma, location is usually a tip-off [11]. Inverted papillomas may occasionally erode the skull base (as may benign polyps), simulating a malignant tumor [3].

Malignant Neoplasms

In sinonasal malignancies, usually CT and MR imaging should be acquired, and these studies should be completed when possible before any type of surgical intervention including biopsy [13–16]. Such imaging may provide excellent information regarding the origin and the extent of the neoplasm as well as the presence of tumor vascularity. Such preoperative imaging may allow optimal localization for

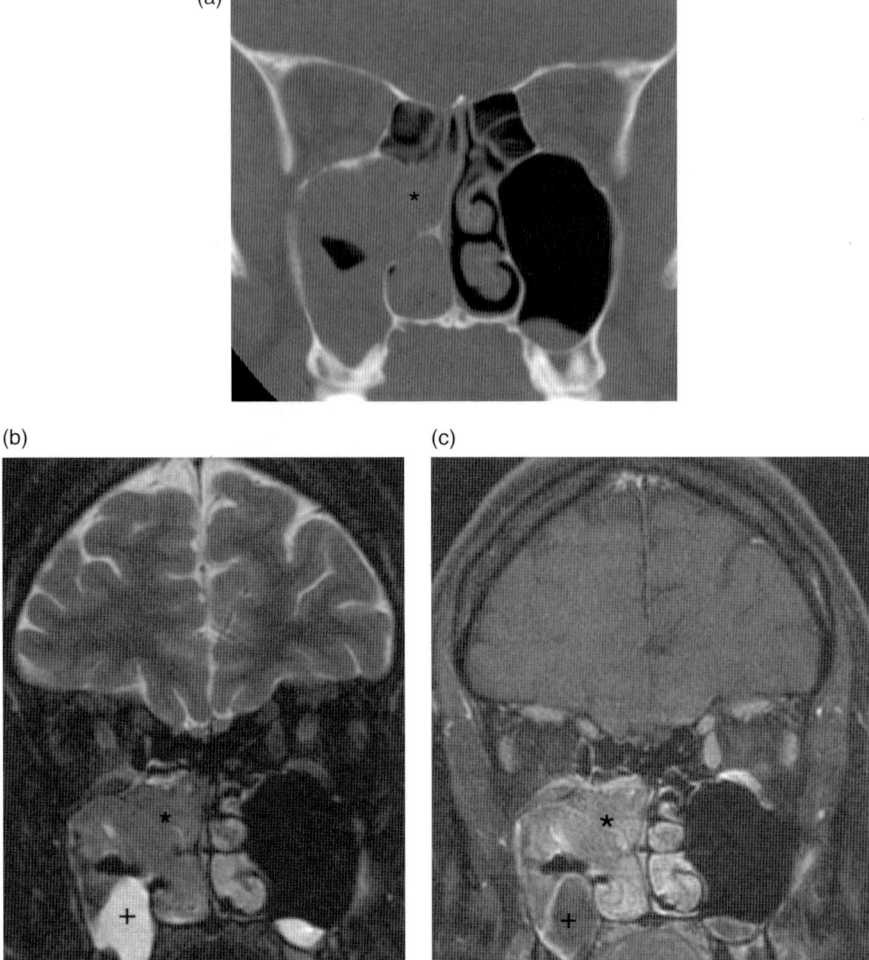

Fig. 10.13 Inverting papilloma in a 35-year-old woman with unilateral nasal stuffiness. (**a**) Coronal CT image shows expansile soft tissue in the right nasal cavity (*), and opacification of the right maxillary sinus. (**b**) Coronal T_2-weighted MR image shows that the mass (*) is similar to brain in signal characteristics and distinguishes the secretions that are bright (+). (**c**) Coronal fat-suppressed enhanced T_1-weighted image shows more solidly enhancing tissue consistent with tumor (*) and the peripheral enhancing secretions (+)

tissue biopsy, and may be extremely useful in preparing and minimizing complications of surgery, including blood loss, in the setting of vascular neoplasms. Tumors extending into the nasal cavity may be amenable to transnasal biopsy. Biopsy may be performed by using endoscopic sinus surgery or by open transcutaneous or transoral procedures.

In sinonasal malignancies, MR imaging distinguishes sinus opacification related to tumor from opacification related to inspissated secretions [5,6]. Most neoplasms may be distinguished from inflammatory conditions by their imaging characteristics as well as their more solid enhancement pattern following intravenous contrast administration (compared to peripheral enhancement in benign inflammatory disease). In addition, T_2-weighted imaging may be helpful, as most malignancies are heterogeneous and intermediate in signal compared to inflammatory secretions that tend to be homogeneously hyperintense (bright). Sinonasal secretions are complex and have variable signal intensity patterns on MR imaging related to the protein concentration and mobile water protons within the secretions [5]. As protein concentration increases, the signal intensity on T_1-weighted imaging changes from hypointense to hyperintense, then to hypointense again. On T_2-weighted images, secretions with low protein content are initially bright; however, as the protein content and viscosity increase, the signal intensity decreases. Fungus is frequently black on T_2-weighted images, mimicking an "aerated sinus." Imaging of sinonasal malignancies must also include high-resolution views of the orbit, skull base, and the intracranial compartment [15,17,18]. Direct extension of tumor or perineural spread of tumor outside the sinonasal cavity and into these important adjacent anatomic locations may occur, with significant impacts upon the patient's operability, the type of resection that will occur, and the necessity for radiation therapy [17,18]. An especially important anatomic location for detection of tumor spread is the pterygopalatine fossa. When tumor from the sinonasal cavity spreads to this anatomic location, extension into the adjacent orbit, infratemporal fossa, skull base, and intracranial compartment may subsequently occur.

(a)   (b)

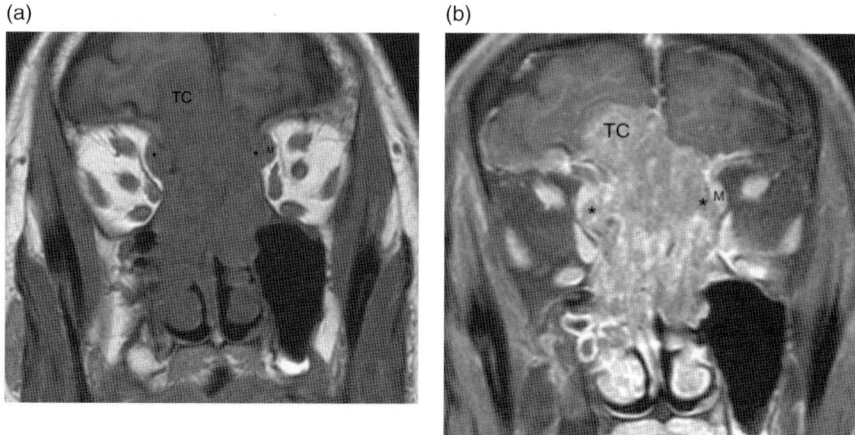

Fig. 10.14 Sinonasal undifferentiated carcinoma with extension through the periorbita and intracranial spread. Coronal unenhanced (**a**) and fat-suppressed enhanced (**b**) T_1-weighted images show a large mass in the bilateral sinonasal cavity. The patient presented with nasal stuffiness. There is extension of tumor through the periorbita (*), and transcranially through the anterior cranial fossa (cribriform plate) into the intracranial compartment (*TC*). *M*, medial rectus muscle

Squamous cell carcinoma is the most common malignancy of the paranasal sinuses and nasal cavity, representing two-thirds of all cancers in this region [13]. Occupational exposures including radium, Thorotrast, and especially nickel are causative factors. The majority of squamous cell carcinomas originate in the maxillary sinus anthrum, the next most common site being the nasal cavity septum [13]. Tumors of minor salivary gland origin such as adenoid cystic carcinoma [14] and melanoma may occur [16]. Adenocarcinomas, lymphoma, undifferentiated carcinomas (Fig. 10.14a,b), esthesioneuroblastomas [15], and sarcomas may also occur in the sinonasal structures. Following squamous cell carcinoma, minor salivary gland tumors and melanomas (which arise from melanocyte rests in the sinonasal mucosa) are the next most common malignancies to affect the nasal cavity [15,16]. Minor salivary gland tumors represent a wide spectrum of histological subtypes including adenoid cystic carcinoma (most common), mucoepidermoid carcinoma, and acinic cell carcinomas. Metastatic disease to the paranasal sinuses is unusual, with renal cell carcinoma most commonly reported.

Summary

Rhinosinusitis is among the most common ailments in the United States. Computed tomography is the most widely utilized imaging modality to assess this as well as other disease processes of the sinonasal cavity. The use of plain film radiographs is relatively obsolete. To understand the pathogenesis of rhinosinusitis and other pathological processes that may affect the paranasal sinuses, some understanding of sinonasal development and anatomy as it pertains to mucociliary clearance is essential. Focused imaging assessment of disease processes in the sinuses is invaluable when used correctly. Indications for performing MR imaging include CT scan findings such as bone destruction or extension of disease outside the sinonasal cavity that raise concern for an aggressive infection or neoplasm. For many lesions, including complicated rhinosinusitis, encephaloceles, and neoplasms, CT and MR imaging play complementary roles.

References

1. Schaeffer JP. The Embryology, Development and Anatomy of the Nose, Paranasal Sinuses, Nasolacrimal Passageways and Olfactory Organs in Man. Philadelphia: Blakiston's, 1920.
2. Zinreich SJ, Kennedy DW, Kuman AJ, et al. MR imaging of normal nasal cycle: comparison with sinus pathology. J Comput Assist Tomogr 1988;12:1014–1019.
3. Som PM, Lawson W, Lidov MW. Simulated aggressive skull base erosion in response to benign sinonasal disease. Radiology 1991;180:755–759.
4. Babbel RW, Harnsberger HR, Sonkens J, et al. Recurring patterns of inflammatory sinonasal disease demonstrated on screening sinus CT. Am J Neuroradiol 1992;13:903–912.
5. Dillon KB, Som PM, Fullerton GD. Hypointense MR signal in chronically inspissated sinonasal secretions. Radiology 1990;174:73–78.
6. Som PM, Shapiro MD, Biller HF, et al. Sinonasal tumors and inflammatory tissues: differentiation with MR. Radiology 1988;167:803–808.

7. Lanzieri CF, Shah M, Krauss D, et al. Use of gadolinium-enhanced MR imaging for differentiating mucoceles from neoplasms in the paranasal sinuses. Radiology 1991;178:425–428.

8. Loevner LA, Yousem DM, Lanza DC, et al. MR evaluation of frontal osteoplastic flaps using autogenous fat grafts to obliterate the sinus. Am J Neuroradiol 1995;16:1721–1726.

9. Kallman JE, Loevner LA, Yousem DM, et al. Heterotopic brain in the pterygopalatine fossa. Am J Neuroradiol 1996;18:176–179.

10. Barkovich AJ, Vandermarch P, Edwards MSB, et al. Congenital nasal masses: CT and MR imaging features in 16 cases. Am J Neuradiol 1991;12:105–116.

11. Woodruff WW, Vrabec DP. Inverted papilloma of the nasal vault and paranasal sinuses: spectrum of CT findings. AJR 1994; 162:419–423.

12. Lasser A, Rothfeld PR, Shapiro RS. Epithelial papilloma and squamous cell carcinoma of the nasal cavity and paranasal sinuses: a clinicopathologic study. Cancer (Phila) 1976;38: 2503–2510.

13. St. Pierre S, Baker SR. Squamous cell carcinoma of the maxillary sinus: analysis of 66 cases. Head Neck Surg 1983;5:508–513.

14. Sigal R, Monnet O, de Baere T, et al. Adenoid cystic carcinoma of the head and neck: evaluation with MR imaging and clinical-pathologic correlation in 27 patients. Radiology 1992;184:95–101.

15. Som PM, Lidov M, Brandwein M, et al. Sinonasal esthesioneuroblastoma with intracranial extension: marginal tumor cysts as a diagnostic MR finding. Am J Neuroradiol 1994;15: 1259–1262.

16. Yousem DM, Li C, Montone KT, et al. Primary malignant melanoma of the sinonasal cavity: MR evaluation. Radiographics 1996;16:1101–1110.

17. Eisen MD, Yousem DM, Loevner LA, et al. Preoperative imaging to predict orbital invasion by tumor. Head Neck Surg 2000;22:456–462.

18. Loevner LA, Sonners AI. Imaging of neoplasms of the paranasal sinuses. Neuroimaging Clin N Am 2004;14 (4):625–646

Chapter 11
Systemic Diseases and Chronic Rhinosinusitis

Christine Reger, Christina F. Herrera, Megan Abbott, and Alexander G. Chiu

Many systemic diseases can cause nasal symptoms, either as an initial presentation or a manifestation later in the disease process. When patients present with nasal symptoms resembling infection—such as purulent nasal discharge, crusting, and congestion—acute rhinosinusitis is likely to be diagnosed. However, when these symptoms persist despite appropriate medical therapy, other etiologies should be considered. In some cases, underlying inflammation of the nasal mucosa causes recurrent or chronic sinusitis, as in nasal polyposis or allergic rhinitis. Less frequently, systemic rather than local conditions are the cause, requiring a more detailed evaluation, comprehensive systemic management, and long-term follow-up [1]. The number of systemic illnesses that can cause nasal symptoms is substantial; only those most commonly affecting the nose and sinuses are discussed here. For purposes of discussion, the diseases have been categorized as follows: autoimmune disorders, infectious processes, and hematologic-oncologic diseases. The discussion of these processes includes common presenting nasal symptoms, physical examination findings, recommended radiographic and serologic testing, and treatment options.

Autoimmune Disorders

Wegener's Granulomatosis

Wegener's granulomatosis is an autoimmune disorder affecting three main organ systems: the head and neck, the lungs, and the kidneys. Pathologically, Wegener's lesions are typically characterized by necrotizing granulomas of small to medium vessels. Although symptoms may vary depending on the system involved, the most frequently reported initial symptom is nasal obstruction; this is often accompanied by purulent drainage, crusting, and, less frequently, epistaxis. These symptoms may temporarily improve when treated with antibiotics and/or steroids but often recur

A.G. Chiu
Department of Otorhinolaryngology, University of Pennsylvania, Philadelphia, PA, USA
e-mail: alexander.chiu@uphs.upenn.edu

E.R. Thaler, D.W. Kennedy (eds.), *Rhinosinusitis*, DOI: 10.1007/978-0-387-73062-2_11,
© Springer Science+Business Media, LLC 2008

after treatment is discontinued. If left untreated, this granulomatous disease can progress to a stage of more generalized vasculitis and systemic Wegener's, making early diagnosis crucial [2]. Contrarily, a patient already diagnosed with Wegener's may have local nasal exacerbations caused by uncontrolled disease or secondary rhinosinusitis. In both scenarios, physical examination findings are similar.

Nasal endoscopic examination of a patient with Wegener's granulomatosis usually reflects granulomatous inflammatory changes. Main characteristics include generalized edema, friable nasal mucosa, erosion of the septum and/or turbinates, sometimes accompanied by a saddle nose deformity, and the presence of purulence and crusting [3]. The destructive process typically starts in the midline region, first affecting the septum and turbinates, before spreading symmetrically to the remainder of the nasal cavity and sinuses. The end result, if left untreated, may be the appearance of a single cavity [2] (Fig. 11.1).

If a granulomatous disease is suspected on nasal exam, an autoimmune workup is indicated. Serologic testing recommended for diagnosis of Wegener's granulomatosis includes measurement of antineutrophil cytoplasmic antibodies with cytoplasmic staining (C-ANCA), which has been found to have good specificity. However, this test lacks sensitivity, making diagnosis of a patient with only nasal symptoms and a negative C-ANCA result challenging. In this case, computed tomography (CT) and magnetic resonance imaging (MRI) can be helpful if the imaging is consistent with granulomatous changes; in particular, evidence of bone destruction combined with new bone formation on CT, along with a fat signal from sclerotic sinus on MRI [2]. In addition, nasal biopsy should be acquired to evaluate for caseating granulomas, vasculitis, and necrosis. Excluded here is the evaluation of lungs and kidneys (chest X-ray for nodular infiltrates, urinalysis for sediment, and positive biopsy of lungs or kidneys), as recommended by the American College of Rheumatology [4].

If Wegener's granulomatosis is suspected or confirmed, a referral to rheumatology is recommended. Treatment of the disease focuses on initial remission, maintenance, and treatment of exacerbations. Remission is usually inducted with

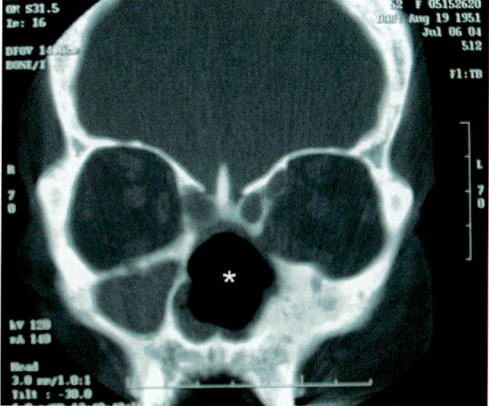

Fig. 11.1 Coronal computed tomography (CT) scan of patient with chronic sinonasal manifestations of Wegener's granulomatosis shows destruction of the midline structures (*)

cyclophosphamide and prednisone; maintenance therapy follows with methotrexate and bactrim; and relapses are typically treated with cyclophosphamide and prednisone as needed [5]. Nasal manifestations in particular may need to be managed with culture-directed antibiotics and oral steroids as indicated by symptoms and nasal examination.

Sarcoidosis

Similar to Wegener's granulomatosis, sarcoidosis is a multisystem autoimmune disorder. Its hallmark pathological characteristic is the presence of noncaseating granulomas with associated granulomatous inflammation, most often originating in the respiratory system. The exact cause of this disease remains unknown. The progression ranges from being self-limited (resolving with no residual damage) to becoming chronic (leading to organ failure if left unmanaged) [6]. Although pulmonary symptoms are usually the main features of the initial presentation, there is frequent nasal involvement. Almost all the patients who develop sarcoidosis in the nasal cavity and paranasal sinuses present with nasal symptoms, either externally or internally. Symptoms typically resemble chronic rhinosinusitis, including anosmia, nasal obstruction, and crusting [1]. However, nasal exam usually differs from examination findings typical of rhinosinusitis alone.

External and intranasal rhinology examination can both show granulomatous changes if sarcoidosis is present. External involvement includes erythema and edema of the nose and adjacent nasolabial area. Intranasal involvement can include: generalized edema of the nasal mucosa, hypertrophy of the turbinates, and submucosal nodules found on the anterior portions of the inferior turbinates and septum [1] (Fig. 11.2). There may also be the appearance of rhinosinusitis caused by secondary infection.

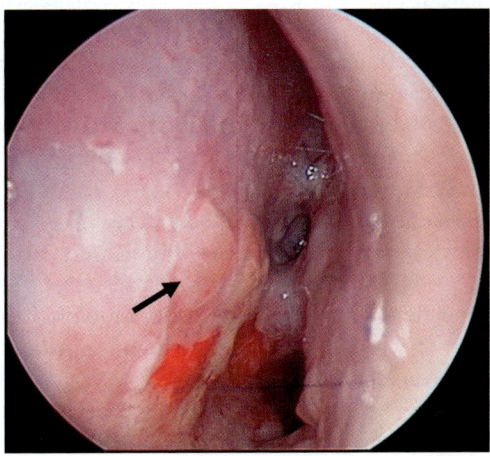

Fig. 11.2 Endoscopic picture of submucosal nodules (*arrow*) within the mucosa of the nasal septum in a patient with sinonasal sarcoidosis

If the symptoms and exam findings previously described are present along with other evidence of sarcoidosis, such as respiratory and constitutional symptoms, an autoimmune evaluation is warranted. Serum angiotensin-converting enzyme (ACE) is elevated in greater than 60% of patients with sarcoidosis. An ACE level can be helpful as a screening tool or for tracking response to treatment, but lacks specificity for diagnostic purposes. Another useful screening tool is a chest X-ray to evaluate for the presence of hilar adenopathy. Chest CT is more useful to detect pulmonary changes if a patient has a normal chest X-ray but sarcoidosis is still suspected [6]. The most definitive method of diagnosis is a tissue biopsy for histological confirmation of noncaseating granulomas, which is the pathological hallmark of sarcoidosis [1,6].

Once sarcoidosis is suspected or confirmed, a referral to rheumatology is recommended. Treatment is controversial, often depending on patient symptoms and staging of the disease. Staging of sarcoidosis is based on the degree of pulmonary disease found on chest radiography, which is outside the scope of this chapter. Ideally, patients in the earliest stage should be observed without therapy because there is a chance of spontaneous remission. As the disease progresses to the second stage, use of oral steroids is considered the cornerstone of treatment. Many different drugs have been utilized in trying to manage later stages of the disease, the most effective being methotrexate and hydroquinone [1,6,7]. As previously mentioned, steroids and antibiotics may be beneficial for exacerbations of nasal symptoms caused by secondary infection.

Cystic Fibrosis

Cystic fibrosis (CF) is an autosomal recessive disorder mainly affecting the respiratory system, with the potential for multiorgan effects including pancreatic insufficiency, intestinal disorders, liver disease, infertility, and nasal polyposis [8,9]. Since the CF gene was identified on chromosome 7 in 1989, more than 800 mutations have been recognized, which can be classified as mild to severe. The classification of CF mutation identified corresponds with the severity of clinical manifestations [9]. The presence of CF mutations has been found to correlate with increased frequency of chronic rhinosinusitis; even carriers of a single CF mutation have a higher prevalence of rhinosinusitis [8].

The presenting symptoms differ according to age of diagnosis and severity of disease: Adults are more likely to have mild disease and present with recurrent respiratory symptoms, whereas children are more likely to have more severe disease with gastrointestinal complications at the onset [9]. Specifically regarding rhinosinusitis, CF patients of any age may have symptoms of recurrent or persistent sinus infection, with or without nasal polyps found on examination. The presence of nasal polyps has been identified as an important parameter for severity of paranasal disease in CF patients [10,11]. Imaging may be useful in determining surgical options for patients CF; while there are a number of reported findings on CT scan, including a mucocele, sinus opacification, and changes in sinus development, the sensitivity and specificity for diagnosing CF in particular have not been determined [10].

The whole clinical picture is used in making the diagnosis of CF, including presence of clinical features, history of CF in a sibling, and a positive newborn screen for immune-reactive trypsin. However, the hallmark for confirmation of the diagnosis is the sweat chloride concentration test [9,12]. If sweat testing is not diagnostic, the defective chloride channel found in epithelial cells of patients with CF can also be identified in raised potential difference across the nasal epithelium. In addition, genetic screening panels can identify CF-causing mutations, but are limited as diagnostic tools due to the large number of possible CF mutations. Absence of identified mutations does not exclude CF, and follow-up testing is recommended if indicated by the clinical picture [9]. Once diagnosed, there are a number of system-specific tools to determine the severity of CF, such as pulmonary and pancreatic function tests [10].

Improving life expectancy in patients with CF is the goal of treatment, as there is no cure. The focus of treatment is mostly on management of pulmonary disease, which is the major cause of morbidity and mortality in CF patients [13]. The following have been recommended by the CF Foundation to improve lung function and decrease frequency and severity of infection in patients with CF:

- Inhaled tobramycin for suppression of *Pseudomonas aeruginosa* infection
- Dornase alpha to reduce airway secretions
- Hypertonic saline inhalation to increase mucociliary clearance
- Oral ibuprofen to slow loss of lung function
- Inhaled beta$_2$-adrenergic receptor agonists

Other medical and surgical treatments not included in the CF Foundation recommendations have been tried with varying degrees of success, including oral and inhaled corticosteroids, leukotriene inhibitors, cromolyn, prophylactic use of oral antistaphylococcal antibiotics, inhaled anticholinergic bronchodilators, and lung transplantation [14].

When specifically treating rhinosinusitis in CF patients, culture-directed antibiotic therapy should be used. The frequent use of antibiotics in this population causes an increased risk of drug resistance. Resistance to specific drugs is typically transient, and patients become susceptible again when antibiotic use is altered [13]. In the case of nasal polyposis, endoscopic sinus surgery may be required when medical therapy fails [11]. Ultimately, patients should be referred to a CF specialty center for definitive diagnosis and management of the disease.

Churg–Strauss Syndrome

Churg–Strauss syndrome (CSS), as defined by the American College of Rheumatology, is a rare and unusual systemic vasculitis characterized by the presence of asthma, eosinophilia, neuropathy, nonfixed pulmonary infiltrates, extravascular eosinophils presenting as vasculitis, and symptoms of chronic rhinosinusitis [15].

Clinically, CSS patients present in one of three phases: the prodromal phase, consistent with adult-onset asthma and chronic rhinosinusitis; the second phase, associated with peripheral eosinophilia; or the third phase, as evidenced by systemic vasculitis involving the neurological, gastrointestinal, cutaneous, cardiac, and/or renal organ systems [15]. Rhinosinusitis is present in 75% of cases of CSS, commonly with symptoms such as nasal congestion and discharge. Nasal endoscopy examination of a CSS patient typically reveals mucosal edema and nasal polyps [16].

Diagnostic serology includes antineutrophil cytoplasmic antibody testing (P-ANCA and C-ANCA, with both perinuclear and cytoplasmic staining patterns), and complete blood count with differential to evaluate for an elevated peripheral eosinophil count. Other inflammatory markers, such as erythrocyte sedimentation rate and C-reactive protein, can be followed to monitor disease activity. Chest imaging should be obtained if pulmonary involvement is suspected [1,17]. If possible, a biopsy of the affected tissue should be obtained for further histological examination. Small necrotizing granulomas, composed of an eosinophilic core surrounded by macrophages, giant cells, and necrotizing vasculitis, are consistent with a diagnosis of Churg–Strauss syndrome [1].

Any suspected case of CSS should be referred to rheumatology for further evaluation and treatment management. The aim of treatment is to limit and control the vasculitis and is best achieved through the tapering of a high dose of systemic steroids. Depending on the severity of disease and response to initial therapy, CSS patients may also be treated with adjuvant regimens including cyclophosphamide, methotrexate, and/or glucocorticoid-sparing agents. Severity of disease is measured through a five-factor score: proteinuria greater than 1 g/day, creatinemia greater than 1.58 mg/dL, cardiomyopathy, gastrointestinal tract involvement, and central nervous system involvement. The greater number of factors present increases the risk for mortality and may necessitate adjuvant immunosuppressant therapy [17].

Relapsing Polychondritis

Relapsing polychondritis is a rare autoimmune disease in which cartilaginous tissues are destroyed. The most common areas affected are the eyes (ocular edema), ears (audiovestibular problems), nose (chondritis), and respiratory system. Regarding otorhinolaryngology, these patients may complain of ear and nasal pain, rhinorrhea, and epistaxis. Nasal exam reveals mucosal inflammation and possibly a saddle nose deformity, resulting from recurrent inflammation and eventual collapse of the nasal cartilage. The auricular effects are similar, producing floppy "cauliflower"-like ears from the destruction of auricular cartilage, while sparing the noncartilaginous earlobe. Other manifestations may include joint pain and effusions, episcleritis and scleritis, wheezing, dyspnea, trachea tenderness, hearing loss, ataxia, vertigo, tinnitus, cardiovascular disease, cerebral vasculitis, glomerulonephritis, skin lesions, fever, and weight loss [18].

Although an erythrocyte sedimentation rate is generally elevated in these patients, there are no consistent sensitive laboratory tests that correlate with relapsing polychondritis. Therefore, diagnosis is made primarily through clinical evaluation [18]. Diagnosis is made by the presence of three of the following six criteria: auricular chondritis, nonerosive seronegative inflammatory polyarthritis, nasal chondritis, ocular inflammation, respiratory chondritis, and audiovestibular damage [19]. A biopsy of affected nasal tissue can further exclude other differential diagnoses and generally reveals a loss of cartilage basophilia with the presence of granulation tissue and fibrosis in later cases [20].

Relapsing polychondritis patients would benefit from referral to a rheumatologist, who would manage the patient's therapy based on the severity of symptoms. Treatment primarily consists of oral corticosteroids. However, disease-modifying and steroid-sparing agents such as methotrexate, azathioprine, and cyclophosphamide may be necessary in more severe cases. In instances where relapsing polychondritis patients are resistant to traditional treatment, autologous stem cell transplantation may be attempted [20].

Lupus

Lupus is an autoimmune connective tissue disorder that is composed of several different subtypes, the most severe being systemic lupus erythematosus (SLE). While a less aggressive form of lupus may only affect superficial tissues, typically SLE affects multiple organ systems [21]. The cause of lupus remains unknown, although the process has been linked to medication use, sun exposure, trauma, surgery, and pregnancy [22]. Rhinosinusitis symptoms may be present with the onset of disease, or later as a result of immunosuppressant therapy [21,23].

In most cases of lupus, the first presenting symptom is the development of a butterfly rash across the malar eminences of the face. The patient may also report oral lesions and vesicular or plaque lesion formation in the head and neck region. Nasal symptoms may resemble that of rhinosinusitis, including nasal congestion and discolored mucus. Nasal endoscopy in a patient present with SLE may reveal granulomatous inflammatory changes with edema, nasal crusting, and possibly septal perforation [22].

If lupus is suspected following a physical examination, autoimmune serologic testing should be done. This workup should include an antinuclear antibody titer (ANA), an anti-double-stranded DNA titer, and an anti-Smith antibody titer (ASA) [24]. All these antibody screens are very specific for SLE; however, a positive result on any one of these tests alone is not diagnostic of SLE. Other serologic test findings may reveal altered C3 and C4 complement protein levels. These levels will be elevated during times of inactive disease and low during periods of symptom flare-ups [4]. In all cases of suspected SLE, correlation of serologic testing with physical examination findings is imperative. Imaging, including the use of MRI and CT, is indicated to evaluate the extent of sinus involvement secondary to infection and cutaneous manifestations [24].

Standard treatment of SLE is generally managed by a rheumatologist and currently includes the use of corticosteroids. Low-dose oral prednisone and nonsteroidal antiinflammatory medications are used to alleviate symptoms of SLE. Antimalarial agents have proven to be effective in treatment of fatigue, arthritis, and arthralgias. Patients presenting with central nervous system, renal, or pulmonary effects of SLE may require high doses of intravenous corticosteroids. Before any medical treatment for SLE, the suspected cause of the disease must be considered. As some medications have been linked to the exacerbation and manifestations of SLE, removal of an offending medication may eliminate symptoms and thereby eliminate the need for immunosuppressive therapy [22]. In those patients for whom immunosuppressive agents are required, monitoring for invasive fungal sinus infections is important. Similarly, with patients who are unresponsive to antibiotic therapy to relieve rhinosinusitis symptoms, fungal infections should be suspected. Fungal infections in patients with SLE receiving immunosuppressants, if left untreated, can lead to life-threatening complications [22,23].

Infectious Processes

Fungal Infections

Fungal infections affecting the sinuses are being identified more and more frequently, which has been attributed to better technology for diagnosing fungal disease and improved treatment for the diseases that increase a patient's susceptibility to fungal infections. Fungal disease can be broadly classified as invasive (fulminant or chronic), noninvasive (saprophytic overgrowth or fungal ball), and allergic (hypersensitivity to fungi). Fulminant invasive fungal infections are most commonly found in immunocompromised hosts, such as patients with leukemia, acquired immunodeficiency, diabetes, or organ transplantation. Noninvasive fungal infections can be found in otherwise immunocompetent patients who have an altered immune system through use of medications such as antibiotics or steroids [25,26]. Similarly, chronic invasive disease usually affects immunocompetent patients, whereas patients with allergic fungal disease are typically atopic.

Each classification of fungal disease can affect the sinuses with varying degree. Chronic invasive and allergic fungal infections involving the sinuses are found most often in the setting of chronic rhinosinusitis not responsive to traditional medical therapy [1]. Noninvasive infections can cause additional symptoms, such as diplopia or headache, as in the case of a fungal mass [25]. (Fig. 11.3). Fulminant invasive fungal infections of the sinuses may start with symptoms of rhinosinusitis that quickly develop into an emergent situation as the spores invade adjacent vasculature and soft tissue of the orbit and cranium, with resultant symptoms including fever, periorbital edema, and mental status changes [27].

Early diagnosis is imperative, especially in the face of fulminant invasive fungal sinusitis. Critical information needed for an accurate diagnosis is ideally obtained through tissue specimens for pathology and microbiology, preferably taken from the affected area before initiation of antifungal treatment. Microbiology cultures can identify the specific fungus involved. This step is crucial not only for a diagnosis

Fig. 11.3 Endoscopic view of a fungal ball (*arrow*) within a sphenoid sinus

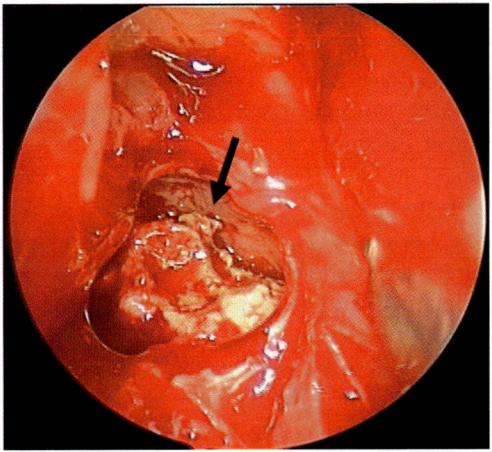

but for treatment decisions as well. Pathology is important not only to confirm the presence of fungal hyphae but to help determine the degree of tissue invasion and identify any associated inflammatory processes [25,27]. Radiologic evidence of fungal disease is another important component of the diagnosis. Specifically, CT scan of the paranasal sinuses is useful in determining the extent of the disease and possible bone destruction. An MRI can also demonstrate fungal disease; the image findings are hypointense on MRI as opposed to being hyperintense on CT [26,27] (Fig. 11.4). Finally, while blood cultures can be used to isolate a specific fungus, in some cases extensive tissue invasion can occur despite negative cultures [26].

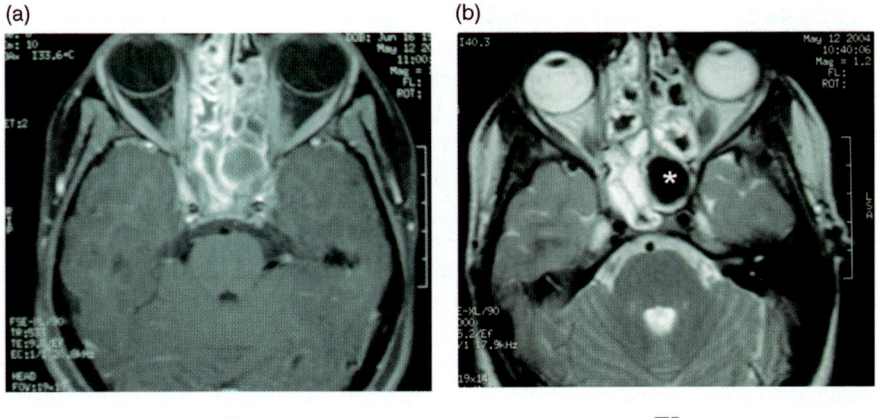

T1   T2

Fig. 11.4 T_1-weighted (a) and T_2-weighted (b) axial magnetic resonance (MR) images of a fungal rhinosinusitis. Note the signal dropout within the left sphenoid sinus on the T_2-weighted image, representative of fungal concretions (*)

When indicated, fungal infections are treated initially with surgical debridement to remove the offending organism, followed by culture-directed antifungal medications. In other cases, surgical intervention is reserved for failure or delayed response to appropriate antifungal therapy [1,27]. The medical management of fungal infections has changed over the past few years. Previously, treatment of fungal strains affecting the sinuses was limited to amphotericin and itraconazole, with the consequent emergence of resistant strains. More recently, another triazole, voriconazole, has been found effective against some fungal strains, specifically *Aspergillus*. Additionally, a new class of antifungal agents, the echinocandins, has been approved for the treatment of fungal infections. Although they are only useful with a limited number of fungal strains, and currently only available in intravenous form, it is thought that these new drugs will play an important role in treating fungus when used in combination with amphotericin formulations or triazoles [26]. All these medications can have serious complications and interactions (for example, the triazoles can all cause liver damage to some extent), and therefore should be used with appropriate monitoring or under the direction of an infectious disease specialist.

Syphilis

Syphilis is a sexually transmitted disease that can be characterized into one of three distinct phases: the primary phase, the secondary phase, or the tertiary phase. The primary phase is evidenced by the presence of a painless, indurated anogenital, oral, or nipple (depending on the site of primary exposure) lesion or chancre as well as regional lymphadenopathy [28]. Due to these mild manifestations, a diagnosis at this time may be missed, allowing for the progression of this disease into the secondary phase. The secondary phase is further divided into early and late stages distinguished by the type of lesion observed and the timing of its appearance. The early stage of secondary syphilis is characterized solely by skin lesions, whereas the late stage begins to affect the mucosa, such as the nose, mouth, palate, lips, tongue, tonsils, and throat [29,30]. A generalized rash can be appreciated, especially on the soles and palms, as well as diffuse lymphadenopathy. Finally, the tertiary phase is evidenced by involvement of the cardiovascular and neurological symptoms, and by the appearance of gummatous lesions, which are granulomatous ulcers that can cause organomegaly and the destruction of supporting structures such as the palate [28]. In this phase, patients are at risk for meningitis, stroke, aortic incompetence, and aortic aneurysm [28,30].

Examination and history findings vary depending on the stage in which the patient seeks medical attention. However, nasal symptoms begin to present in late secondary syphilis, worsening as the patient progresses to the tertiary syphilis phase. Nasal endoscopic exam can reveal several types of nasal lesions, described as either annular, frambesiform, or pustular [29]. Annular lesions are papular in nature and can present as a single papule or merge into patches, whereas frambesiform lesions are hypertrophic, raspberry-like growths filled with serous material and have a foul odor. Last, the pustular lesions begin as vesicles, containing a minimal amount of pus, eventually rupturing into ulcerations [29]. As the disease progresses into the tertiary phase, septal perforation or collapse may occur [28].

The means of diagnosis varies depending on the stage in which the patient presents but is made through a combination of serologic and histological findings. Serologic testing generally includes the rapid plasma reagin test (RPR) or the venereal disease research laboratory test (VDRL). However, these tests may require some time to become positive, and in cases of suspected primary syphilis it is prudent to also run either a treponemal enzyme immunoassay immunoglobulin-M (EIA IgM) test or a fluorescent antibody absorption (FTA-abs) test, which are more sensitive at this time [28]. At any phase, histological examination of any lesions or lymph node aspirate should take place using either dark-field microscopy (DFM) or direct fluorescent antibody stain (DFA) for identification of the *Treponema pallidum* spirochete [28].

Treatment consists of benzathine penicillin G, to be administered intramuscularly at 2.4 megaunits as a single dose in patients who have had symptoms for less than a year, and at 2.4 megaunits intramuscularly once a week for two or three doses for those with symptoms for more than a year. Alternatives for those with penicillin allergies include doxycycline, one 100-mg tablet twice a day for 2 weeks; tetracycline, one 500-mgtablet four times a day for 2 weeks; or azithromycin, one 500-mg tablet once daily for 1 week [28].

Mycobacterium

Mycobacterial infection of the nasal and paranasal cavities is a very rare condition that can be quite challenging to diagnose and treat. *Mycobacterium* is the genus of bacteria that is typically responsible for tuberculosis infections. Tuberculosis can cause acute or chronic rhinosinusitis, although the incidence is rare. Atypical mycobacterial infections, such as *Mycobacterium mageritense*, are more likely to be found with rhinosinusitis than tuberculosis. Mycobacterial infections are more common in patients with advanced human immunodeficiency virus (HIV) infection or leprosy; however, they have been isolated in otherwise healthy individuals and therefore need to be considered with persistent nasal and paranasal disease [1,31].

Patients with mycobacterial rhinosinusitis typically present with complaints of nasal congestion, mucopurulent nasal discharge, and dental and facial discomfort. Nasal endoscopic exam may reveal mucopurulent sinus secretions, significant inflammatory changes of the nasal and paranasal sinus mucosa, and nasal crusting [1]. Diagnosis is made by isolation of the offending mycobacterium on culture. In the case of mycobacterial rhinosinusitis, the offending organism is often not initially isolated histopathologically [1]. Sinus secretions should be sent for bacterial culture and Gram stain, with acid-fast testing done if indicated on Gram stain [32].

As with other forms of bacterial rhinosinusitis, treatment often begins empirically with antibiotics. For infection and symptoms to resolve, the appropriate antibiotics must be selected for the particular microbe [32]. The complexity of identification of

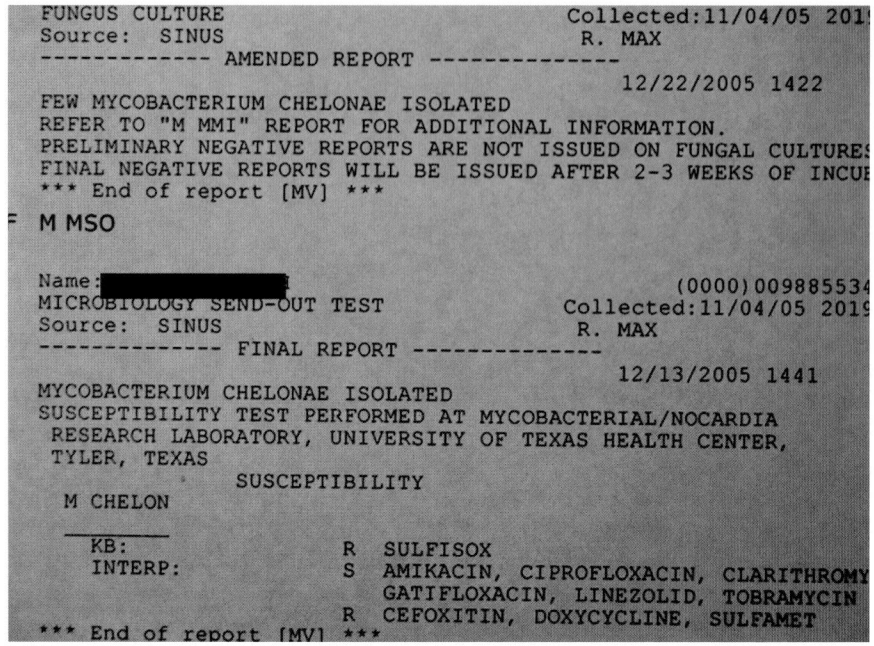

Fig. 11.5 Culture results in a patient later diagnosed with immunodeficiency, showing the growth of atypical *Mycobacterium* in a sinusitis otherwise refractory to traditional antibiotics

these microbes requires that treatment be driven by culture results to avoid development of resistant strains of *Mycobacterium*[1,32,33] (Fig. 11.5). An infectious disease specialist may be consulted in this scenario, especially in the rare occurrence of tuberculin infection.

Rhinoscleroma

Caused by *Klebsiella rhinoscleromatis*, rhinoscleroma is a rare chronic infection characterized by the formation of granulomatous nasal masses [34]. Rhinoscleroma patients present in one of three classic stages. The first stage, or the atrophic stage, is evidenced by symptoms and endoscopy findings mimicking rhinosinusitis, such as nasal obstruction, rhinorrhea, purulent discharge, and crusting. This is followed by the hypertrophic stage, where nasal nodules begin to form, eventually leading to the destruction of nasal cartilage. Finally, the sclerotic stage is marked by extensive fibrosis and scarring [1]. Although this condition primarily affects the nose, with nasal symptoms present in 95% to 100% of rhinoscleroma patients, other sites of involvement have been reported including the sinuses, eustachian tubes, mouth, larynx, trachea, bronchi, nearby skin, and even the brain, causing destruction and stenosis in these sites [34]. As a result, voice hoarseness, as well as hearing and vision loss, may result if this condition is not effectively managed [35].

Rhinoscleroma is minimally contagious, transmitted through prolonged exposure, and is more likely to be found in the rural areas of Central Europe, the Middle East, Central and South America, Asia, and tropical Africa [34,35]. It is therefore prudent to ask suspected patients about any recent extended travel in these areas.

Diagnosis is made through a combination of a positive culture as well as histopathological examination of a biopsy of the affected nasal tissue [34]. The classic biopsy findings compatible with rhinoscleroma include Mikulicz cells, macrophages containing large amounts of bacteria-filled vacuoles, and Russell bodies, spherical structures found in the cytoplasm of plasma cells. The culture with sensitivity serves to further support the diagnosis as well as to later direct therapy, although less than 70% of cultures come back positive for the *Klebsiella rhinoscleromatis* bacterium [1,34].

Treatment includes the use of extended courses of culture-directed antibiotics lasting between 1 and 3 months. Some antibiotics commonly used for rhinoscleroma include flouroquinolones such as ciprofloxacin and levofloxacin, clindamycin, rifampin, and tetracycline [34]. Surgical debridement may also be needed in cases of significant nasal stenosis [35].

Hematologic-Oncologic Illnesses

Neoplasms

Distinguishing neoplasms from other infectious and inflammatory processes causing persistent symptoms of rhinosinusitis is an important role for rhinologists [36]. While the source may be one of the atypical infectious and autoimmune disorders outlined in earlier sections of this chapter—such as syphilis, fungus, and Wegener's granulomatosis—neoplasms should also be part of the differential diagnosis. Neoplasms are either benign, as is usually the case in inverted papillomas, or malignant. Malignant neoplasms of the nasal cavity and paranasal sinuses can be broadly categorized as epithelial, including squamous cell, transitional cell, adenoid cystic and adenocarcinomas; nonepithelial, including lymphoid tumors, reticular tumors, and sarcomas; or metastatic cancer [37].

Neoplasms of the nasal cavity or paranasal sinuses should be ruled out in a patient with prolonged symptoms of rhinosinusitis recalcitrant to conventional therapy or with persistent unilateral symptoms. The clinical picture of most sinonasal tumors lacks specificity, with symptoms resembling more benign processes, including nasal obstruction, nasal discharge, epistaxis, rhinitis, anosmia, facial pain, and/or neuropathies [36,38]. Physical examination of the nasal cavity may reveal an intranasal mass, septal destruction, mucosal ulceration, necrosis, destruction of sinus walls, or the presence of an oronasal fistula [38] (Fig. 11.6).

As with most malignant processes, early diagnosis is crucial for a favorable prognosis. A biopsy is required for determination of histopathology. An adequate specimen is imperative, which is sometimes difficult to obtain for reasons of nasal anatomy or the possible presence of necrosis. Multiple biopsies may be needed for

Fig. 11.6 Endoscopic picture
of a malignant sinonasal
lesion within the right nasal
cavity (*). Notice the friable
and fleshy nature of the
lesion, an adenoid cystic
carcinoma of the ethmoid
sinus

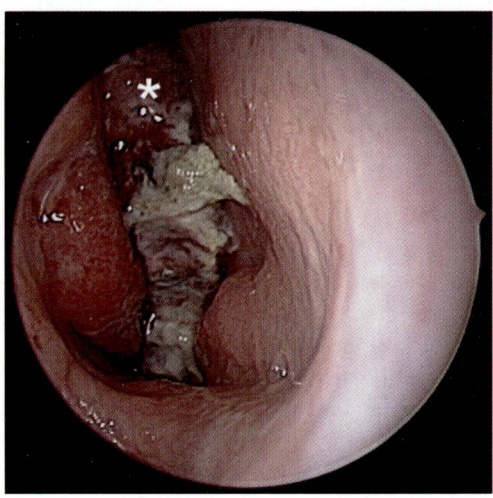

an accurate diagnosis [36–38]. Some studies suggest sending all tissue removed
from the nasal cavity or paranasal sinuses for routine histopathology, including nasal
polyps [39]. Also included in the diagnostic workup of neoplasms are radiologic
images (initially MRI and CT scans), which are useful for determining the amount
of local disease present and helping to stage tumors [36,38] (Fig. 11.7).

(a)   (b)

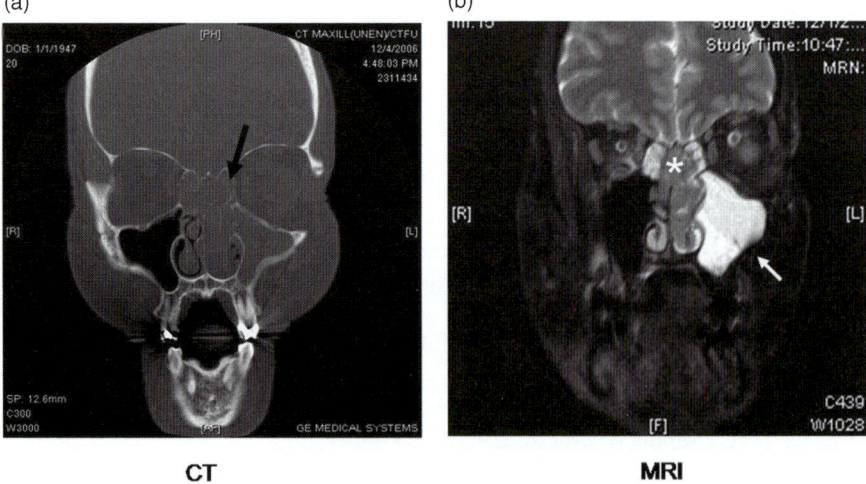

CT   MRI

Fig. 11.7 CT (*left*) and magnetic resonance imaging (MRI, *right*) views of a malignant mucosal
melanoma of the left nasal cavity. Notice that, on CT scans, differentiating this malignant lesion
from nasal polyps can be difficult. The bony erosion of the superior septum hints of an aggressive lesion (*arrow*). The corresponding T_2-weighted MRI shows a solid mass (*) extending to the
anterior skull base and retained secretions within the left maxillary sinus (*arrow*)

Once a rhinologic neoplasm is identified, management is usually determined by a team of health care providers, including otorhinolaryngologists, radiation oncologists, hematology oncologists, and neuroradiologists. Depending on the malignant process involved and the extent of disease, treatment options include surgical resection, chemotherapy, and radiotherapy; each may be used as adjunct or monotherapy [36,38].

Hereditary Hemorrhagic Telangiectasia

Although the clinical picture of hereditary hemorrhagic telangiectasia (HHT), also known as Rendu–Osler–Weber syndrome, does not resemble typical chronic rhinos-inusitis in terms of symptoms, it is a chronic systemic syndrome that affects the nasal mucosa and has, therefore, been included in this discussion.

HHT is an inherited autosomal dominant disease that is characterized by recurrent epistaxis, mucocutaneous telangiectases, and visceral arteriovenous malformations [40]. It is an age-dependent condition, with most patients presenting with symptoms by age 21. Genetic mutations cause the formation of thin-walled and dilated submucous postcapillary venules, eventually resulting in the development of arteriovenous shunts or telangiectases [41]. These vascular anomalies can appear in any organ, with 90% of HHT patients demonstrating them in their nasal mucosa, 85% exhibiting them on their skin (Fig. 11.8), 75% presenting with liver arteriovenous malformations, and up to 33% showing evidence of gastrointestinal telangiectases [40]. Other possible sites of involvement include the lungs, urethra, brain, spinal column, retina, kidney, prostate, and spleen. Clinical signs and symptoms vary depending on the severity and sites of the telangiectases and arteriovenous malformations, ranging from cosmetic considerations on the skin to bleeding at the

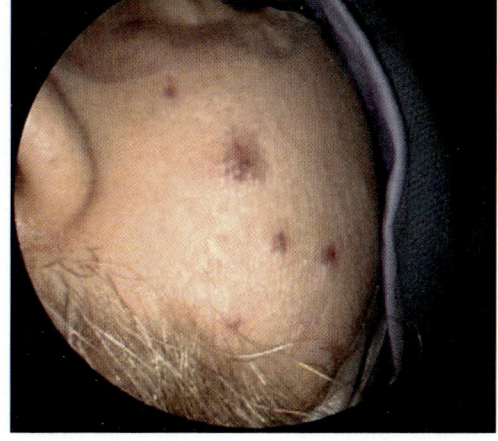

Fig. 11.8 Picture of arteriovenous (AV) malformations in the skin of the cheek of a patient with hereditary hemorrhagic telangiectasia

mucosal sites, symptoms of congestive heart failure with liver involvement, and seizures with cerebral vascular malformations [40].

Nosebleeds are the most common complaint of these patients and severely affect their quality of life [42]. On nasal endoscopy, multiple telangiectases can be observed (Fig. 11.9). They have been described as superficial dilated vascular structures found along the nasal mucosa [42]. Crusting from dried blood may also be seen. On general physical examination, telangiectases can be appreciated on the face, especially on the lips, oral cavity, and fingers [1]. A thorough history should include a family history significant for nosebleeds; the severity and frequency of the patient's nosebleeds; and the need for intervention for previous nosebleeds, such as nasal packing, cauterization, iron supplementation, or blood transfusions.

Diagnosis of HHT is made based on the presence of at least two of the following criteria: recurrent nosebleeds; multiple telangiectases, especially at the lips, in the nose, and in the oral cavity; the presence of visceral arteriovenous malformations; or a positive first-degree family history of HHT [43]. If there is a suspicion of HHT, the patient should be referred to an HHT center where a multidisciplinary approach can be made for further testing and screening. These centers include geneticists, radiologists, hematologists, psychiatrists, otolaryngologists, dermatologists, cardiologists, and pulmonologists, touching on each aspect of HHT [40].

Although there is currently no cure for this condition, interventions should be performed to control the patient's symptoms and prevent the complications that are associated with the arteriovenous malformations and telangiectases [40]. In terms of the symptom of recurrent epistaxis, several treatments may be selected based on the severity of the nosebleeds: these include (in order of treatment for mild recurrent nosebleeds to severe nosebleeds) the use of water-based nasal lubricants and environmental humidity, administration of topical estrogen/progesterone preparations,

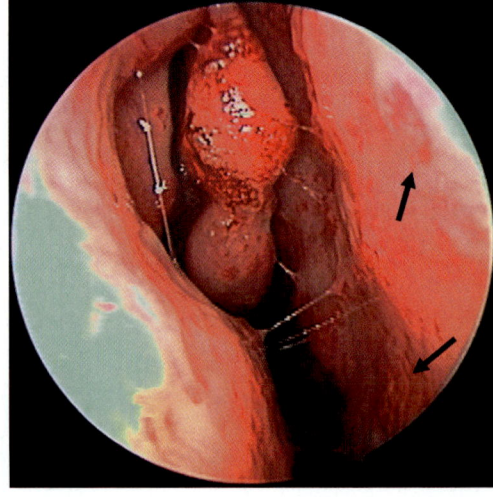

Fig. 11.9 Endoscopic picture of the right nasal cavity of a patient with hereditary hemorrhagic telangiectasia. There are multiple lesions along the anterior septum (*arrows*) and middle turbinate

chemical cauterization, bipolar electrocoagulation, laser therapy, embolization of nasal arteries, and septodermoplasty. As a last resort, the Young's procedure can be performed, which involves the closure of the nostrils [40,41].

Human Immunodeficiency Virus (HIV)

HIV is an immune-altering infection that causes increased vulnerability to potentially fatal illnesses, including opportunistic infections and malignancies. Specific to otolaryngology, approximately 80% of HIV-infected patients present with head and neck symptoms [44]. These patients have an increased risk of rhinosinusitis, both acute and recurrent. Studies suggest this increased incidence of rhinosinusitis is related to decreased CD4 counts, increased IgE production, and prolonged mucociliary transport time inherent to HIV-infected patients. Specifically, CD4 counts less than 200/mm [3] have been associated with resistant and chronic rhinosinusitis, whereas excessive IgE leads to IgE-mediated allergic rhinitis. In addition, delayed mucociliary clearance, which is usually chronic and thought to be irreversible, has been identified as a major factor of recurrent rhinosinusitis in the HIV-infected population [44–46].

Head and neck symptoms of patients with HIV infection, in order of prevalence, include oropharyngeal complaints, neck edema, and rhinologic and otologic complaints [44]. The rhinologic complaints are consistent with symptoms of rhinosinusitis: anosmia, nasal congestion, purulent discharge, fever, and facial pain and pressure. Physical examination findings on nasal exam are also consistent with those found with rhinosinusitis but are also more likely to include epistaxis and associated cervical lymphadenopathy [44,45].

Because of the head and neck manifestations, HIV infections are often diagnosed by otolaryngologists [44]. Centers for Disease Control (CDC) guidelines indicate that all patients with an opportunistic illness consistent with HIV infection should be HIV tested and counseled. Enzyme immunoassay (EIA) is the most widely used serologic test for detecting HIV-1 antibody. If this test is found reactive for HIV-1 antibody, a supplemental test is done for increased specificity, the most common of which is the Western blot [47]. If rhinosinusitis is present, a nasal culture should be sent for bacterial, fungal, and AFB (acid-fast bacilli) pathogens to aid in the selection of medical therapy. As with other disease processes, radiographic imaging is useful in determining the extent of involvement, with MRI or CT being the most sensitive. The majority of HIV-infected patients with rhinosinusitis have posterior sinus involvement; the severity of disease found on imaging is inversely related to CD4 counts [46].

Patients diagnosed with HIV are typically managed by a health care provider specializing in HIV treatment. Treatment usually includes highly active antiretroviral therapy (HAART), often as a combination of antiretroviral drugs to increase chances of successfully altering viral replication [48]. Along with antiretroviral treatment, patients may need medications for prophylaxis and/or comorbidities related to their immunocompromised state. Regarding otolaryngologic manifestations, treatment varies depending on the pathogen isolated and may include antifungal therapy, antituberculous treatment, culture-directed antibiotics, and even chemotherapy and/or radiation therapy if applicable for malignancy [44]. Rhinosinusitis in patients with HIV infection can be difficult to eradicate, requiring the use of long-term oral or intravenous antibiotics. Surgery is indicated if medical therapy fails; in particular, functional endoscopic sinus surgery is useful in this scenario [44,46]. Additionally, preventative measures—such as use of guaifenesin, nasal irrigations, and the pneumococcal vaccine—have all been shown to have some benefit with HIV-related rhinosinusitis [49–51].

Substance Abuse: Cocaine

Although substance abuse is not generally thought of as a systemic disease contributing to rhinosinusitis, the symptoms and manifestations of substance abuse can mimic those of granulomatous sinus disease and those of rhinosinusitis. Specifically, nasal inhalation of cocaine is a form of substance abuse that directly affects the nasal and sinus cavities. Localized destruction of the nasal and sinus cavities is a direct result of the vasoconstrictive effects of inhaled cocaine. Vasoconstriction is directly followed by vasodilation of the mucosa and chronic tissue ischemia, resulting in atrophy of the surrounding tissue and increased susceptibility for anaerobic infection. Chronic vasoconstriction and tissue ischemia from intranasal cocaine abuse leads to tissue necrosis, resulting in extensive erosion of the nasal and sinus cavities [52].

Patients often present with complaints of nasal and facial pain, nasal congestion, epistaxis, and discolored or malodorous nasal discharge. Endoscopic exam may reveal septal perforation, hard palate perforation, necrosis of the nasal septum, and nasal crusting [52]. Necrosis and destruction of the nasal septum may extend to total loss of the nasal septum, saddle nose formation, and atrophy of the nasal turbinates. Not as commonly, patients may also complain of visual disturbances, including diplopia or blurred vision, accompanied by severe headaches and eye swelling (Fig. 11.10); this complaint may be indicative of sinuorbital involvement and should be further evaluated using nuclear magnetic resonance imaging [53].

To more fully evaluate nasal cavity destruction, a CT scan should be performed. Tissue destruction can mimic that of granulomatous disease. Therefore, workup should include serologic testing to determine if the destruction of the nasal mucosa results from a granulomatous disease process or from localized tissue necrosis secondary to substance abuse. Intranasal substance abuse is often not reported by patients; therefore, serology testing should include autoimmune screening as well as serum drug screening. Tissue biopsy of the nasal mucosa or nasal septum may reveal granulation tissue with inflammatory cells and may show extensive bacterial overgrowth. However, pathology will show no evidence of neoplasm or granuloma formation in patients where nasal and sinus cavity destruction is caused by intranasal substance abuse [52,54]. Subsequent to mucosal damage, secondary bacterial sinusitis is quite common [52]. Typically, the offending organism is found to be staphylococcus or streptococcus and may be identified through bacterial culture of nasal secretions [55,56].

Fig. 11.10 Endoscopic picture of a patient complaining of left eye pain who had a history of previous sinus surgery. The white powdered substance located within the left maxillary sinus is crushed narcotics, which the patient was routinely snorting

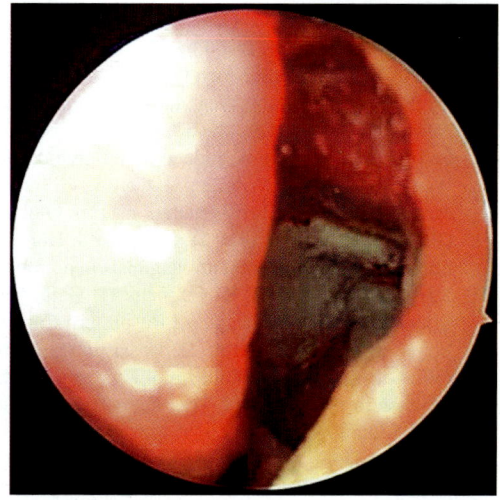

Patients found to have a history of cocaine use should be referred to drug counseling. In patients in whom extensive erosion and necrosis of the nasal septum and nasal mucosa is identified, surgical intervention may be indicated [52]. Treatment for the rhinosinusitis symptoms typically includes the use of steroids and culture-directed antibiotic therapy [53,55], but many of these treatment paradigms have suboptimal results unless the patient ceases use of intranasal cocaine.

Conclusion

Historically, the terms lethal midline granuloma or idiopathic midline destructive disease have been used to describe the process of progressive inflammation and necrosis of the nasal cavity and paranasal sinuses. Although still useful for establishing a broad differential, these all-inclusive terms have been replaced by the specific pathogens involved [36]. Current research and improved technology have given us the knowledge and tools needed to better diagnose occult otorhinolaryngologic processes. Therefore, the differential for persistent rhinosinusitis needs to include, but not be limited to, the autoimmune, infectious, and hematologic-oncologic systemic diseases described in this chapter.

References

1. Tami TA. Granulomatous diseases and chronic rhinosinusitis. Otolaryngol Clin N Am 2005;38:1267–1278.
2. Lloyd G, Lund VJ, Beale T, et al. Radiology in focus: rhinologic changes in Wegener's granulomatosis. J Laryngol Otol 2002;116: 565–569.
3. Woywodt A, Haubitz M, Haller H, et al. Wegener's granulomatosis. Lancet 2006;367: 1362–1366.

4. Lagnese ME, Dhaliwal G. Case report: an initial diagnosis of Wegener's granulomatosis in an 82-year-old woman. Hosp Phys 2007;52:33–36.
5. Leavitt RY, Fauci AS, Bloch DA, et al. The American College of Rheumatology 1990 criteria for the classification of Wegener's granulomatosis. Arthritis Rheum 1990;33:1101–1107.
6. Newman LS, Rose CS, Maier LA. Sarcoidosis. N Engl J Med 1997;337:1124–1234.
7. Cox CE, Davis-Allen A, Judson MA. Sarcoidosis. Med Clin N Am 2005;89:817–828.
8. Wang X, Kim J, McWilliams R, Cutting G. Increased prevalence of chronic rhinosinusitis in carriers of a cystic fibrosis mutation. Arch Otolaryngol Head Neck Surg 2005;131:237–240.
9. Gilljam M, Ellis L, Corey M, Zielenski J, Durie P, Tullis E. Clinical manifestations of cystic fibrosis among patients with diagnosis in adulthood. Chest 2004;126:1215–1224.
10. Jorissen M, De Boek K, Cuppens H. Genotype-phenotype correlations for the paranasal sinuses in cystic fibrosis. Am J Respir Crit Care Med 1999;159:1412–1416.
11. Young M, Gould J, Upton, G. Nasal polyposis in children with cystic fibrosis: a long-term follow-up study. Ann Otol Rhinol Laryngol 2002;111:1081–1086.
12. Rosenstein B, Cutting G. The diagnosis of cystic fibrosis: a consensus statement. J Pediatr 1998;132:589–595.
13. Ratgen F, Doring G. Seminar: cystic fibrosis. Lancet 2003;361:681–689.
14. Flume P, O'Sullivan B, Robinson K, et al. Cystic fibrosis pulmonary guidelines: chronic medications for maintenance of lung health. Am J Respir Crit Care Med 2007;176:957–969.
15. Abril A, Calamia KT, Cohen MD. The Churg Strauss syndrome (allergic granulomatous angiitis): review and update. Semin Arthritis Rheum 2003;33:106–114.
16. Pagnoux C, Gulpain P, Guillevin L. Churg-Strauss syndrome. Curr Opin Rheumatol 2007;19:25–32.
17. Keogh KA, Specks U. Churg-Strauss syndrome. Semin Respir Crit Care Med 2006;27: 148–157.
18. Rapini RP, Warner NB. Relapsing polychondritis. Clinics Dermatol 2006;24:482–485.
19. Liu CM, Hata TR, Swinyer L, et al. Morphology: relapsing polychondritis. Int J Dermatol 2003;42:707–708.
20. Kent PD, Michet CJ, Luthra HS, et al. Relapsing polychondritis. Curr Opin Rheumatol 2004;16:56–61.
21. D'Cruz DP, Khamashta MA, Hughes GRV. Systemic lupus erythematosis. Lancet 2007;369:587–596.
22. Rothfield N, Sontheimer R, Bernstein M. Lupus erythematosis: systemic and cutaneous manifestations. Clinics Dermatol 2006;24:348–362.
23. Gungor A, Adusumilli V, Corey J. Fungal sinusitis: progression of disease in immunosuppression. Ear Nose Throat J 1998;77:207–212.
24. Mandava P, Chaljub G, Patterson K, et al. MR imaging of cavernous sinus invasion by mucormycosis: a case study. Clin Neurol Neurosurg 2001;103:101–104.
25. Mylona S, Tzavara V, Ntai S, et al. Chronic invasive sinus aspergillosis in an immunocompetent patient: a case report. Dentomaxillofacial Radiol 2007;36:102–104.
26. Kauffman CA. Fungal infections. Proc Am Thorac Soc (PATS) 2006;3:35–40.
27. Iwen PC, Rupp ME, Hinrichs SH. Invasive mold sinusitis: 17 cases in immunocompromised patients and review of the literature. Clin Infect Dis 1997;24:1178–1184.
28. Goh BT. Syphilis in adults. Sex Transm Dis 2005;81:448–452.
29. Baughn RE, Musher DM. Secondary syphilitic lesions. Clin Microbiol Rev 2005;18: 205–216.
30. Hamlyn E, Marriott D, Gallagher RM. Secondary syphilis presenting as tonsillitis in three patients. J Laryngol Otol 2006;120:602–604.
31. Wallace RJ, Brown-Elliott BA, Hall L, et al. Clinical and laboratory features of *Mycobacterium mageritense*. J Clin Microbiol 2002;40:2930–2935.
32. Cincik H, Ferguson BJ. The impact of endoscopic cultures on care in rhinosinusitis. Layngoscope 2006;116:1562–1568.

33. Griffith DE. Therapy of nontuberculous mycobacterial disease. Curr Opin Infect Dis 2007;20:198–203.
34. Hart CA, Rao SK. Rhinoscleroma. J Med Microbiol 2000;49:395–396.
35. Yilmaz M, Aydil U, Vural C, et al. Simultaneous occurrence of nasal and cervical rhinoscleroma. J Otolaryngol 2006;35:206–208.
36. Chain JR, Kingdom TT. Non-Hodgkin's lymphoma of the frontal sinus presenting as osteomyelitis. Am J Otolaryngol 2006;28:42–45.
37. Thompson LD. Mini-symposium: head and neck pathology—sinonasal carcinomas. Curr Diagn Pathol 2006;12:40–53.
38. Al-Hakeem DA, Fedele S, Carlos R, et al. Extranodal NK/T-cell lymphoma, nasal type. Oral Oncol 2007;43:4–14.
39. Chen S, Wu CS, Chan K, et al. Primary sinonasal non-Hodgkin's lymphoma masquerading as chronic rhinosinusitis: an issue of routine histopathological examination. J Laryngol Otol 2003;117:404–407.
40. Sabbà C. A rare and misdiagnosed bleeding disorder: hereditary hemorrhagic telangiectasia. J Thromb Haemost 2005;3:2201–2210.
41. Kühnel TS, Wagner BH, Schurr CP, et al. Clinical strategy in hereditary hemorrhagic telangiectasia. Am J Rhinol 2005;19:508–513.
42. Geisthoff UW, Sittel C, Plinkert PK. Contact endoscopic findings in hereditary hemorrhagic telangiectasia. Head Neck 2005;28:56–63.
43. HHT Foundation International. Hereditary Hemorrhagic Telangiectasia page. Available at: http://www.hht.org/index.php. Accessed July 12, 2007.
44. Prasad HK, Bhojwani KM, Shnoy V. HIV manifestations in otolaryngology. Am J Otolaryngol 2006;27:179–185.
45. Milgrim LM, Rubin JS, Small CB. Mucociliary clearance abnormalities in the HIV-infected patient: a precursor to acute sinusitis. Larnygoscope 1995;105:1202–1208.
46. Godofsky EW, Zinreich J, Armstrong M, et al. Sinusitis in HIV-infected patients: a clinical and radiographic review. Am J Med 1992;93:163–170.
47. Centers for Disease Control. Revised Recommendations for HIV testing of Adults, Adolescents, and Pregnant Women in Health-Care Settings page. Available at: http://www.cdc.gov/mmwr/preview/mmwrhtml/rr5514a1.htm. Accessed July 12, 2007.
48. Yeni PG, Hammer SM, Hirsch MS, et al. Treatment for adult HIV infection: 2004 recommendations of the International AIDS Society-USA panel. JAMA 2004;292:251–265.
49. Wawrose SF, Tami TA, Amoits CP. The role of guaifenesin in the treatment of sinonasal disease in patients infected with the human immunodeficiency virus. Laryngoscope 1992;102:1225–1228.
50. Tomooka LT, Murphy C, Davidson TM. Clinical study and literature review of nasal irrigation. Laryngoscope 2000;110:1189–1193.
51. Shafinoori S, Ginocchio CC, Greenberg AJ, et al. Impact of pneumococcal conjugate vaccine and the severity of winter influenza-like illnesses on invasive pneumococcal infections in children and adults. Pediatr Infect Dis J 2005;24:10–16.
52. Talbott JF, Gorti GK, Koch RJ. Midfacial osteomyelitis in a chronic abuser: a case report. Ear Nose Throat J 2001; 80:738–743.
53. Neugebauer P, Fricke J, Neugebauer A, et al. Sinuorbital complications after intranasal cocaine abuse. Strabismus 2004;12:205–209.
54. Leibovitch I, Khoramian D, Goldberg RA. Severe destructive sinusitis and orbital apex syndrome as a complication of intranasal cocaine abuse. Am J Emerg Med 2006;24:499–501.
55. Gordon RJ, Lowy FD. Bacterial infection in drug users. N Engl J Med 2005;353:1945–1954.
56. Klutmans J, van Belkum A, Verburgh H. Nasal carriage of Staphylococcus aureus: epidemiology, underlying mechanisms, and associated risks. Clin Microbiol Rev 1997;10:505–520.

/

Chapter 12
Reactive Airway Disease and the Management of Samter's Triad

Roxanne S. Leung, Rohit K. Katial, and Todd T. Kingdom

It has become increasingly clear that respiratory inflammation affects both the upper and lower airways. Recent investigation has established both epidemiologic and pathophysiological links between allergic rhinitis (AR), chronic rhinosinusitis (CRS), chronic rhinosinusitis with nasal polyposis (CRSwNP), and asthma. Physicians who frequently diagnose and manage patients with upper airway diseases, such as AR and CRS, encounter patients with asthma or concurrent lower respiratory disease. Conversely, physicians primarily addressing lower airway diseases encounter patients with significant sinonasal diseases that may be quite relevant to the patients' overall conditions. Physicians such as family medicine specialists, pulmonary specialists, allergists, internists, and otolaryngologists must design treatment protocols, and expectations, based on this current understanding of the role that respiratory inflammation plays in the development of upper and lower airways diseases.

Patients with nasal polyps remain one of the more challenging groups of patients to manage. The precise pathogenesis of nasal polyp formation remains poorly defined; however, chronic paranasal sinus mucosal inflammation appears to be the underlying driving force behind its development. A wide range of etiologies have been proposed and include chronic bacterial infection, atopy, fungal infection, environmental factors, genetic factors, and viral infection. Aspirin-exacerbated respiratory disease (AERD)—also referred to as Samter's triad—represents a subset of patients with severe recalcitrant nasal polyposis and asthma in the setting of sensitivity to aspirin. The underlying pathophysiology appears to be dysregulation in the eicosanoid metabolism pathway leading to increased production of cysteinyl leukotrienes and decreased levels of prostaglandins [1]. Treatment of this patient group is targeted at controlling both upper and lower airways diseases in a multi-modal fashion. Because their disease is more severe and difficult to control, the patient with AERD presents a greater challenge to the treating physician when compared to the "typical" CRS patient with or without nasal polyps.

T.T. Kingdom
Department of Otolaryngology, University of Colorado Health Sciences Center, Aurora, CO, USA
e-mail: todd.Kingdom@uchsc.edu

E.R. Thaler, D.W. Kennedy (eds.), *Rhinosinusitis*, DOI: 10.1007/978-0-387-73062-2_12,   187

The objective of this chapter is to review the contemporary approach to diagnosing and treating patients with AERD or Samter's triad. Our current understanding of the epidemiology and pathogenesis of CRS and reactive airway disease is also reviewed. Finally, current protocols and clinical outcomes for the medical and surgical management of this complex disease process are reviewed.

Reactive Airway Disease and the Unified Airway

Asthma and AR are both highly prevalent diseases. In the United States, asthma affects more than 20 million people [2], whereas AR affects about 30 million [3]. Often, these two diseases coexist. Asthma is reported in up to 40% of patients with AR, and AR occurs in 30% to 80% of asthmatics [4]. Although coincidence does not prove causality, this strong epidemiologic link suggests that these two diseases may be related. Furthermore, both AR and asthma are related in a temporal, physiological, histopathological, and therapeutic fashion [4]. The concept that both upper and lower airways are tightly linked has been coined "The One Airway Hypothesis."

Temporal Association

Although not universal, most patients develop AR before the onset of asthma. Atopy as defined by positive skin test, if developed in early childhood (by age 8 to 10 years), was found to be a risk factor for the development of asthma [5]. In a prospective 23-year follow-up of 690 college students with no evidence of asthma, those students who initially reported nasal symptoms developed asthma at a rate threefold more often than those students without rhinitis [6]. Moreover, perennial rhinitis has been found to be an independent risk factor for asthma [7].

Physiological Relationship

Clearly, the upper and lower airways are connected in an anatomic fashion; however, the mechanism whereby one affects the other is under considerable debate. Nonspecific stimuli to the nasal passages, such as cold air, histamine, or methacholine, can also result in bronchoconstriction. In the case of cold air, the lower airway response can be blocked by either disruption of the afferent reflex through local anesthesia or suppression of the efferent reflex by an anticholinergic agent [8]. Together, these data suggest the existence of a reflex between the nasal mucosa and airway smooth muscle.

One hallmark of asthma is increased sensitivity to inhaled methacholine or histamine, and this is termed *airways hyperresponsiveness*. Patients with seasonal AR, even in the absence of asthma, demonstrate increased airways hyperresponsiveness, which is especially marked if tested during their allergy season [9]. Corren et al. performed a double-blind, randomized, placebo-controlled study of patients with a history of asthma exacerbated after the onset of seasonal AR symptoms. Once the subjects displayed nasal symptoms in response to a nasal allergen challenge, they underwent several measures of lung function. Although there was no evidence of airflow obstruction, these patients did exhibit increased airways hyperresponsiveness to methacholine [10].

Postnasal drip is a common complaint among patients with AR, and aspiration of nasal secretions is a possible mechanism whereby rhinitis could aggravate asthma. Bardin et al. placed radiolabeled material in the maxillary sinuses of patients with rhinosinusitis or rhinosinusitis and asthma, and although they could detect signals in the nasopharynx, esophagus, and lower gastrointestinal (GI) tract, the label could not be found in the lower airways when imaged 24 h later [11]. Thus, the notion that nasal secretions are aspirated into the lower airways and directly trigger lower airway disease is inadequate in explaining this phenomenon.

Histopathology

The histopathological appearance of AR and asthma are similar in some regards and different in others. The upper and lower airways are contiguous structures that are lined by pseudostratified epithelium, with columnar ciliated cells that rest upon a basement membrane. Inflammation is common to both the upper and lower airways, and both demonstrate an infiltrate rich in eosinophils, mast cells, and T cells. However, other pathological changes characteristic of asthma are not found in the nasal mucosa of those with AR. Increased thickness of the reticular layer of the basement membrane—one possible manifestation of airway remodeling in asthmatics—is not found in nasal biopsy specimens of patients with AR. Furthermore, in asthma, desquamation of the respiratory epithelium is common, whereas in AR the epithelium tends to remain intact [12]. Last, the mechanism of obstruction in both the upper and lower airways differs widely. The nasal subepithelium is rich in vascular structures, and once it is perturbed, nasal congestion ensues. In contrast, bronchoconstriction of the lower airways is caused by contraction of airway smooth muscle, which is absent in the upper airway.

Therapeutic Association

Early studies suggested that treatment of AR may improve asthma symptoms. After 4 weeks of treatment with intranasal budesonide, 37 children with asthma and chronic perennial allergic rhinitis demonstrated attenuation of exercise-induced asthma and a decrease in asthma symptoms [13]. Welsh et al. [14] found improvement in asthma symptoms in ragweed allergic patients treated with intranasal beclomethasone diproprionate or flunisolide. Further studies also demonstrated reduction in airways hyperresponsiveness after treatment of AR with intranasal corticosteroids [15,16]. One could argue that the improvement of asthma symptoms was simply a result of deposition of intranasally administered corticosteroid into the lung. However, Watson et al. disproved this by following radiolabeled beclomethasone and finding that less than 2% was deposited in the lung [16]. They argue that the improvement in asthma symptoms and airways hyperresponsiveness is the result of improvement of nasal inflammation, rather than the direct, local effect of corticosteroid. Overall, several studies have reached the same conclusion: treatment of AR with intranasal corticosteroids improves bronchial hyperresponsiveness, but does not improve lung function [10,15,16]. Adams et al. performed a retrospective cohort study of patients with asthma and an upper airways condition (which they defined as either rhinitis, rhinosinusitis, or otitis media) and found that treatment with intranasal corticosteroids significantly decreased asthma exacerbations treated in the emergency room [17]. On the other hand, treatment of asthma may improve AR. As a proof-of-concept study, Greiff et al. demonstrated that in nonasthmatics with seasonal allergic rhinitis, inhaled budesonide improves nasal symptoms and lowered both nasal eosinophil and peripheral eosinophil counts [18].

Perhaps one of the most compelling pieces of evidence that link both the upper and lower airways was observed in the Preventive Allergy Treatment study (PAT). Children with allergic rhinitis were randomized to either a 3-year course of subcutaneous immunotherapy (SIT) or symptomatic control [19]. Now, after 10 years of follow-up, far fewer patients in the SIT-treated group developed asthma, compared to the control group, resulting in an odds ratio of 2.48 [20].

Aspirin-Exacerbated Respiratory Disease (Samter's Triad)

Epidemiology

The association between asthma, nasal polyposis, and aspirin sensitivity has been observed for almost a century, but this syndrome gained more widespread recognition after publication of the work of Max Samter in 1968 [21]. Thereafter, this syndrome has been known as Samter's triad. Although several different names and acronyms have been used to identify Samter's triad, throughout this chapter we use aspirin-exacerbated respiratory disease, or AERD.

It is difficult to determine the prevalence of aspirin sensitivity in asthmatics by history alone, and estimates range widely. On the one hand, a patient who has never been challenged with an aspirin or nonsteroidal antiinflammatory drug (NSAID) will not be able to report a reaction. In other instances, patients may not recognize the link between aspirin or NSAID ingestion and exacerbation of their asthma, which may explain the lower estimates of aspirin sensitivity in asthmatics when obtained by survey compared to prospective aspirin challenge [1]. In a meta-analysis of several studies that used oral aspirin challenge to prove the diagnosis of aspirin sensitivity in asthmatics, the combined prevalence was 21% in adults and 5% in children (ages 0–18 years) [22]. The potential pool of patients is further enriched if also diagnosed with nasal polyposis or chronic rhinosinusitis; in this subset of patients, the prevalence of aspirin sensitivity was reported to be as high as 30% to 40% [1].

Pathophysiology

First, special mention should be made that AERD is not a true allergy. The term allergy should be reserved for an antigen-specific IgE-mediated hypersensitivity reaction. Certainly, patients can develop true allergy to aspirin, but the mechanism of action and subsequent treatment is quite different than in AERD. Instead, AERD is characterized by an intense eosinophilic and mast cell inflammatory process. The initiating insult has yet to be found, but some theories include viral infection, exposure to air pollution, or tobacco smoke [1]. Aspirin itself has not been implicated as the instigating factor for this inflammatory process, as it is ongoing before the first aspirin-induced reaction.

Patients with AERD often react to aspirin and several NSAIDs. Because these agents all share the ability to block the enzyme cyclooxygenase (COX), especially COX-1, one theory proposes that alterations in the balance of downstream mediators lead to the phenotype of AERD. The pathway for arachidonic metabolism, and the effect of aspirin, are outlined in Fig. 12.1. Membrane phospholipids are metabolized by phospholipase A_2 into arachidonic acid. Through the action of the enzyme 5-lipoxygenase, arachidonic acid is further metabolized into several lipid products known as leukotrienes. Through the action of the enzyme cysteinyl leukotriene C_4 synthase, the three cysteinyl leukotrienes (cysLT) LTC_4, LTD_4, and LTE_4 (and previously called the "slow-reacting substance of anaphylaxis") are produced. As overproduction of leukotrienes can be a result of upregulated synthesis, several groups have looked at polymorphisms in the gene encoding leukotriene C_4 synthase.

Although there was an association between one single nucleotide polymorphism and risk of AERD in a Polish population, this finding could not be reproduced in an American population [23,24]. Regardless of the mechanism of upregulation, high levels of these leukotrienes are responsible for the following actions: bronchoconstriction of the airways, stimulation of mucous production, and recruitment of inflammatory cells into the airway [25].

Most AERD patients have elevated baseline levels of these products, as measured by urinary excretion of leukotriene E_4, and once challenged with aspirin, these levels are pushed even higher [26]. Elevated cysLT levels have also been identified in patients with CRSwNP, regardless of AERD status. Thus elevated expression of cysLTs has been implicated in the pathogenesis of polypoid rhinosinusitis. Additional research has demonstrated increased expression of the cysteinyl leukotriene 1 receptor ($cysLT_1$) on leukocytes infiltrating nasal mucosa from patients with AERD and nasal polyps; after treatment with aspirin desensitization, those receptors are downregulated [27]. Thus, both increased cysLT synthesis and increased receptor expression may contribute to the pathogenesis of this process.

Arachidonic acid can also be metabolized through a separate pathway by the enzyme cyclooxygenase to produce prostaglandins (PG) (see Fig. 12.1). One prostaglandin in particular, PGE_2, has been shown to block both aspirin-induced bronchospasm and the rise in urine leukotriene E_4 [28]. Although PGs have a wide array of actions, PGE_2 works as an antiinflammatory mediator by downregulating

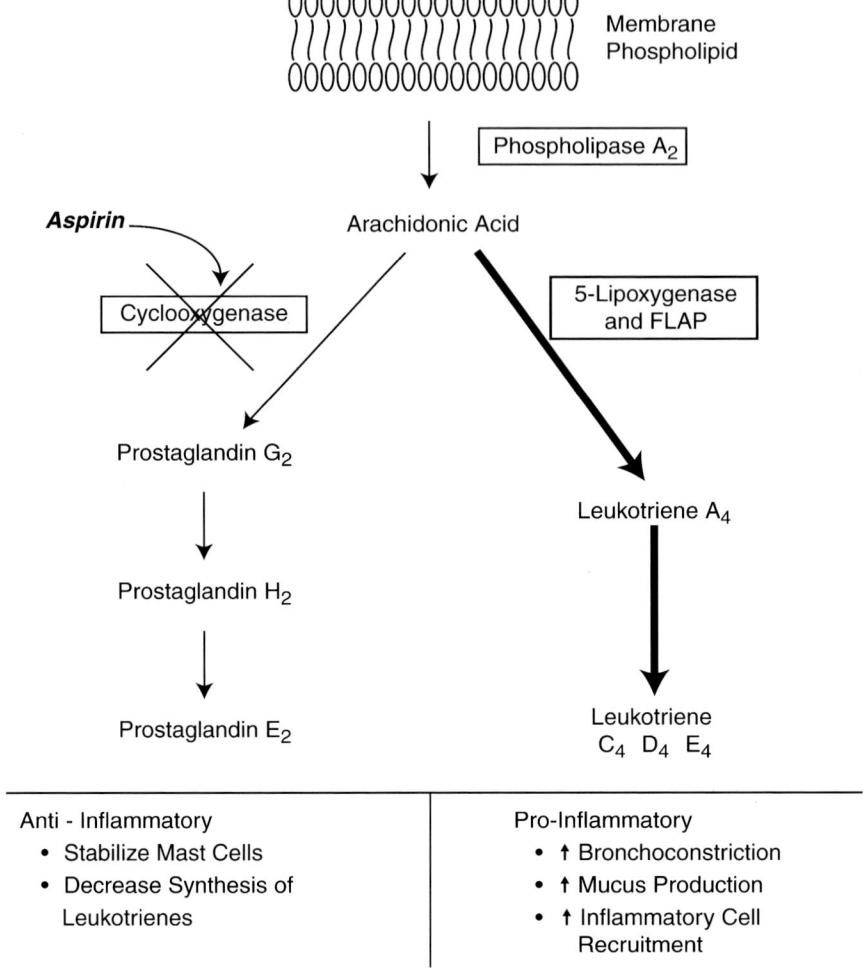

Fig. 12.1 Possible mechanism of aspirin-exacerbated respiratory disease (AERD). Arachidonic acid is metabolized into both proinflammatory and antiinflammatory mediators. Cyclooxygenase normally converts arachidonic acid to prostoglandin G_2, and through a number of other enzymatic reactions, produces prostaglandin E_2. This mediator in turn acts to dampen the inflammatory response by increasing stability of mast cells and decreasing synthesis of proinflammatory leukotrienes. Aspirin is a nonreversible inhibitor of cyclooxygenase and works to functionally push the arachidonic cascade in favor of the leukotrienes by blocking the production of prostaglandin E_2

the production of leukotrienes. In essence, it works as an inhibitor of the inflammatory response. In patients with AERD, production of PGE_2 is impaired, and it is the relative lack of PGE_2 that appears equally important in the pathophysiology of AERD. Also, PGE_2 further works to stabilize mast cells. Therefore aspirin, a nonreversible inhibitor of cyclooxygenase, may work to push the arachidonic cascade in favor of the leukotriene pathway, at least in a functional manner, thus augmenting the proinflammatory response.

Ongoing research continues to explore the relationship between cysLT and PG synthesis in the pathogenesis of AERD. Recent work performed on nasal polyp tissue in patients with AERD has demonstrated differential COX-2 expression and activity [29–31]. Dysregulation of COX-2 would presumably lead to decreased PGE_2 synthesis and subsequent lowering of the antiinflammatory effects. These data combined with increased cysLT expression in this patient group suggest the relative "balance" between cysLT and PG synthesis is the more important factor in this process. Thus, the absolute expression of the cysLTs is not as important as the balance between their proinflammatory effects, relative to the antiinflammatory actions of the PGs. So perhaps the expression of AERD is the result of more proinflammatory signal (leukotriene), less antiinflammatory signal (PGE_2), more receptor ($cysLT_1$), and subsequent augmentation of downstream signaling pathways.

Assessment and Diagnosis

As already discussed, history alone is not sufficient to make the diagnosis of AERD. However, there are several red flags in the history that may identify which patients are more likely to have true AERD [1]:

- Severe asthma attack requiring emergency room intervention soon after ingestion of any COX-1 inhibitor
- History of severe asthma attack, on more than one occasion, after ingestion of different COX-1 inhibitors

The best way to assess a patient for AERD is through aspirin challenge, as there are currently no reliable, validated in vitro surrogates. Aspirin challenge can be done a number of different ways, depending on the route of administration and the challenge drug.

In the United States, oral administration is most common. We perform challenges in our procedure unit, under close supervision. In contrast to traditional immunotherapy, antihistamines are not given before challenge. We also avoid bronchodilator use the morning of the procedure as this may confound interpretation of a drop in lung function during the procedure. Patients are asked to continue with all their other medications.

Patients are then challenged with one or more doses of aspirin, depending on their clinical history. Lung function and symptoms are followed after each dose. A positive challenge is called after a significant drop in forced expiratory volume in 1 s (FEV_1), and/or the appearance of naso-ocular symptoms. In Europe, aspirin lysine is used in both bronchial and nasal challenges; however, because it is not approved for use in human subjects by the U.S. Food and Drug Administration (FDA), it is not available for use in the United States.

Management of Samter's Triad

Medical Therapy

Avoidance of COX-1 inhibitors is paramount. Patients need to be especially careful of any over-the-counter medications that may contain aspirin or other NSAIDs. For example, some Alka-Seltzer products contain 325 to 500 mg aspirin. In contrast to the cross-reactivity of COX-1 inhibitors, COX-2 inhibitors have been shown to be remarkably safe. Several studies have shown, with greater than 95% confidence, that these agents can be used in patients with AERD [32]. Acetaminophen, on the other hand, is a weak COX-1 inhibitor. Patients with AERD can usually tolerate doses up to 650 mg. However, at the higher dose of 1000 mg, 20% of patients may have a reaction [33].

As patients with AERD have markedly elevated leukotrienes, therapy to block production or action of these mediators would seem to be a logical strategy. In the United States, there are two types of antileukotriene therapy approved by the FDA for use in the treatment of asthma. The first, zileuton (Zyflo), is an inhibitor of the 5-lipoxygenase (5-LO), and partially blocks conversion of arachidonic acid to leukotriene A_4 (Fig. 12.2). In our practice, we prescribe zileuton at a dosage of 600 mg four times a day. We check a baseline liver function profile, then check every month for 3 months, then every 2 to 3 months thereafter. Zileuton can cause a rise in alanine aminotransferase (ALT) in 2% of patients, and it is contraindicated in patients with active liver disease. Montelukast (Singulair 10 mg daily) and zafirlukast (Accolate 20 mg twice daily) are examples of the second class of antileukotriene therapy. They act downstream of zileuton and work by competitively binding to the $cysLT_1$ receptor (see Fig. 12.2). In practice, clinical effects of these treatments seem to vary widely.

The use of antileukotriene therapy in the management of CRSwNP is an off-label treatment strategy increasingly used by clinicians. These medications do not have approved indications for use in the treatment of upper respiratory disease, with the exception of montelukast, which has been approved for allergic rhinitis. Well-controlled data examining the use of these medications for patients with nasal polyps are lacking. Dahlen at al. reported improvement in smell, rhinorrhea, and nasal congestion in 40 patients with AERD, asthma, and nasal polyps receiving 16 weeks of zileuton compared to controls [34]. In 2000, Parnes and Chuma reported their experience with zafirlukast (26 patients) and zileuton (10 patients) in the management of nasal polyposis. Overall, they reported 72% subjective improvement and 50% objective improvement or stabilization. Significant limitations of this study include lack of a control group, AERD status was not defined, and outcome measures were not rigorous [35]. Ragab et al. looked at the use of montelukast as an add-on therapy to topical and inhaled corticosteroids in patients with asthma and nasal polyps, with and without AERD [36]. They found subjective and objective improvement in asthma and nasal polyps, but independent of AERD status. They concluded that their findings were consistent with a subgroup of nasal polyp and asthma patients in whom leukotriene receptor antagonists are effective. Overall,

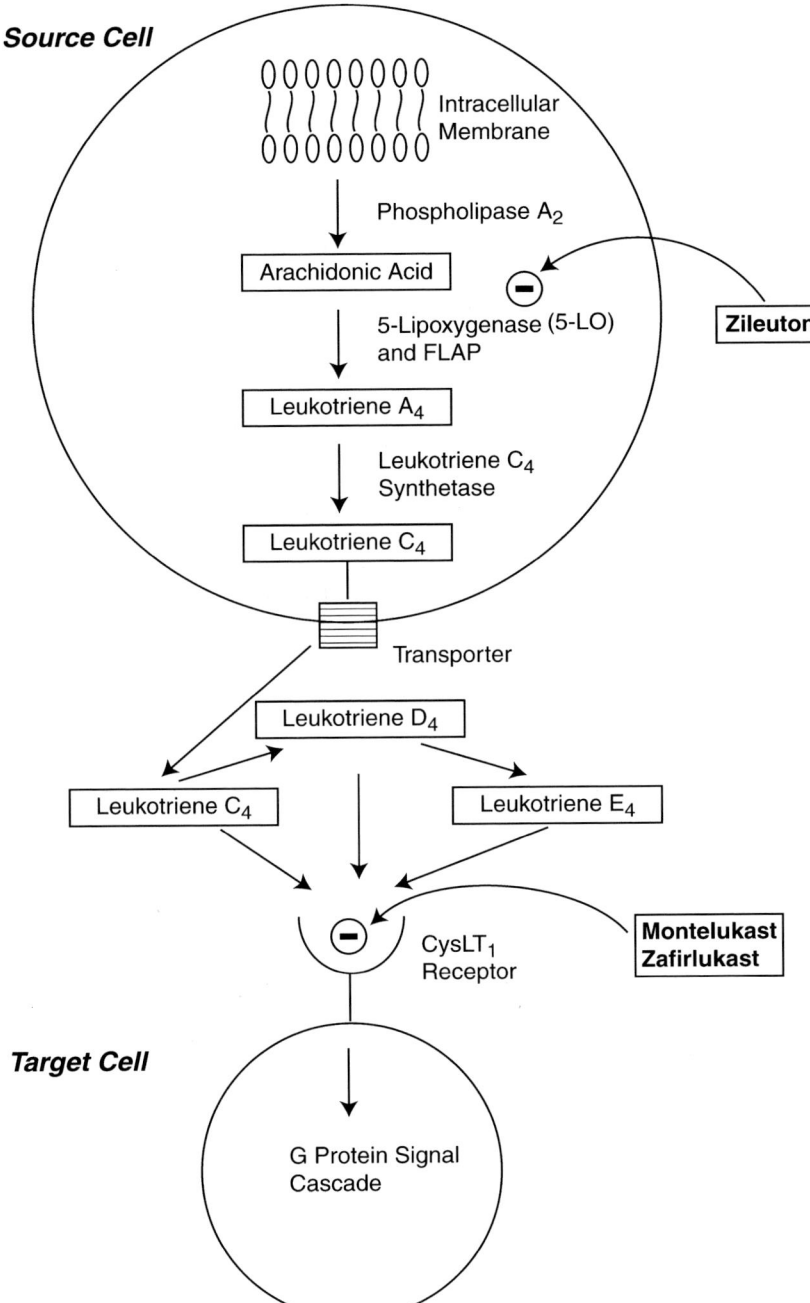

Fig. 12.2 Antileukotriene therapy. Zileuton partially blocks conversion of arachidonic acid to LTA$_4$ by interfering with the enzyme 5-lipoxygenase (5-LO). Montelukast and zafirlukast block the action of leukotriene C$_4$, D$_4$, and E$_4$ by competitive binding to the cysteinyl leukotriene receptor 1 (CysL1 receptor)

antileukotriene medications appear to have a role in the management of select patients with nasal polyposis. Clinical experience has shown that response is variable, but side effects are usually minimal.

As discussed previously, inflammation of the upper airway may contribute to poor control of the lower airway. We recommend aggressive treatment of polyposis with high-dose intranasal steroids, nasal saline rinses, and selective use of oral corticosteroids. Currently, mometasone furoate monohydrate is the only intranasal steroid with an FDA indication for the treatment of nasal polyposis. In refractory cases, systemic corticosteroids of variable duration may be required to control disease and improve quality of life. Antibiotics are reserved for acute bacterial exacerbations of sinonasal disease, but should be used selectively. Treating the underlying mucosal inflammation is the most important step in patient management. Too often antimicrobial medications are prescribed as the sole therapy in patients with hyperplastic or polypoid rhinosinusitis.

Treatment of an acute aspirin-induced lower respiratory reaction is best treated with nebulized albuterol. Repeat doses can be given every 5 to 10 min until improvement of symptoms. Laryngeal edema is treated with either subcutaneously injected epinephrine or inhaled racemic epinephrine. Nasal congestion responds to topical decongestants such as oxymetazolone. Oral antihistamines may also be helpful. In the event of severe symptoms, intubation, mechanical ventilation, and intensive care monitoring are appropriate.

Aspirin Desensitization

Aspirin desensitization should be considered as add-on therapy in patients not adequately controlled with traditional medical management, or in those patients who require aspirin or NSAID treatment for other medical conditions.

Desensitization to aspirin not only allows the patient to safely take aspirin, but also allows them to tolerate therapeutic doses of other cross-reacting NSAIDs. During aspirin desensitization, patients are given successive doses of aspirin, escalated in an incremental fashion much like in an aspirin challenge. In essence, the first part of the desensitization is the aspirin challenge. During an aspirin challenge, patients are given doses of aspirin until symptomatic (in our experience, at the dose of 81 mg or 162 mg) the procedure is stopped, and the patient is given a diagnosis of AERD. In contrast, the desensitization protocol pushes past this "threshold" dose to take the patient into a tolerant state.

As significant, severe asthma exacerbations may occur, patients should be well informed of the risks of the procedure. Also, patients should have stable, controlled asthma before the procedure. If necessary, patients are often given a 7-day course of prednisone before the procedure. The morning of the procedure, patients are placed on continuous monitoring (pulse oximetry and cardiac monitor) and IV access is established. Aspirin desensitization protocols have been previously published, and our protocol is similar [37]. A dedicated nurse is assigned to the care of the patient, and the treating physician should always be available to assess any reaction. Adequate cardiopulmonary resuscitation equipment should be on hand at all times.

Once patients are successfully desensitized, they are instructed to take 650 mg aspirin twice daily to maintain their desensitized state. Patients remain refractory to aspirin-induced reactions for 48 h after their last dose, and slowly over the next 2 to 5 days return to their original, sensitized state in the absence of continued aspirin (ASA) therapy [38].

In an attempt to increase the safety of aspirin desensitization, several studies have investigated the effect of pretreatment with different pharmacologic agents, given just before desensitization. Antileukotriene therapy, and in most cases montelukast (10 mg), has been shown to block half the cases of aspirin-induced asthma reaction, and in the remaining half it attenuates the response. This treatment has also been shown to "shift" the response from the lower airway to the upper airway alone, so the overall rate of positive reaction remains unchanged [39,40].

Long-term results of aspirin desensitization are favorable. After the first 6 months of treatment, several clinical markers were shown to be significantly better: fewer sinus infections, improved sense of smell, and improved nasal and asthma symptoms. After at least 1 year of follow-up, not only were these benefits sustained, but the authors reported improvements in several other clinical markers: fewer sinus operations, fewer hospitalizations for asthma, and fewer emergency department visits for asthma. Corticosteroid use, including intranasal, inhaled, and oral systemic, were all diminished after at least 1 year of treatment, compared to the baseline. Overall, 87% of patients who completed at least a year of treatment improved. A total of 14% of patients could not complete treatment because of side effects, most commonly gastric pain [41].

In summary, aspirin desensitization is an effective, yet underutilized treatment, and should be considered in patients with AERD that is not adequately controlled with medical management, including both topical corticosteroid and antileukotriene therapy. The following categories of patients should be considered for desensitization treatment [1]:

1. Patients with AERD, moderate to severe asthma, and/or intractable nasal congestion
2. Patients with AERD whose asthma is not adequately controlled
3. Patients with AERD and recurrent nasal polyp formation
4. Patients with AERD who are systemic corticosteroid dependent
5. Patients with AERD who require aspirin for other diseases

Surgical Management

Endoscopic sinus surgery (ESS) remains the treatment of choice for medically refractory CRS with and without nasal polyposis. Since its introduction in the 1980s, ESS has undergone review, reassessment, and substantial refinement confirming its role in the management of CRS. When considering a wide range of patient subgroups, overall success rates have been reported to range from 85% to 97% [42–46]. It is widely believed that the CRS patient with nasal polyps carries a more significant burden of disease; namely, increased severity of nasal congestion and obstruction, disturbance in olfaction, and more extensive objective stage of disease [47]. It has also been suggested that the presence of nasal polyps is predictive of worse surgical outcome and poor response to therapy. Recent reports in the literature, however, have reexamined this issue in more detail and now provide more information to guide management decisions and expected outcomes in patients with nasal polyposis.

The published outcomes that are data specific to the management of nasal polyps in the patient with AERD remain limited. In contrast, recent published prospective data have demonstrated the benefits of ESS in patients with and without nasal polyps [48,49]. Poetker et al. reported on the subjective and objective outcomes of 43 polyp and 76 non-polyp patients undergoing ESS [50]. In this study all patients, regardless of polyp status, had significant improvement in both subjective and objective parameters. Despite worse preoperative and postoperative CT and endoscopy scores, patients with polyps showed a greater degree of improvement than patients without polyps. These authors did not comment on the presence of AERD or examine the impact of ESS on asthma. Nonetheless, these data support the beneficial role of ESS in select patients with CRS and nasal polyps refractory to medical therapy.

A number of authors have investigated the impact of surgical treatment of CRS on asthma, with both improvement [51–54] and equivocal [55] outcomes reported. Although these reports included some patients with AERD, none focused on this patient group or had large enough cohorts to comment in detail. Recently, the first prospective randomized study examining the impact of medical and surgical treatment of CRS on asthma was published [56]. These authors examined subjective and objective outcomes in 43 patients with CRS with and without nasal polyps and concomitant asthma randomized to medical or surgical treatment. Asthma symptoms, control of asthma, FEV_1, peak flow, exhaled nitric oxide, medication use, and hospitalization at 6 and 12 months were recorded. The authors reported overall improvement in asthma control following both treatment modalities; no differences were demonstrated based on the presence of nasal polyps. Thus the authors concluded treatment of CRS benefits concomitant asthma. Although historically a source of much debate, these published data suggest ESS favorably impacts asthma outcomes in carefully selected patients with and without nasal polyps.

Assessing the impact of ESS on patients with AERD and nasal polyps remains problematic, largely because published data are limited. Nakamura et al. prospectively evaluated the impact of traditional and endoscopic sinus surgery on 22 patients with AERD [57]. Overall, patients benefited from surgical interventions, although validated outcomes measures were not used and no comparison group was included. Other reported data are of limited value due to their retrospective design. McFadden et al. retrospectively reviewed 80 patients with AERD undergoing ESS and reported improvements in sinus symptoms and asthma disease with reduced postoperative steroid use [58]. Once again, a comparison group was not included. Some authors have reported no benefit from ESS in the AERD patient group. Amar et al.

retrospectively reviewed 18 patients with AERD undergoing ESS and compared them to patients with CRS without AERD [59]. These authors reported AERD patients had greater postoperative medication use, increased need for revision surgery, and a lesser degree of symptomatic improvement when compared to patients without AERD. Batra et al. retrospectively examined the impact of ESS of 17 patients with nasal polyps and steroid-dependent asthma (9 with AERD) and reported the impact of surgery was less pronounced in the AERD patient cohort [60]. However, the small sample size and study design limit the clinical applications of these data.

Robinson et al. recently published a prospective study examining the impact of AERD on the outcomes of ESS in a small cohort of patients [61]. They utilized validated disease-specific quality-of-life (QOL) measurement instruments and objective parameters to assess outcomes in 19 patients with AERD after ESS and compared this group to 104 patients without AERD. Nasal polyps were present in 74% of the AERD cohort and 30% of the ASA-tolerant group. Mean follow-up was 17.7 months. The patients with AERD had significantly worse preoperative CT and endoscopy scores. After ESS, statistically significant improvements in endoscopy scores and QOL measures were demonstrated for the AERD group. Interestingly, improvement did not significantly differ by AERD status. This important study shows that similar proportions of AERD patients and ASA-tolerant patients demonstrate subjective and objective improvements in sinonasal outcomes after ESS.

The impact of ESS on asthma outcomes in patients with AERD is even less well defined. Two published studies have attempted to explore this issue. Nakamura et al. retrospectively evaluated the asthma component in patients with AERD 1 year after ESS [57]. These authors reported improvements in 91% of patients subjectively and based on pulmonary function testing. However, follow-up was only 1 year and a comparison group was not included. More recently, Loehrl et al. published their retrospective review of 31 patients with AERD who had undergone ESS [62]. This retrospective study used a standardized survey and had a mean follow-up of 10 years. Overall, 94% of patients reported long-term postoperative improvement in their asthma symptoms, and 68% reported additional improvement beyond the first postoperative year. Emergency department visits and inpatient hospitalizations decreased for this cohort. The weakness of this study, however, is the lack of a control group and the retrospective design. Nonetheless, these data suggest a potential benefit in asthma outcomes in patients with AERD undergoing ESS for CRS, similar to the data in asthmatics without AERD.

Our knowledge of CRS with and without nasal polyposis, and in particular AERD, has advanced tremendously. Refinement in surgical technique and a deeper understanding of the pathophysiology have moved us beyond the time when polypectomy was believed to exacerbate, or even cause, asthma attacks [63]. The surgical management of nasal polyposis, including patients with AERD, has progressed from withholding operations to studies demonstrating the benefit of surgical management. Published data suggest that surgical intervention may lead to improved outcomes for both sinonasal and asthma symptoms. Patients with AERD and nasal polyposis represent a complex cohort of patients who require multimodality therapy for optimal control of upper and lower airways disease. The benefits of ESS in this patient group appear validated, and thus surgical management must be considered a viable adjunctive option when making management decisions.

Conclusions

We now appreciate some of the complex interactions between the upper and the lower airways. As discussed, the inflammatory processes in CRS, AR, and asthma are linked in a number of ways. As patients often present with more than one of these diseases in concert, a comprehensive, multimodal approach is warranted. One key to controlling the ongoing inflammation is to be mindful of the contribution the upper airway can have to the lower airway, and vice versa.

In the subset of patients with AERD, management is especially challenging. As we learn more, the balance of proinflammatory leukotrienes and antiinflammatory prostaglandins appears to be important in the pathogenesis of the disease. Agents targeted at disruption of the leukotriene pathway seem to be effective in some patients. Aspirin desensitization is a specialized procedure that allows patients with AERD to safely tolerate aspirin and other cross-reacting NSAIDs. The benefits of aspirin therapy include better control of both upper and lower airway diseases, and should be considered as add-on therapy for those patients not controlled with traditional medical management. Equally, ESS should be considered as part of the patient's overall disease management. Once considered controversial or even detrimental, ESS is now thought to contribute to better control of sinonasal and asthma disease. Taken as a whole, a combined medical and surgical approach—with collaboration from family medicine specialists, pulmonary specialists, allergists, internists, and otolaryngologists—should lead to better patient clinical outcomes.

References

1. Stevenson DD, Szczeklik A. Clinical and pathologic perspectives on aspirin sensitivity and asthma. J Allergy Clin Immunol 2006; 118:773–786.
2. National Health Interview Survey, National Center for Health Statistics, Centers for Disease Control and Prevention, 2005. Available at http://www.cdc.gov/asthma/nhis/05/data.htm. Accessed August 1, 2007.
3. Allergies in America: a landmark survey of nasal allergy sufferers. Available at: http://www.myallergiesinamerica.com/. Accessed August 1, 2007.
4. Simons FER. Allergic rhinobronchitis: the asthma-allergic rhinitis link. J Allergy Clin Immunol 1999;104:534–540.
5. Peat JK, Salome CM, Woolcock AJ. Longitudinal changes in atopy during a 4-year period: relation to bronchial hyperresponsiveness and respiratory symptoms in a population sample of Australian schoolchildren. J Allergy Clin Immunol 1989;85:65–74.
6. Settipane RJ, Hagy GW, Settipane GA. Long-term risk factors for developing asthma and allergic rhinitis: a 23 year follow-up study of college students. Allergy Proc 1994;15:21–25.
7. Leynaert B, Bousquet J, Neukirch, et al. Perennial rhinitis: an independent risk factor for asthma in nonatopic subjects. J Allergy Clin Immunol 1999;104:301–304.
8. Fotanari P, Burnet H, Zattara-Hartmann MC, et al. Changes in airway resistance induced by nasal inhalation of cold dry, dry, or moist air in normal individuals. J Appl Physiol 1996;81:1739–1743.

9. Gerblich AA, Schwartz HJ, Chester EH. Seasonal variation of airway function in allergic rhinitis. J Allergy Clin Immunol 1986;77:676–681.

10. Corren J, Adinoff AD, Irvin CG. Changes in bronchial responsiveness following nasal provocation with allergen. J Allergy Clin Immunol 1992;89:611–618.

11. Bardin PG, Van Heerden MMB, Jourbert JR. Absence of pulmonary aspiration of sinus contents in patients with asthma and sinusitis. J Allergy Clin Immunol 1990;86:82–88.

12. Chanez P, Vignola AM, Vic P, et al. Comparison between nasal and bronchial inflammation in asthmatic and control subjects. Am J Respir Crit Care Med 1999;159:588–595.

13. Henriksen JM, Wenzel A. Effect of an intranasally administered corticosteroid (budesonide) on nasal obstruction, mouth breathing, and asthma. Am Rev Respir Dis 1984;130: 1014–1018.

14. Welsh PW, Stricker WE, Chu CP, et al. Efficacy of beclomethasone nasal solution, flunisolide, and cromolyn in relieving symptoms of ragweed allergy. Mayo Clin Proc 1987;62:125–134.

15. Forensi A, Pelucchi A, Gherson G, et al. Once daily intranasal fluticasone proprionate (220 mcg) reduces nasal symptoms and inflammation but also attenuates the increase in bronchial responsiveness during the pollen season in allergic rhinitis. J Allergy Clin Immunol 1996;98:274–282.

16. Watson WTA, Becker A, Simons ER. Treatment of allergic rhinitis with intranasal corticosteroids in patients with mild asthma: effect on lower airway responsiveness. J Allergy Clin Immunol 1993; 91:97–101.

17. Adams RJ, Fuhlbigge A, Finkelstein JA, et al. Intranasal steroids and the risk of emergency department visits for asthma. J Allergy Clin Immunol 2002;109:636–642.

18. Greiff L, Andersson M, Svensson C, et al. Effects of orally inhaled budesonide in seasonal allergic rhinitis. Eur Respir J 1998;11:1268–1273.

19. Moller C, Dreborg S, Ferdousi H, et al. Pollen immunotherapy reduces the development of asthma in children with seasonal rhinoconjunctivitis (the PAT-Study). J Allergy Clin Immunol 2002;109:251–256.

20. Valovirta E, Jacobsen L, Niggemann B, et al. A 3-year course of subcutaneous specific immunotherapy results in long-term prevention of asthma in children. Ten-year follow-up on the PAT-study. J Allergy Clin Immunol 2006;117:721.

21. Samter M, Beers RF. Intolerance to aspirin. Ann Intern Med 1968;68:975–983.

22. Jenkins C, Costello J, Hodge L. Systemic review of prevalence of aspirin-induced asthma and its implications for clinical practice. BMJ 2004;328:434–437.

23. Sanak M, Simon H-U, Szczeklik A. Leukotriene C_4 synthase promoter polymorphism and risk of aspirin-induced asthma. Lancet 1997;350:599–600.

24. Van Sambeek R, Stevenson DD, Baldsaro M, et al. 5'-Flanking region polymorphism of the gene encoding leukotriene C4 synthase does not correlate with the aspirin-intolerant asthma phenotype in the United States. J Allergy Clin Immunol 2000;106:72–76.

25. Drazen JM. Leukotrienes as mediators of airway obstruction. Am J Respir Crit Care Med 1998;158:S193–S200.

26. Sanak M, Kielbasa B, Bochenek G, et al. Exhaled eicosanoids following oral aspirin challenge in asthmatic patients. Clin Exp Allergy 2004;34:1899–1904.

27. Sousa AR, Parikh A, Scadding G, et al. Leukotriene-receptor expression on nasalmucosal inflammatory cells in aspirin-sensitive rhinosinusitis. N Engl J Med 2002;347:1493–1499.

28. Sestini P, Armetti L, Gambaro G, et al. Inhaled PGE_2 prevents aspirin induced bronchoconstriction and urinary LTE_4 excretion in aspirin-sensitive asthma. Am J Respir Crit Care Med 1996;153:572–575.

29. Pujols L, Mullol J, Alobid I, et al. Dynamics of COX-2 in nasal mucosa and nasal polyps from aspirin-tolerant and aspirin-intolerant patients with asthma. J Allergy Clin Immunol 2004;114:814–819.

30. Mullol J, Fernandez-Morata JC, Roca-Ferrer J, et al. Cyclooxygenase 1 and cyclooxygenase 2 expression is abnormally regulated in human nasal polyps. J Allergy Clin Immunol. 2002;109:824–830.

31. Owens J, Shroyer K, Kingdom TT. Expression of cyclooxygenase and lipoxygenase enzymes in nasal polyps of aspirin sensitive and aspirin tolerant patients. Arch Otolaryngol Head Neck Surg 2006;132:579–587.

32. Simon RA. Treatment of patients with respiratory reactions to aspirin and nonsteroidal anti-inflammatory drugs. Curr Allergy Asthma Rep 2004;4:139–143.

33. Settipane RA, Shrank PJ, Simon RA, et al. Prevalence of cross-sensitivity with acetaminophen in aspirin-sensitive asthmatic subjects. J Allergy Clin Immunol 1995;96:480–485.

34. Dahlen B, Nizankowska E, Szczeklik A, et al. Benefits from adding the 5-lipoxygenase Inhibitor zileuton to conventional therapy in aspirin-intolerant asthmatics. Am J Respir Crit Care Med 1998;157:1187–1194.

35. Parnes SM, Chuma AV. Acute effects of antileukotrienes on sinonasal polyposis and sinusitis. Ear Nose Throat J 2000;79:18–20.

36. Ragab S, Parikh A, Darby YC, et al. An open audit of montelukast, a leukotriene receptor antagonist, in nasal polyposis associated with asthma. Clin Exp Allergy 2001;31:1385–1391.

37. Macy E, Berstein JA, Castells MC, et al. Aspirin challenge and desensitization for aspirin-exacerbated respiratory disease: a practice paper. Ann Allergy Asthma Immunol. 2007;98:172–174.

38. Pleskow WW, Stevenson DD, Mathison DA, et al. Aspirin desensitization in aspirin sensitive asthmatic patients: clinical manifestations and characterization of the refractory period. J Allergy Clin Immunol 1982;69:11–19.

39. White A, Stevenson D, Simon R. The blocking effect of essential controller medications during aspirin challenges in patients with aspirin-exacerbated respiratory disease. Ann Allergy Asthma Immunol 2005;95:330–335.

40. Berges-Gimeno MP, Simon RA, Stevenson DD. The effect of leukotriene-modifier drugs on aspirin-induced asthma and rhinitis reactions. Clin Exp Allergy 2002;32:1491–1496.

41. Berges-Gimeno MP, Simon RA, Stevenson DD. Long-term treatment with aspirin desensitization in asthmatic patients with aspirin-exacerbated respiratory disease. J Allergy Clin Immunol 2003;111:180–186.

42. Levine HL. Functional endoscopic sinus surgery: evaluation, surgery, and follow-up of 250 patients. Laryngoscope 1990;100:79–83.

43. Kennedy DW. Prognostic factors, outcomes, and staging in ethmoid sinus surgery. Laryngoscope 1992;102:1–18.

44. Senior BA, Kennedy DW, Tanabodee J, et al. Long-term results of functional endoscopic sinus surgery. Laryngoscope 1998;108:151–157.

45. Metson RB, Gliklich RE. Clinical outcomes in patients with chronic sinusitis. Laryngoscope 2000;110(suppl 94):24–28.

46. Poetker DM, Smith TL. Adult chronic rhinosinusitis: surgical outcomes and the role of endoscopic sinus surgery. Curr Opin Otolaryngol Head Neck Surg 2007;15:6–9.

47. Banerji A, Piccirillo JF, Thawley SE, et al. Chronic rhinosinusitis patients with polyps or polypoid mucosa have a greater burden of illness. Am J Rhinol 2007;21:19–26.

48. Smith TL, Mendolia-Loffredo S, Loehrl TA, et al. Predictive factors and outcomes in endoscopic sinus surgery for chronic rhinosinusitis. Laryngoscope 2005;115:2199–2205.

49. Ragab SM, Lund VJ, Scadding G. Evaluation of the medical and surgical treatment of chronic rhinosinusitis: a prospective, randomized, controlled trial. Laryngoscope 2004;114:923–930.

50. Poetker DM, Mendolia-Loffredo S, Smith TL. Outcomes of endoscopic sinus surgery for chronic rhinosinusitis associated with sinonasal polyposis. Am J Rhinol 2007;21:84–88.

51. Nishioka GJ, Cook PR, Davis WE, et al. Functional endoscopic sinus surgery in patients with chronic sinusitis and asthma. Otolaryngol Head Neck Surg 1994;110:494–500.

52. Palmer JN, Conley DB, Dong RG, et al. Efficacy of endoscopic sinus surgery in the management of patients with asthma and chronic sinusitis. Am J Rhinol 2001;15:49–53.

53. Senior BA, Kennedy DW, Tanabodee J, et al. Long-term impact of functional endoscopic sinus surgery on asthma. Otolaryngol Head Neck Surg 1999;121:66–68.

54. Dhong HJ, Jung YS, Chung SK, et al. Effect of endoscopic sinus surgery on asthmatic patients with chronic rhinosinusitis. Otolaryngol Head Neck Surg 2001;124:99–104.
55. Goldstein MF, Grundfast SK, Dunsky EH, et al. Effect of functional endoscopic sinus surgery on bronchial asthma outcomes. Arch Otolaryngol Head Neck Surg 1999;125:314–319.
56. Ragab S, Scadding GK, Lund VJ, et al. Treatment of chronic rhinosinusitis and its effects on asthma. Eur Respir J 2006;28:68–74.
57. Nakamura H, Kawasaki M, Higuchi Y, et al. Effects of sinus surgery on asthma in aspirin triad patients. Acta Otolaryngol (Stockh) 1999;119:592–598.
58. McFadden EA, Woodson BT, Fink JN, et al. Surgical management of aspirin triad sinusitis. Am J Rhinol 1997;11:263–270.
59. Amar YG, Frenkiel S, Sobol SE. Outcome analysis of ESS for chronic sinusitis in patients having Samter's triad. J Otolaryngol 2000;29:7–12.
60. Batra PS, Kern RC, Tripathi A, et al. Outcome analysis of ESS in patients with nasal polyps and asthma. Laryngoscope 2003;113:1703–1706.
61. Robinson JL, Griest S, James KE, et al. Impact of aspirin intolerance on outcomes of sinus surgery. Laryngoscope 2007;117:825–830.
62. Loehrl TA, Ferre RM, Toohill RJ, et al. Long-term asthma outcomes after endoscopic sinus surgery in aspirin triad patients. Am J Otolaryngol Head Neck Med Surg 2006;27:154–160.
63. Francis C. The prognosis of operations of nasal polypi in cases of asthma. Practitioner 1928;123:272–278.

Chapter 13
Pediatric Perspectives of Rhinosinusitis

Lisa Elden and Lawrence W.C. Tom

Embryology And Anatomic Considerations

The paranasal sinuses begin to develop during the third week of gestation and continue to grow throughout early childhood and adolescence (Fig. 13.1). Two mesenchymal grooves develop along the lateral wall of the nasal cavity that become the inferior turbinate, the middle meatus, and the inferior meatus. The ethmoido-turbinate mesenchymal folds develop superiorly to give rise to the middle and superior turbinates. Once the turbinates are established, the sinuses begin to develop. During the third month of gestation, the maxillary sinus arises as an ectodermal outpocket from within the region of the middle meatal groove developing laterally. At birth, the cavity of the maxillary sinus is relatively small, with dimensions 7 × 4 × 4 mm. The sinus cavity continues to grow inferiorly and posteriorly and does not become level with the floor of the nose until age 12 years after the adult teeth have erupted [1]. As a result, the tooth buds are at increased risk during certain surgical procedures in young children. The anterior ethmoid sinus is also present at birth and is composed of small air cells that multiply as the child grows. The sphenoid and the frontal sinuses become apparent between the ages of 3 and 7 and between 6 and 13 years of age, respectively. Both these sinuses continue to grow into adulthood. Clinically, complications related to sinusitis tend to occur when sinuses are undergoing increased phases of growth. Younger children with sinusitis (ages 2–5 years) are more likely to develop complications related to the spread of disease from the ethmoid to the adjacent orbit through the thin bony partition (lamina papyrcea), resulting in orbital complications. Alternatively, older children (especially adolescents) are more likely to have intracranial complications when infection spreads from their developing frontal sinuses (and less commonly from their sphenoid sinuses) to the brain and surrounding tissues.

L. Elden
Department of Otorhinolaryngology, Head and Neck Surgery, University of Pennsylvania School of Medicine,The Children's Hospital of Philadelphia, Philadelphia, PA, USA
e-mail: elden@email.chop.edu

E.R. Thaler, D.W. Kennedy (eds.), *Rhinosinusitis*, DOI: 10.1007/978-0-387-73062-2_13,
© Springer Science+Business Media, LLC 2008

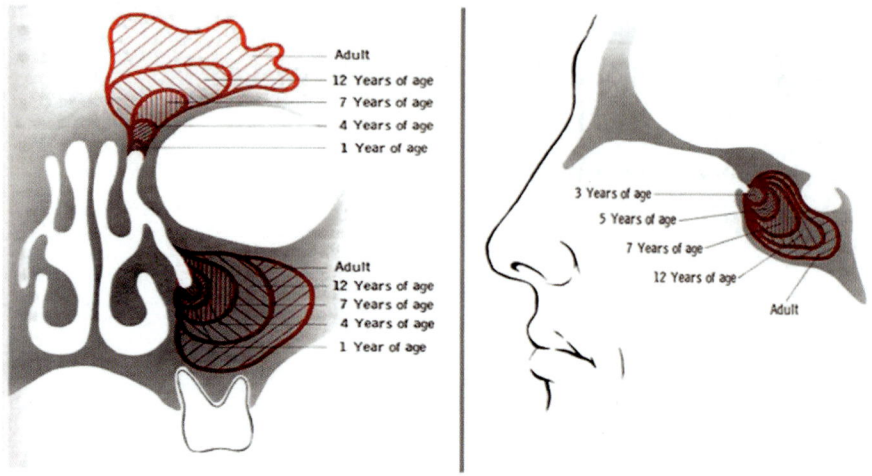

Fig. 13.1 Development of sinuses throughout childhood. (Reproduced from Naumann HH. Surgery of the paranasal sinuses. In: Naumann HH, ed. Head and Neck Surgery, vol. 1. Philadelphia: Saunders, 1980, pp 390–391, with permission.)

Physiology

Of the four pairs of paranasal sinuses (the maxillary, ethmoid, frontal, and sphenoid sinuses), all drain into the middle meatus via the infundibulum, except the posterior ethmoid and sphenoid, which drain into the superior meatus (Fig. 13.2). Anatomically, the infundibulum, the anterior ethmoid air cells, and uncinate comprise the ostiomeatal complex. The cilia in the columnar lining of the normally sterile sinuses carry the blanket of mucus toward the sinus ostia and function to keep the sinus free

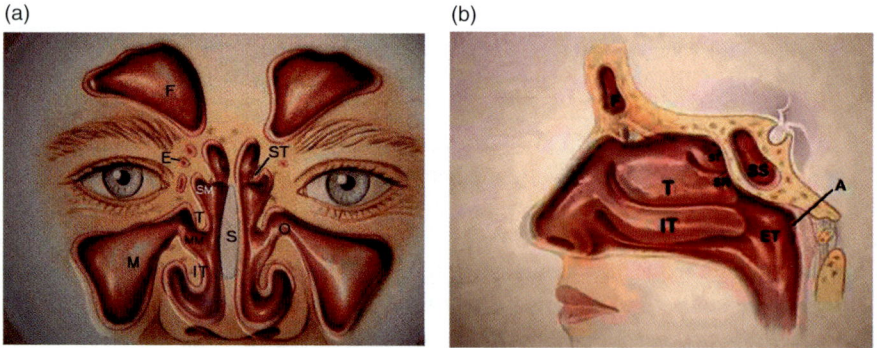

Fig. 13.2 Anatomy of sinuses. (**a**) *F*, frontal sinuses; *E*, ethmoid sinuses; *M*, maxillary sinuses; *O*, maxillary sinus ostium; *ST*, superior turbinate; *T*, middle turbinate; *IT*, inferior turbinate; *SM*, superior meatus; *MM*, middle meatus; *S*, septum. (**b**) *SS*, sphenoid sinus; *SR*, sphenoethmoidal recess; *ET*, eustachian tube orifice; *A*, adenoids. (Reproduced with kind permission of Astra Pharmaceuticals. Images courtesy of sinuses.com © 1997–2007 by Wellington S. Tichenor, M.D.)

of bacteria and debris. When there is a functional or mechanical obstruction of the ostia, negative pressure develops, oxygen is absorbed, and colonizing nasopharyngeal and nasal bacteria are aspirated into the sinus. When the volume of bacteria reaches a critical number, the sinus becomes inflamed and then infected. The most common causes of mucosal edema that result in sinusitis in children are upper respiratory tract infections (URTIs) (80%) and allergies (10%–20%). Anatomic anomalies that also can obstruct drainage pathways are similar to those anomalies found in adults, including Haller cells (ethmoid air cells located on the inferior orbital walls), concha bullosa (pneumatized middle concha within the middle turbinate), septal deviation, turbinate hypertrophy, and uncinate anomalies [2].

Definitions

Rhinosinusitis (RS) is defined as symptomatic inflammation of the paranasal sinuses and nasal cavity by bacteria or viruses. Bacterial RS is classified into categories by duration: acute RS (ARS) lasts 10 days to 3 weeks, subacute RS lasts 3 weeks to 3 months, and chronic RS (CRS) lasts more than 3 months. Recurrent RS is defined as four or more episodes in 1 year, each episode lasting longer than 7 days with complete clearance between episodes [3] Children with chronic or recurrent disease can usually be treated with antibiotic or allergy therapies to reduce the edema that leads to functional obstruction; however, sinus surgery is necessary in some cases to correct obstructing anomalies or enlarge natural sinus drainage pathways to prevent ongoing disease. Unlike children with normal mucociliary blankets, children with congenital cilia anomalies (ciliary dyskinesia or cystic fibrosis) are less likely to benefit from surgical procedures that widen natural openings and, instead, need procedures that promote gravity-dependent drainage of the sinus contents into the nasal cavity and provide larger sinus openings for mechanical irrigation.

Prevalence

Most infections that cause nasal discharge are viral and involve the respiratory epithelium of the nose and sinuses. In contrast to adults, who develop viral upper respiratory tract infections (URTIs) two to three times per year, children typically develop three to eight viral URTIs per year [4]. Of those with viral rhinosinusitis, only 0.5% to 13% of patients develop bacterial rhinosinusitis, but up to 80% of children with bacterial sinusitis will have had a preceding viral infection [5–7]. Among all age groups, bacterial sinusitis remains the fifth most common reason that antibiotics are prescribed in the United States [7]. The majority of these patients are children, because the peak incidence of both viral and bacterial sinusitis occurs between the ages of 2 and 6 years. Younger children are at greater risk of being chronically colonized with pathogenic and resistant bacteria that can lead to sinusitis, partly because they are exposed to bacteria from other children in daycare or school situations and also because adenoid tissue is more prominent at younger ages.

Children with recurrent and chronic sinusitis have been found to have more pathogenic bacteria in their adenoid pad [8].

Differential Diagnosis of Rhinosinusitis

Approximately 10% to 20% of children have allergic rhinitis that may mimic the symptoms or predispose children to bacterial ARS. Dust mite and mold allergies are common and can result in yearlong symptoms; but many children with allergies have more seasonal variations in their symptoms. Nonspecific nasal congestion is a frequent symptom in children who have allergies, but the presence of sneezing and itchy eyes may help to differentiate allergy from bacterial ARS. Adenoid hypertrophy and recurrent adenoiditis are most common from 3 to 6 years of age and can also cause symptoms similar to those seen with ARS. Foreign bodies are another cause of nasal discharge, which is usually unilateral in nature, causing foul-smelling discharge that resolves when the foreign body is removed. Unilateral choanal atresia or stenosis can also cause chronic mucopurulent discharge that may not be detected until early school age. Children with bilateral choanal atresia usually present at birth with breathing difficulties and have had surgical repair before sinus symptoms become evident. In adolescents, tumors such as nasopharyngeal carcinoma and, less often, angiofibromas should be considered, especially when unilateral nasal signs and symptoms fail to respond to antibiotics (Table 13.1).

Risks of ARS and CRS

Bacterial RS in children usually follows recent viral URTIs, or allergies, or is exacerbated by adenoid hypertrophy. Less common causes include anatomic anomalies

Table 13.1 Differential diagnosis: common conditions that mimic rhinosinusitis (RS) in children

Diagnosis	Differentiating Factors
ALLERGIC RHINITIS	Itchy, red eyes Seasonal variation
ADENOID HYPERTROPHY	Persistent snoring with or without apnea Peak age 3–7 years
FOREIGN BODY IN NOSE	Younger children or developmentally delayed Unilateral foul-smelling discharge
CHOANAL ATRESIA/STENOSIS	Unilateral: • Chronic discharge varying from mucus to purulent material • Inability to breathe through affected nostril Bilateral: • Chronic bilateral discharge • Often presents during infancy with periodic oxygen desaturation and failure to thrive

(see above) and certain environmental factors, such as increased exposure to other children in daycare settings and chronic nasal inflammation caused by secondhand smoke. Swimming can cause inflammation from chronic chlorine exposure, which predisposes the child to bacterial RS, whereas diving (from a board or SCUBA diving) more often results in acute inflammation and trauma that especially impacts the frontal sinuses. Dental infections are rare causes of sinusitis in children as compared to adults. Children with anatomic nasal or midface anomalies—such as Crouzon's syndrome, Apert's syndrome, or Treacher Collins' syndrome—are at risk for RS.

More unusual causes of sinusitis occur in children who have been intubated with nasotracheal or nasogastric tubes (18%–32% of these children develop RS) [9]. Chronically ill children at risk are those who have underlying immunodeficiencies, including transient or congenital antibody deficiencies, human immunodeficiency virus (HIV), or complement disorders. Finally, gastroesophageal reflux disease (GERD) is more prevalent in children with CRS and has been shown to contribute to the development of sinusitis in some children. Polyps are rarely found in children and, if present, require genetic screening and diagnostic testing for cystic fibrosis (CF). Most children with CF who have homozygous recessive genotypes eventually develop signs of CRS, but they tend to be less symptomatic than healthy children with chronic RS. Only 10% of CF children have polyps compared with 50% in adults or teenagers [10]. Genetic testing for CF is recommended in otherwise healthy children with CRS because a significant number are heterozygous for 1 of the 16 mutations that account for 85% of CF alleles in the general population (7% with CF mutation with CRS versus 2% with CF mutation in asymptomatic patients) [10]. Many authors believe that these children have a more mild variation of CF.

Diagnostic Tests

Diagnosis Bacterial ARS

The diagnosis of bacterial ARS is usually made clinically. However, it is difficult to differentiate viral from bacterial RS because the symptoms are similar. Patients with viral RS follow a fairly predictable course, starting with several days of clear nasal discharge, followed by symptoms of sneezing and congestion that usually are accompanied by low-grade fever, facial fullness, and later cough and sore throat. The nasal discharge usually changes from mucoid to purulent after several days, and then the patient improves clinically as the viral infection spontaneously resolves within 5 to 7 days [11]. The presence of purulent discharge is not strongly predictive of a bacterial infection unless it can be localized to the middle meatus. The discharge usually results from breakdown products derived from nasal mucous glands and neutrophils, and less from the presence of bacteria and their by-products. Several groups have described guidelines to help clinicians identify symptoms more likely to predict presence of ARS: [12] these include the presence of purulent discharge from the *os* or nasopharynx, nasal obstruction, and facial pain or pressure of the face, periorbita, or head. However, these diagnostic predictors are less helpful in the management of pediatric ARS because children have difficulty describing specific symptoms that localize pain to the sinuses, especially when the pain is unilateral or when it is referred to the teeth or cheek. Children are more likely to present with nonspecific symptoms and signs including cough, halitosis, low-grade fever, and purulent rhinorrhea (Table 13.2). In adults or children, the most important factor that is used to differentiate viral from bacterial disease is the duration of symptoms (minimum, 7–10 days) or the presence of worsening symptoms after 5 days [1,12]. Unusually severe symptoms or signs of extranasal symptoms, including facial or eye swelling, are more suggestive of aggressive bacterial infection or complications that should be addressed promptly. In contrast to adults, children are also more likely to develop secondary infections that may cause the clinician to overlook ARS, including otitis media, asthma exacerbations, or bronchitis.

Clinical Examination

Although palpation of the cheek over the sinus may be helpful in identifying sinus related pain in adults, young children rarely cooperate enough for this sign to be helpful. Instead, direct examination with an otoscope (or nasal speculum in an older child) is more likely to reveal signs such as swelling and inflammation or abundant purulent material localized to the region of the middle meatus. Examination of the oropharynx may also reveal purulent discharge from the nose or adenoid. Routine cultures obtained from the nose or nasopharynx do not correlate with those from maxillary sinus aspirates. Directed middle meatal cultures are more accurate, but play a limited role in children because it is difficult to obtain a noncontaminated specimen. These cultures should be considered in sedated or anesthetized children in the intensive care setting or for those who are undergoing surgery for other procedures such as adenoidectomy.

Imaging Studies

Radiographic imaging studies used to diagnose sinusitis include plain sinus films, lateral neck films, coronal computed tomography (CT), and magnetic resonance sinus imaging (MRI) (Table 13.3). Of these studies, lateral neck films are the

Table 13.2 Most common features of pediatric acute rhinosinusitis

SYMPTOMS AND SIGNS	Cough, halitosis, low-grade fever, purulent rhinorrhea
DURATION	Acute rhinosinusitis (ARS) more likely when signs/symptoms present more than 7–10 days or worsen after 5 days
CLINICAL SIGNS	Otoscopic or nasal speculum most helpful to identify purulent material within the middle meatus/nasopharynx

Table 13.3 Considerations regarding the use of radiographic imaging studies for RS in children

Suspected Acute RS	
LATERAL NECK PLAIN FILM	Identifies adenoid disease as coexisting or primary etiology Inexpensive
PLAIN SINUS FILMS	Less accurate than in adults (smaller cavities), rarely used in practice
COMPUTED TOMOGRAPHY (CT) OF SINUSES	Most accurate, but expensive Higher dose of radiation concerning False-positive rate high unless following: • Mucosal thickening greater than 4 mm • Air-fluid level present • Complete opacification of a sinus cavity Consider if: • Concerns about anatomic anomaly • Concerns about tumor/polyps • Complications suspected • Need to rule out uncertain disease

least expensive and often help to identify adenoid hypertrophy, which can result in symptoms that mimic RS. The American Academy of Pediatrics (2001) guideline recommends that sinus radiographs (plain or CT) not be used as a routine clinical adjunct to diagnose ARS in children 6 years of age or younger, because clinical history predicts outcome of imaging studies with 88% accuracy in that age group [7,13]. However, they may be considered in older children (over 6 years of age) because the accuracy is closer to 70% in this group. Sinus CTs may also help to distinguish bacterial ARS from other nonbacterial upper respiratory infections, but false-positive rates are high when relying on information from CT alone. Specifically, Gwaltney et al demonstrated that up to 77% of patients with symptoms of the common cold (and no evidence of acute bacterial RS) had occlusion of the ethmoid infundibulum and 87% had abnormalities of the maxillary sinus that usually cleared within 2 weeks without antibiotics [14]. These sites are also the more commonly affected by bacterial infections, so unless specific findings are present—including complete opacification of a sinus, air-fluid levels within the sinus, or mucosal thickening greater than 4 mm—then CT is less helpful in directing the physician as to who may need antibiotics [5,15,16]

Sinus CT should be obtained when the child is severely ill or when complications of disease are suspected. It is important to order both coronal and axial views of the sinuses and surrounding tissues (with contrast) to assess the sinuses, brain, and orbit. Sinus and brain MRI is more helpful in determining the extent and the nature of extranasal complications when disease spreads from the sinuses to the brain. However, they are less helpful than CT in demonstrating bone defects, and they exaggerate mild mucosal thickening.

Diagnosis of Chronic/Recurrent RS

In contrast to children with ARS, sinus CT is more useful in patients with uncertain diagnoses to rule out chronic diseases. It is also helpful in children with histories of chronic sinusitis to determine effectiveness of treatment (usually following a 3- to 6-week course of topical nasal steroids and antibiotics) and to identify the presence of anatomic anomalies, polyps, or tumors that can be contributing to sinus disease. CT will define the anatomy if endoscopic sinus surgery is to be performed.

Microbiology

In children, the normal bacteria that colonize the nose and nasopharynx are most commonly responsible for infection of the sinuses. The bacteria are the same responsible as those for otitis media and bronchitis in children: they include *Streptococcus pneumoniae* (30%–60% of clinical isolates), nontypable *Haemophilus influenzae* (20%–30%), and *Moraxella catarrhalis* (12%–20%) [3,6,17]. Heptavalent pneumococcal conjugate vaccine (PCV 7) has been effective in lowering the rate of *S. pneumoniae* infections in some regions, but this bacterium continues to be the most clinically significant. It is more likely to cause severe infections and is less likely to clear spontaneously compared with *H. influenzae* and *M. catarrhalis*. Resistance patterns vary widely across the nation. Overall, approximately 15% of *S. pneumoniae* strains are intermediately penicillin resistant and 25% are highly penicillin resistant. Fewer strains are resistant to multiple drugs [18]. In contrast to *S. pneumoniae*, the *H. influenzae* vaccine has greatly reduced the rate of infection of invasive *Haemophilus influenzae* B, which is more likely to result in meningitis or bacteremias, but has not changed the rate of infections from nontypable *H. influenzae* that is responsible for infections affecting the sinuses, ear, and upper bronchi. In some regions, infections from nontypable *H. influenzae* have become more common than those from *S. pneumoniae*. Rates of resistance among *H. influenza* and *M. catarrhalis* also vary regionally, with up to 30% to 40% of *Haemophilus* and nearly 100% of *Moraxella* producing beta-lactamase enzymes, but many of these infections clear spontaneously [6,7].

Pathogens resistant to first-line antibiotics are more likely to colonize the nose and nasopharynx during the winter and during periods of viral URI, especially in children who are in daycare settings [12]. In contrast to adults, 16% of children with bacterial ARS have been found to have concurrent streptococcus pyogenes group A pharyngeal infections, and this pathogen accounts for up to 3% to 7% of pediatric sinusitis [6,7,19]. Other less common pathogens responsible for acute bacterial RS include other aerobic streptococcus species, *Staphylococcus aureus*, and mixed gram-negative and gram-positive bacteria.

The same bacteria responsible for ARS usually cause chronic infections in children (*Streptococcus pneumoniae*, *H. influenzae*, and *M. catarrhalis*). However, CRS can also be caused by anaerobic bacteria (peptostreptococcus species, prevotella species, and fusobacterium species), mixed gram-negative bacteria (including

Klebsiella pneumoniae, *Escherichia coli*, and *Pseudomonas aeruginosa*), and gram-positive bacteria (*Staphylococcus aureus* that may be methicillin resistant).

In children with CF, common bacteria (*S. pneumoniae*, *H. influenzae*, and *M. catarrhalis*), streptococcus group A, and anaerobes more likely cause ARS/CRS, but cultures should be considered in those patients with recalcitrant disease to identify less common organisms such as *Pseudomonas* [20,21].

Rationale for Treatment of ARS

Similar to children with otitis media, there is debate as to whether children with acute bacterial RS should be treated with antibiotics because the infection clears spontaneously in 40% to 67% of children [3,6,18,22]. Therapy is empiric in most cases because cultures are not easily obtained. A meta-analysis of six randomized trials in the Cochrane database, comparing placebo or decongestant treatment with antibiotics in children with nasal discharge lasting longer than 10 days and radiographic evidence of rhinosinusitis, revealed only moderate benefits in those treated with antibiotics. In this study, the number of children needed to treat before one child benefited from antibiotics compared with observation was one in eight children; however, the risks of side effects from antibiotics (mostly diarrhea and rashes) were relatively low (1 in 30 episodes) [11,18,23]. Effective antibiotic therapy does appear to reduce time with symptoms. Despite the modest treatment benefit, very few (19%–40%) clinicians surveyed in various studies withhold antibiotic treatment, even in infants with only scant nasal discharge [1,24]. Studies have not been done to determine if treatment reduces the likelihood of developing chronic sinusitis or other secondary infections, especially acute otitis media (AOM).

Treatment Strategies

Antibiotic Therapy for ARS/Recurrent ARS

Two separate guidelines have been published that propose similar treatment regimens for children with ARS [5,7,13]. Both groups stress the need to treat *S. pneumoniae* as a primary goal and the need to monitor therapy, as there is an expected failure rate of treatment that may reach 10% to 20% when first-line therapy is used. In most cases of mild to moderate disease, less expensive first-line agents—such as amoxicillin in higher doses (80–90 mg/kg per day) in non-penicillin-allergic patients, or TMP-SMX or macrolide antibiotics in children with type 1 hypersensitivity allergy to penicillins—are as clinically effective and cost effective as the more expensive cephalosporins. Children younger than 2 years of age with mild disease who have not been recently treated with antibiotics or who do not attend daycare may be treated with the usual dosage of amoxicillin, as there is less likelihood that resistant strains of *S. pneumoniae* are present [3,6,7]. Higher dosages of amoxicillin appear to be fully adequate in eradicating intermediate and fully resistant *S. pneumoniae*, but do not cover multidrug-resistant strains. In children who fail to respond to initial therapy designed to address *S. pneumoniae,* or for those in daycare or who live in regions where beta-lactamase-producing *H. influenzae* or *M. catarrhalis* are prevalent, second- and third-generation cephalosporins or amoxicillin/clavulinate with higher doses of amoxicillin are more likely to be effective therapies. The amoxicillin/clavulinate can be used in special preparations to raise the dose of amoxicillin (80–90 mg per kg per day) but keep the dose of clavulinate at standard levels (6.4 mg per kg per day) to avoid gastrointestinal irritation as can occur with high levels of clavulinate. Specific second- and third-generation cephalosporin antibiotics should be reserved to treat sicker children or those with chronic disease. These drugs are more likely to have excellent activity against all the major pathogens with better coverage against beta-lactamase-producing bacteria, including cefpodoxime proxetil (10 mg/kg/day daily), cefprozil (30 mg/kg/day in two divided doses), cefuroxime axetil (30 mg/kg/day in two divided doses) [3], and cefdinir (14 mg/day daily) [3,6,17]. More specific recommendations may be found in Table 13.4 based on the Sinus and Allergy Health Partnership guideline recommendations for initial antibiotic therapy that categorizes treatment options based on severity of disease: mild disease (with and without a history of use of antibiotics in

Table 13.4 Orbital complications of rhinosinusitis

Stage	Complication	Clinical Signs	Management Options
Stage 1	Preseptal cellulitis	• Eyelid swelling, erythema, normal extraocular mobility, normal vision	• IV antibiotics
Stage 2	Orbital cellulitis	• Edema extends into orbit	• IV antibiotics
Stage 3	Subperiosteal abscess	• Subperiosteal purulent collection usually within medial aspect of orbit • Restricted extraocular mobility • Vision usually normal	• IV antibiotics • With or without surgical drainage of sinus and orbit (endoscopic or open approach)
Stage 4	Orbital abscess	• Purulent collection within orbit • Restricted extraocular mobility, proptosis, chemosis, decreased vision	• IV antibiotics • Surgical drainage of orbit (ophthalmology) and sinuses (ENT)
Stage 5	Cavernous sinus thrombosis	• Similar to orbital abscess except findings usually bilateral • Meningeal irritation frequently seen	• IV antibiotics • Surgical drainage of sinuses (ENT) and brain (neurosurgery)

the previous 4–6 weeks) or moderate disease (regardless of use of recent antibiotics) and allergy to antibiotics (type 1 and non-type 1 hypersensitivity) (see Table 13.4). The guidelines do not address severe disease or those with complications. Most children improve after several days of starting antibiotics, but a full 10- to 14-day course is recommended to eradicate disease.

Antibiotics for CRS/Treatment Failure

Treatment failures usually occur because resistant, but common organisms are present, and less commonly occur because unusual organisms are present. Cultures are helpful in identifying appropriate antibiotic therapy. As stated previously, second- and third-generation antibiotics are good choices when beta-lactamase-producing organisms are present. Clindamycin is most effective for highly penicillin-resistant *S. pneumoniae*, but does not adequately cover *H. influenzae* or *M. catarrhalis*. Clindamycin is also more helpful in treating chronic sinusitis caused by *S. aureus* and anaerobes [25].

Fluoroquinolones including levofloxacin, moxifloxacin, and gatifloxacin are some of the most effective oral therapies to cover resistant *S. pneumoniae* and beta-lactamase-producing organisms, but are not indicated in children younger than 18 years of age because of potential effects on bone growth. In children, these fluoroquinolone agents should be reserved for those with moderate to severe infections or for those with CF who are more likely to have bacterial infections caused by unusual organisms, such as *Pseudomonas*, to reduce the chance of promoting resistance. Duration of therapy is 3 to 4 weeks for those children with CRS.

Supplemental medications that have been used to help clear secretions and reduce edema have not been shown to decrease the duration of disease, but may help control symptoms of congestion; these include nasal saline, nasal steroids, and short courses of topical decongestant (phenylephrine hydrochloride or oxymetazoline hydrochloride) that stimulate alpha-adrenergic receptors. The decongestants should be used for a maximum of 3 to 5 days to reduce the likelihood of rebound symptoms. The use of systemic decongestants is not recommended in children because they increase the risk of irritability and hyperactivity. Antihistamines may help in children with allergies, but are not recommended for relief of symptoms in children with ARS who are not atopic because they increase viscosity of mucus and decrease likelihood of drainage. Older corticosteroid nasal preparations including dexamethasone and betamethasone are not recommended for use in children, but newer agents such as beclomethasone dipropionate, triamcinolone acetonide, flunisolide, budesonide, fluticasone propinonate, and mometasone furoate have fewer side effects. Specifically, systemic effects that can suppress growth or affect the hypothalamic-pituitary-adrenal axis are much less likely to occur with the newer agents, unless used concurrently with other steroids such as pulmonary steroids [26]. Although the nasal steroids were initially designed to treat allergic rhinitis, they have also been found to be effective when used in the acute setting of RS to treat sneezing, rhinorrhea, itching, and congestion. Symptomatic relief of symptoms can be seen within 7 to 8 h after starting the nasal steroids, but efficacy may not be maximal until 2 weeks later.

Surgical Therapy

When ARS becomes recurrent or chronic (failing to respond to first-line medical management, including allergy control and oral antibiotics), adenoidectomy should be considered regardless of the size of the pad because it can serve as a reservoir for pathogenic bacteria. If purulent discharge is present in the middle meatus, cultures should be obtained at the same time to determine if unusually resistant bacteria are present. Using this protocol, one study demonstrated that 90% of children had complete resolution of symptoms and only 10% needed functional endoscopic sinus surgery (FESS) [27]. FESS should be reserved as the last step in management of recurrent or chronic RS, unless tumor or complications of RS are present. The goal of FESS is to relieve obstruction of the ostiomeatal complex (OMC); and FESS has been shown to restore the normal mucociliary blanket that may have become dysfunctional from chronic infection. Children are less likely than adults to have sphenoid or frontal sinus disease and usually improve with limited FESS procedures that address the OMC only. In contrast to most adults, young children may not tolerate postoperative debridement that is important for maximal benefit of the original procedure, so a second staged procedure to debride inflammatory tissue is sometimes needed. Debate exists as to whether performing FESS early in life can modify the growth of the facial skeleton. Piglets that had unilateral FESS at young ages have been shown to have 60% reduction in growth of the ethmoid and maxillary sinuses on the operated side compared with that on the nonoperated side when reevaluated at adult ages [28]. However, cephalometric measurements of the facial and nasal skeleton of adult patients with CF who had sinus procedures at young ages did not vary from those who had surgery later in life or from those who never had the procedures [29].

Special Considerations in Managing RS in Children

Before considering surgery in children with recurrent or chronic sinusitis, a complete evaluation should be done to identify predisposing risks or conditions that may be responsible for the disease. This evaluation should include CF testing (including sweat tests to identify patients with the disease and genetic screening to identify carriers of the heterozygous gene that appears to predispose children to chronic sinusitis). Furthermore, children should undergo allergy testing. Basic immune function testing may be helpful in instances when multiple coexisting infections are frequently present, such as bronchitis and otitis media. The more common immune defects include immunoglobulin subclass deficiencies (especially IgA deficiency) or lack of immune response to previously administered PCV 7 or *H. influenzae* type B vaccines that can be corrected with supplemental boosters. The workup should include quantitative immunoglobulin studies (IgG, IgA, IgM, IgE, and IgG subclasses) and functional antibody assays before and after immunization, including those to pneumonia, tetanus, and diphtheria. Other less common immune causes that can be congenital or acquired include hypo- or agammaglobulinemia and HIV. Serum complement studies should be considered in chronically ill patients. Less often, gastroesophageal reflux disease (GERD) should be considered as a cause of chronic nasal inflammation, especially in children with histories of stomach discomfort and chronic throat clearing. The most sensitive test to identify acid reflux is a 24-h pH probe. Ciliary dyskinesia is more likely to be present in patients who also have recurrent otitis media and bronchitis. Cilia anomalies can be confirmed by in vivo testing with saccharin clearance testing, in vitro with ciliary beat frequency, and by testing ultrastructure by electron microscopy [30].

Although fungal infections are rare in children, they should be considered in cases of refractory disease failing to respond to medical and surgical therapy, and strongly considered in children with poor cellular immunity, which includes children with immune disorders including HIV, complement disorders, or those who are neutropenic from chemotherapy. The most common invasive fungal infections include mucomycosis and *Aspergillus*, which usually occur in children with impaired immune systems (see Chapter 14). More benign fungal infections include mycetoma or fungal balls, but these rarely occur in children. These allergic responses to fungus and mucin are treated with topical or systemic steroids and by surgically debulking the debris within the sinus, allowing for improved aeration.

Complications

Children who develop worsening symptoms while on medication or who have extranasal signs and symptoms should be evaluated for complications of sinusitis that can be local, but usually extend to involve the orbit or brain (including meningitis and subdural, epidural, or intraparenchymal abscesses).

Local Complications

The most common local complications include mucoceles and soft tissue facial infections. Mucoceles rarely obstruct the normal drainage pathways and are usually followed conservatively. Local soft tissue infections can involve the region near the forehead or periorbital region. These infections usually resolve with appropriate antibiotic therapy, but must be monitored closely as they could be related to underlying more severe infections including "Pott's puffy tumor" of the forehead or periorbital cellulitis. Pott's puffy tumor is a subperiosteal abscess of the frontal bone that occurs when the bone develops osteomyelitis following frontal sinusitis. Surgical drainage of the abscess and frontal sinus is usually necessary.

Systemic Complications

In children, orbital complications (OC) are the most common systemic complications and have been classified into five stages by Chandler based on grades of severity that help to guide treatment protocols (see Table 13.4). OC are more common in younger children (especially toddlers), who are more likely to develop ethmoid disease that breaks through the lamina papyracea either by direct spread or via hematogenous spread through veins. A child with fever and eyelid erythema or edema should be evaluated for possibility of OC (see Table 13.4). The clinical evaluation should include ophthalmologic consultation if proptosis, restriction of mobility, or vision changes are found or suspected. In most instances, diagnosis can be confirmed with CT of sinuses with contrast. If the infection is confined to the preseptal region or only cellulitis is found within the orbit, then the child may be treated with topical decongestants and IV antibiotics (either broad-spectrum third-generation cephalosporins or Unasyn to cover both *S. pneumoniae* and invasive *H. influenzae*) (Fig. 13.3). Although some controversy exists, many children have been safely treated with a trial of medical therapy for subperiosteal abscess (Chandler class 3) before considering surgical drainage (Fig. 13.4) [1,31,32]. Medical management alone should only be considered if there is no significant restriction in gaze and vision is normal. If the child's condition does not improve or worsens within 24 to 48 h of starting treatment, then the child should undergo surgical drainage. Antibiotic therapy should be chosen to address the more common bacteria, but if surgery is required, then cultures should be obtained to identify more unusual organisms. More recent studies have demonstrated that these abscesses can be safely drained endoscopically (intranasal ethmoidectomy with direct drainage through the lamina papyracea) instead of by the traditional external ethmoidectomy approach using a facial incision (Lynch approach) near the medial orbit [33]. Orbital abscesses require

(a)   (b)

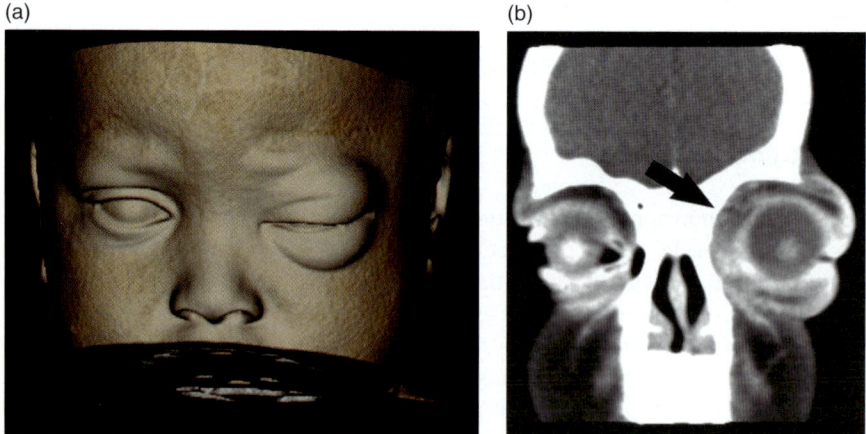

Fig. 13.3 (**a**) Reconstructed image of left (L) medial periorbital cellulitis. (**b**) Axial computed tomography (CT) of left (L) medial periorbital abscess (*arrow*)

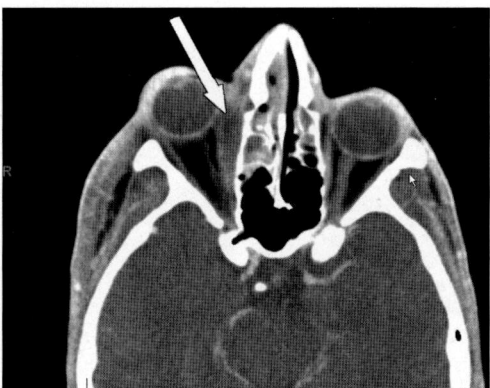

Fig. 13.4 Axial CT of right (R) medial periorbital abscess (*arrow*) and partial opacification of ethmoids bilaterally

joint surgery by otolaryngology to drain the sinus and ophthalmology to drain and monitor the orbit. Cavernous sinus thrombosis caused by sinusitis results in septic thrombosis of the cavernous sinus that can result in blindness, intracranial abscess, or death. In addition to broad-spectrum antibiotics, joint neurosurgical and sinus drainage procedures are needed to drain the infection and control the spread of the disease.

Less common periorbital abscesses have been described that occur in the superior orbit arising from frontal sinusitis, requiring drainage through extended Lynch incisions. It is also possible to have infections/abscesses based laterally in the orbit, but these usually arise from an infected lacrimal gland and are usually caused by *S. aureus*, and, less often, *S. pneumoniae*.

In contrast to OC, intracranial complications are more common in adolescents and usually arise (Fig. 13.5) from infections of the frontal sinus or from the sphenoid sinus. The risk of intracranial complications from acute sinusitis is 3% in children, similar to the 3.7% seen in adults [34]. The majority (67%) of patients with intracranial abscesses (and 5% of children with community-acquired bacterial meningitis) have had preceding frontal or sphenoid sinusitis [35]. Subdural abscesses are more common than epidural or intraparenchymal infections.

Children with intracranial complications have more subtle symptoms than those with periorbital complications (POC). They tend to present with complaints of headaches and fever; some also have signs of meningeal irritation. The diagnosis is confirmed by either CT or MRI of the brain and sinus with contrast. Patients with intracranial infections require broad-spectrum antibiotics that cross the blood–brain barrier and cover aerobic bacteria (especially *S. pneumoniae* and *S. aureus*) and anaerobic bacteria (especially *Streptococcus milleri*). Antibiotic choices should include third-generation cephalosporins (Cefotaxime or Ceftriaxone) along with Vancomycin to cover gram-positive organisms and, less often, Impipenem or Flagyl to cover anaerobic bacteria. Neurosurgical and ENT drainage of the sinuses are

(a)   (b)

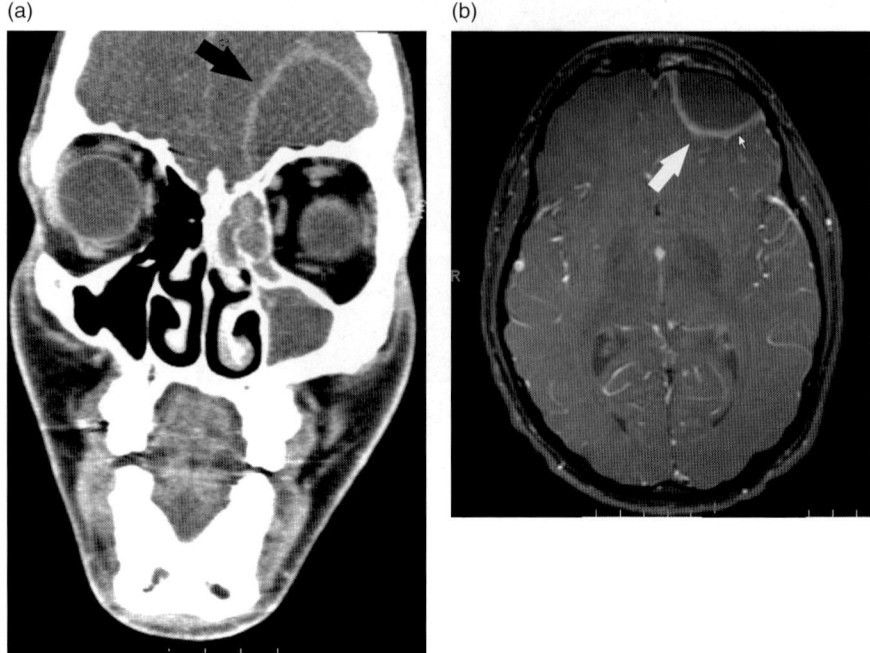

Fig. 13.5 (**a**) Coronal CT image of brain with enhancement: left (L) frontal brain abscess (*arrow*) and opacified sinuses on left (L). (**b**) Axial MRI with contrast demonstrating left (L) frontal abscess (*arrow*)

usually performed at the same time. Except for very small intracranial collections, craniotomy is usually necessary along with endoscopic drainage of the sinuses.

Meningitis is a complication of sinusitis that may be underreported because of unrecognized sinusitis. Children with obvious sinus disease (opacified sinus or air-fluid levels on CT or MRI) should have drainage procedures if they fail initial IV antibiotic.

Isolated sphenoid sinusitis can lead to severe headaches with or without fever and, less commonly, result in vision changes. It is most common in adolescent males. Given the proximity of the sinus to the brain and increased risk of intracranial spread, these children require close observation, aggressive antibiotic therapy (usually intravenous), and prompt surgical drainage of the sinus if they fail to improve after 24 to 48 h of therapy.

Summary

1. The diagnosis of bacterial AR in children should be made based on clinical grounds, but CT should be considered if the child is very ill or if extranasal complications are suspected.

2. Duration of symptoms is the most important factor in differentiating viral from bacterial disease.
3. When bacterial RS is suspected, antibiotics should be chosen that address *S. pneumoniae* and be given in appropriately higher doses to cover penicillin-resistant strains. Follow-up evaluation is recommended if the patient fails to improve, because there is a 10% to 20% expected failure rate when less invasive beta-lactamase-producing bacteria such as *H. influenzae* and *M. catarrhalis* are responsible for the disease.
4. Children with chronic or recurrent sinusitis who fail to respond to medical therapy should undergo CT (coronal cuts) to locate the location and nature of the persistent disease or to identify anatomic anomalies or tumors.
5. Full evaluation should be done prior to elective surgery to identify coexisting adenoid hypertrophy or allergy, to rule out basic immune abnormalities (especially failure of the child to have been adequately immunized with the *S. pneumoniae* vaccine), and to determine if the child has the genes for cystic fibrosis (including homozygous and heterozygous states). Treatment of identified abnormalities should be considered before sinus surgery, including adenoidectomy, allergy control, and booster vaccination.
6. CT and/or MRI with contrast imaging of the sinuses and orbit and brain should be obtained in ill children who have severe disease, and the child should be promptly referred to appropriate specialists if orbital or neurological signs of complication are present.

References

1. Sobol SE. Management of acute sinusitis and its complications. In: Pediatric Otolaryngology: The Requisites in Pediatrics. Philadelphia: Mosby Elsevier, 2007:118–128.
2. Willner A, Choi SS, Vezina LG, Lazar RH. Intranasal anatomic variations in pediatric sinusitis. Am J Rhinol 1997;11(5):355–360.
3. Brook I, Gooch WM III, Jenkins SG, et al. Medical management of acute bacterial sinusitis. Recommendations of a clinical advisory committee on pediatric and adult sinusitis. Ann Otol Rhinol Laryngol 2000;109(suppl):2–20.
4. Sinus and Allergy Health Partnership: Antimicrobial treatment guidelines for acute bacterial rhinosinusitis. Otolaryngol Head Neck Surg 2000;123(suppl 1, pt 2):S1–S32.
5. O'Brien KL, Dowell SF, Schwartz B, et al. Acute sinusitis: principles of judicious use of antimicrobial agents. Pediatrics 1998;101:174–177.
6. Conrad DA, Jenson HB. Management of acute bacterial rhinosinusitis. Curr Opin Pediatr 2002;14:86–90.
7. American Academy of Pediatrics Subcommittee on Management of Sinusitis and Committee on Quality Improvement. Clinical practice guideline: management of sinusitis. Pediatrics 2001;108(3):798–808.
8. Lee D, Rosenfeld RM. Adenoid bacteriology and sinonasal symptoms in children. Otolaryngol Head Neck Surg 1997;116:301–307.
9. Talmor M, Li P, Barie PS. Acute paranasal sinusitis in critically ill patients: Guidelines for prevention, diagnosis and treatment. Clin Infect Dis 1997;25:1441–1446.
10. Wang X, Kim J, McWilliams R, Cutting GR. Increased prevalence of chronic rhinosinusitis in carriers of a cystic fibrosis mutation. Arch Otolaryngol Head Neck Surg 2005;131(3): 237–240.

11. Morris P, Leach A. Antibiotics for persistent nasal discharge (rhinosinusitis) in children. Cochrane Database of Systemic Reviews 2002;4:CD001094.
12. Sinus and Allergy Health Partnership. Antimicrobial treatment guidelines for acute bacterial rhinosinusitis. Otolaryngol Head Neck Surg 2004;130(suppl):1–45.
13. Expert Panel on Pediatric Imaging. Sinusitis in the pediatric population: ACR Appropriateness Criteria. Reston, VA: American College of Radiology, 1999.
14. Gwaltney JM Jr, Phillips CD, Miller RD, Riker DK. Computed tomographic study of the common cold. N Engl J Med 1994;330:25–30.
15. Gwaltney JM Jr. Acute community-acquired sinusitis. Clin Infect Dis 1996;23:1209–1223.
16. Hickner JM, Bartlett JG, Besser RE, et al. Principles of appropriate antibiotic use for acute rhinosinusitis in adults: background. Ann Intern Med 2001;134:498–505.
17. Poole MD, Jacobs MR, Anon JB, Marchant CD, Hoberman A, Harrison CJ. Antimicrobial guidelines for the treatment of acute bacterial rhinosinusitis in immunocompetent children. Int J Pediatr Otorhinolaryngol 2002;63:1–13.
18. Rosenfeld RM, Andes D, Bhattacharyya N, Cheung D, Eisenberg S, Ganiats TG, Gelzer A, Hamilos D, , Hudgins PA, Jones S, Krouse HJ, Lee LH, Mahoney MC, Marple BF, Mitchell JP, Nathan R, Shiffman RN, Smith TL, Witsell DL. Clinical practice guideline: adult sinusitis. Otolaryngol Head Neck Surg 2007;137:S1–S31.
19. Wald ER. Expanded role of group A streptococci in children with upper respiratory infections. Pediatr Infect Dis J 1999;18:663–665.
20. Shapiro ED, Milmoe GJ, Wald ER, Rodnan JB, Bowen AD. Bacteriology of the maxillary sinuses in patient with cystic fibrosis. J Infect Dis 1982;146:589–593.
21. Hui Y, Gaffney R, Crysdale WS. Sinusitis in patients with cystic fibrosis. Eur Arch Otorhinolaryngol 1995;252:191–196.
22. Garau J, Dagan R. Accurate diagnosis and appropriate treatment of acute bacterial rhinosinusitis: minimizing bacterial resistance. Clin Ther 2003;25(7):1936–1951.
23. Ip S, Fu L, Balk E, Chew P, Devine D, Lau J. Update on acute bacterial rhinosinusitis. Evid Rep Technol Assess (Summ) 2005;124:1–3.
24. Schwartz B, Bell DM, Hughes JM. Preventing the emergence of antimicrobial resistance. A call for action by clinicians, public health officials, and patients. JAMA 1997;278:944–945.
25. Bussey MF, Moon RY. Acute sinusitis. Pediatr Rev 1999;20(4):142.
26. Scadding GK. Corticosteroids in the treatment of pediatric allergic rhinitis. J Allergy Clin Immunol 2001;108:S59–S64.
27. Buchman CA, Yellon RF, Bluestone CD. Alternative to endoscopic sinus surgery in the management of pediatric chronic rhinosinusitis refractory to oral antimicrobial therapy. Otolaryngol Head Neck Surg 1999;120(2):219–224.
28. Mair EA, Bolger WE, Breisch EA. Sinus and facial growth after pediatric endoscopic sinus surgery. Arch Otolaryngol Head Neck Surg 1995;121(5):547–552.
29. Van Peteghem A, Clement PA. Influence of extensive functional endoscopic sinus surgery (FESS) on facial growth in children with cystic fibrosis. Comparison of 10 cephalometric parameters of the midface for three study groups. Int J Pediatr Otorhinolaryngol 2006;70(8):1407–1413.
30. White CB, Foshee WS. Upper respiratory tract infections in adolescents. Adolesc Med 2000;11(2):225–249.
31. Chandler JR, Langenbrunner DJ, Stevens ER. The pathogenesis of orbital complications in acute sinusitis. Laryngoscope 1970;80:1414–1428.
32. Arjmand EM, Lusk RP, Muntz HR. Pediatric sinusitis and subperiosteal orbital abscess formation: diagnosis and treatment. Otolaryngol Head Neck Surg 1993;109:886–894.
33. Froehlich P, Pransky SM, Fontaine P, et al. Minimal endoscopic approach to superiosteal orbital abscess. Arch Otolaryngol Head Neck Surg 1997;123:280–282.
34. Lerner DN, Choi SS, Zalzal GH, Johnson DL. Intracranial complications of sinusitis in childhood. Ann Otol Rhinol Laryngol 1995;104:288–293.
35. Glickstein JS, Chandra RK, Thompson JW. Intracranial complications of pediatric sinusitis. Otolaryngol Head Neck Surg 2006;134:733–736.

Chapter 14
Spectrum of Fungal Sinusitis

Kevin C. Welch and James N. Palmer

Fungi are diverse and ubiquitous organisms. Their spores are frequently respired and can be found throughout the nose and sinuses. Generally, the human immune system is naturally equipped to eliminate these airborne invaders; however, in approximately 10% of patients, fungal spores and elements become manifest as disease. The manifestation of disease within the nose and paranasal sinuses varies widely from the benign to the utterly malignant and fatal.

Fungal infections of the paranasal sinuses can be broadly divided into two categories based on the histopathological diagnosis of tissue invasion. For the purposes of this chapter, fungal disease is either noninvasive or invasive [1,2]. The primary manifestations of noninvasive disease are the development of fungal balls or allergic fungal sinusitis (AFS). Invasive fungal sinusitis occurs either as an acute, rapidly progressive sinusitis or in a chronic fashion.

This chapter outlines the diagnosis and treatment of the various forms of fungal sinusitis. A summary of forms of fungal sinusitis can be found in Table 14.1.

Noninvasive Fungal Sinusitis

Characteristics of Fungus

The fungal species typically responsible for noninvasive human infections are divided into two categories based upon their morphological appearance: yeasts and molds. Yeasts are typically round, budding, and reproduce asexually by fission. Molds amalgamate into colonies typified by interwoven hyphae; they produce spores, which can be sexual or asexual. These fungi responsible for noninvasive disease are usually dematiaceous (dark colored) or hyaline (lightly colored) species, are ubiquitous in nature, and typically demonstrate septate hyphal forms. Dematiaceous species responsible for noninvasive disease include members of the

J.N. Palmer
Department of Otorhinolaryngology – Head and Neck Surgery, University of Pennsylvania Health System, Philadelphia, PA, USA
e-mail: james.palmer@uphs.upenn.edu

E.R. Thaler, D.W. Kennedy (eds.), *Rhinosinusitis*, DOI: 10.1007/978-0-387-73062-2_14,   223
© Springer Science+Business Media, LLC 2008

Table 1 Classification and features of fungal sinusitis

	Clinical Features	Culture/Biopsy	Imaging	Treatment
Noninvasive				
Fungal Ball	• Isolated sinus disease • Crumbly, dirt-like mass in sinus • Underlying mucosal inflammation	• Tightly packed fungal hyphae • No tissue invasion	• CT with differential density and/or possible bony erosion • MRI T1 hypodense mass; does not enhance	• Endoscopic removal and thorough irrigation
Allergic Fungal Sinusitis	• Unilateral or bilateral • Polyposis • Tenacious allergic mucin • Recurrence	• Rare fungal hyphae (branching, septate) • Eosinophilic infiltration	• CT with unilateral or bilateral involvement • Bony expansion/erosion • Differential density	• Endoscopic sinus surgery • Oral and nasal corticosteroids • Immunotherapy • +/− Oral antifungal therapy
Invasive				
Acute Invasive	• Immunocompromised or diabetic host • Pale or necrotic appearing mucosa/skin • Anesthesia of affected sinonasal areas • Altered vision if orbital involvment	• Aseptate 90-degree branching fungal hyphae invading tissue and blood vessels; necrotic tissue highest yield	• CT not very specific • MRI demonstrating necrotic tissue that doesn't enhance with contrast • MRI elucidates brain or orbital involvement	• Emergent surgical debridement • Amphotericin-B intravenously • +/− posaconazole therapy long-term
Chronic Invasive	• Immunocompromised or diabetic host • Pale or necrotic appearing mucosa/skin • Anesthesia of affected sinonasal areas	• Aseptate 90-degree branching fungal hyphae invading tissue and blood vessels; necrotic tissue highest yield • Noncaseating granulomas rarely	• MRI demonstrating necrotic tissue that doesn't enhance with contrast • MRI elucidates brain or orbital involvement	• Surgical debridement • Amphotericin-B intravenously • +/− posaconazole therapy long-term • itraconazole in granulomatous forms

following genera: *Bipolaris*, *Curvularia*, *Pseudallescheria*, *Penicillium*, *Fusarium*, and *Alternaria*. Hyaline molds seen in noninvasive disease are typically members of *Aspergillus*.

Fungal Balls

Fungal balls present in the setting of an immunocompetent host with chronic rhinosinusitis (CRS) or the patient with recurrent acute rhinosinusitis of one sinus, typically the maxillary sinus [2]. Symptoms related to fungal balls are nonspecific, or may not even be present. Physical examination with rigid endoscopy reveals a spectrum of disease that ranges from mild edema to frank polyposis with mucopurulence in the patient with concomitant CRS or AFS. Intraoperatively, fungus balls appear as focal lesions that are gritty, dirt like, and vary in color depending upon the fungal elements.

Diagnosis

Imaging of the paranasal sinuses will show unilateral or single sinus disease that, with the exception of a differential density, is often nonspecific. As previously mentioned, the intraoperative findings (Fig. 14.1) confirm the diagnosis when characteristic isolated sinus lesions are identified that often must be scraped or flushed from the sinus. Although the offending agents are typical dematiaceous or hyaline species, often cultures are unrevealing [2,3]. On microscopic examination, densely packed septated fungal hyphae are typically identified. Underlying sinonasal mucosa may demonstrate an influx of leukocytes with evidence of chronic inflammation.

Treatment

Therapy for fungal balls is aimed at elimination of disease and restoration of sinus ventilation and outflow, performed through endoscopic techniques. Extirpation of the fungal ball typically results in a cure, and recurrence rates are minimal [3]. Systemic or topical antifungal medications are not indicated.

Allergic Fungal Sinusitis

Allergic fungal sinusitis is a form of CRS that was initially recognized in 1976 by Safirstein and colleagues, [4] who described a condition of CRS, nasal polyposis, and aspergillus in a patient with allergic bronchopulmonary aspergillosis (ABPA). Later, in 1981, Millar and coworkers [5] reported on a series of patients with CRS and cultures demonstrating *Aspergillus* and their similarities to patients with ABPA, a pulmonary manifestation of hypersensitivity to *Aspergillus* species associated with asthma, peripheral eosinophilia, and elevated IgE. Progressively, an entity of CRS associated with allergies to *Aspergillus* species was described. These patients were

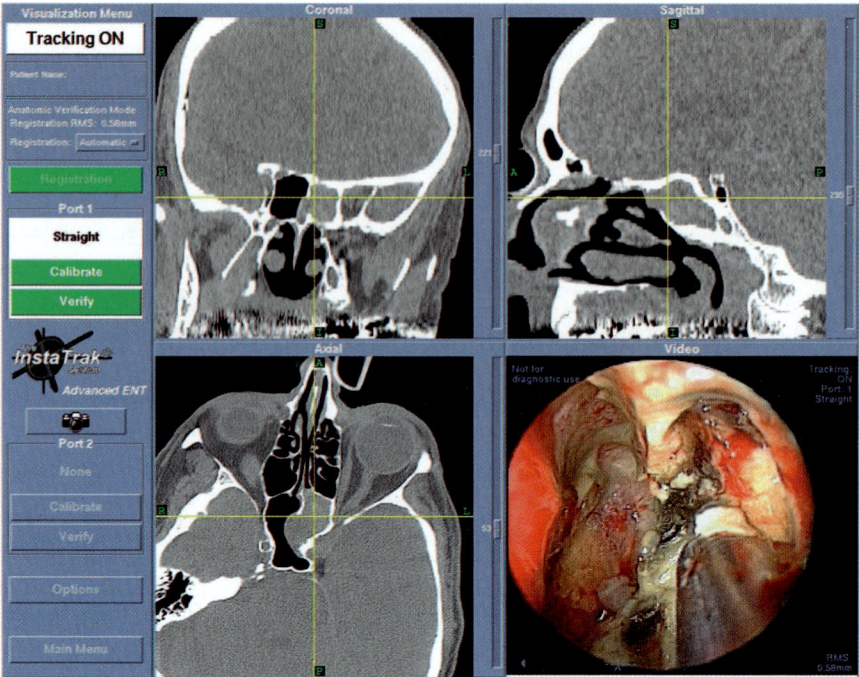

Fig. 14.1 A patient presented with vertex headaches and a unrevealing nasal endoscopy. After computed tomography (CT) and magnetic resonance imaging (MRI) scans were obtained, the patient was brought to the operating room for a sphenoid biopsy. A fungal ball was identified intraoperatively

known to be refractory to conventional medical and surgical therapy; however, they were also known for their high recidivism.

Diagnosis

Clinically, patients with AFS were characterized by nasal polyposis; asthma; peripheral eosinophilia; eosinophilic mucus demonstrating Charcot–Leyden crystals; type I hypersensitivity or atopic disease; and characteristic computed tomographic (CT) findings that included evidence of CRS, calcifications or differential density within the sinus, and often erosion of bone. The proposed mechanism for AFS involves the abnormal immune response to fungal antigens through an IgE-mediated response and through the influx of eosinophils via inflammatory pathways. The resulting inflammation and edema lead to ostial obstruction and stasis of secretions. This clinical scenario was recognized by Bent and Kuhn, [6] who proposed five major criteria for the diagnosis of AFS based on a series of 15 patients with overlapping clinical features: (1) nasal polyposis, (2) evidence of atopic disease or type I hypersensitivity to common fungal agents, (3) eosinophilic mucus without fungal invasion, (4) characteristic CT findings (opacified sinuses, unilateral disease, bony

Fig. 14.2 Features of allergic
fungal sinusitis on computed
tomography. Note the erosion
of normal landmarks and
bony features of the paranasal
sinuses and the differential
density noted in the lesion.
These are characteristics of
allergic fungal sinusitis

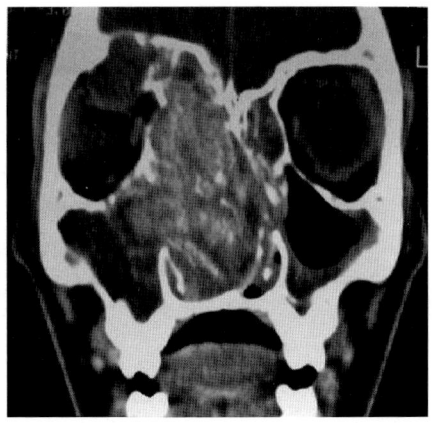

abnormalities, and differential density; Fig. 14.2), and (5) a positive fungal smear. Associated factors included other common, but not always identifiable, conditions such as asthma, peripheral eosinophilia, fungal culture, and bone erosion on CT examination.

Key factors in the diagnosis rested in identification of high levels of IgE in peripheral blood samples, positive skin end-titration, prick testing, or radioallergosorbent test to fungal antigens, and the demonstration of fungi on Grocott's methenamine silver (GMS) staining in a background of eosinophilic mucus.

Despite criteria for the diagnosis of AFS, much controversy exists in the literature about how many of the major criteria established by Bent and Kuhn [6]. are required to meet the diagnosis. Rather, do patients present with "typical" and "atypical" forms of AFS? This question arises when patients present with the clinical features of AFS but do not demonstrate evidence of fungal growth on culture or on smears, or who fail to demonstrate IgE-mediated fungal allergy. This question has led investigators [7–10] to propose that AFS exists on a spectrum of disease that is central to the eosinophil. Ferguson [7] performed a detailed analysis of the literature regarding AFS and has noted differences in the clinical presentation of certain patients with features of AFS yet who lack fungal growth or IgE-mediated fungal allergy. Although all patients presented with CRS, eosinophilia, and characteristic findings on CT, patients with *eosinophilic mucin rhinosinusitis* presented more frequently with bilateral disease, aspirin-sensitive asthma, and IgG deficiencies, in contrast to patients with AFS. The role of IgE in AFS was thought to be fundamental to its diagnosis; however, a demonstrable role for IgE, both local and peripheral, in eosinophilic mucin rhinosinusitis and *nonallergic eosinophilic fungal sinusitis* is less clear. Collins et al. [11] demonstrated local production of IgE in sinonasal mucosa in patients with AFS and highlighted its importance in disease pathogenesis. Carney and colleagues [8]. looked at sinonasal mucosa in patients with AFS, nonallergic eosinophilic fungal sinusitis, and CRS. Peripheral IgE counts were raised in AFS, but they were unelevated in nonallergic eosinophilic fungal sinusitis. However, IgE cell counts within sinonasal mucosa were elevated in all three types of patients when compared to control patients. It was clear from this review that while IgE was not significantly elevated in peripheral counts, local IgE production may play a role in the pathogenesis of all forms of eosinophilic rhinosinusitis. The exact role for IgE-mediated disease in the spectrum of eosinophilic rhinosinusitis has yet to be elucidated.

To add a twist to the issue, a study [12] performed at the Mayo Clinic sampled patients with CRS and healthy volunteers for fungus. Approximately 96% of patients with CRS demonstrated positive fungal cultures. More interestingly, 100% of healthy volunteers demonstrated fungal colonization. This finding serves only to cloud the role of fungus in paranasal sinus disease.

Therapy

The comprehensive management of AFS begins with the surgical extirpation [2,13,14] of the diseased sinuses to reduce the gross fungal load. Surgery should be conducted in an atraumatic manner using the principles of functional endoscopic sinus surgery, which permit restoration of the natural drainage pathways of the diseased sinuses. Intraoperative cultures are taken, which may help to confirm the diagnosis and to assist in the treatment of any overlying bacterial infection. Allergic mucin (Fig. 14.3) is aspirated and may be sent for confirmation of the typical sheets of eosinophils and Charcot–Leyden crystals. The postoperative management of the patient with AFS is critical to increasing the time interval between operative events, as recurrence of disease is common.

Evidence for the use of systemic corticosteroids in the treatment of AFS stems from experience gained in their use for ABPA. Waxman et al. [15] proposed the use of system corticosteroids for AFS based upon its clinical and histolog-

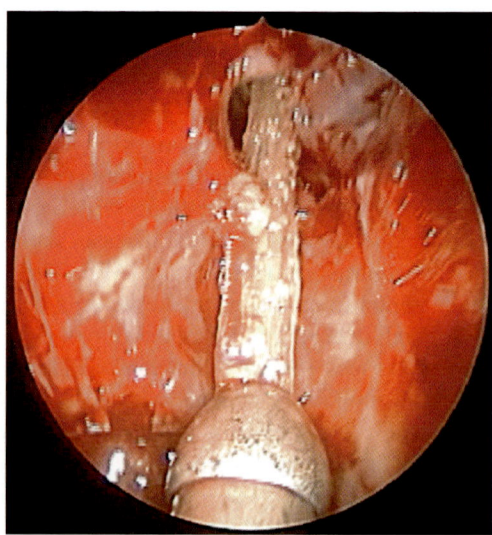

Fig. 14.3 Endoscopic view of a patient with allergic fungal sinusitis. Note the tenacious allergic mucin that typifies this disease

ical picture, which is similar to ABPA. Although no prospective, double-blinded, placebo-controlled studies have been conducted to evaluate the efficacy of systemic and topical corticosteroids in the treatment of AFS, many retrospective studies and case series have demonstrated significantly improved outcomes when they are deployed. Schubert and colleagues [16] retrospectively evaluated 67 patients with AFS. Patients who were administered corticosteroids, at the rate of 0.5 mg/kg/day for 2 weeks followed by a taper, were observed to have fewer revision surgeries and recurrences at 1 year. This study, however, is confounded by the coadministration of immunotherapy and antihistamines. Kuhn and Swain [13] deployed a similar starting dose and used the Kupferberg et al. [17] mucosal grading scales to evaluate the outcomes of postoperative patients with AFS, and when patients achieved a score of 0 (no edema, no allergic mucin) for 6 months, they were converted to topical corticosteroids at two- to threefold the allergic rhinitis dosing. Recurrences were noted within 6 months after ceasing systemic corticosteroids. In another study performed by Kinsella and coworkers, [18] 8 of 15 patients who were not treated with postoperative systemic corticosteroids developed recurrences. In 7 of 15 patients who did not develop recurrence, 4 of those received postoperative corticosteroids. Marple and colleagues [14] recommend a comprehensive management algorithm for the treatment of AFS that involves surgery, adjuvant systemic corticosteroids, saline irrigation, and immunotherapy.

The rationale for immunotherapy in the treatment of AFS stems from the successful treatment of allergic rhinitis in patients with allergies to similar dematiaceous species. Proponents of immunotherapy [19,20] site a number of studies demonstrating improved outcomes when immunotherapy is deployed. In a large study involving 60 patients, Bassichis and colleagues [21] compared outcomes in 36 patients receiving immunotherapy to outcomes in 24 patients who did not receive immunotherapy. Primary outcomes were office visits that necessitated interventions and revision surgery. Patients who did not receive immunotherapy on average required 1.7 more office visits and were more likely to require revision surgery (33% versus 11%). Folker et al. [22] recorded that patients with AFS treated with immunotherapy in addition to surgery reported improved quality of life. Additionally, Mabry and colleagues [23] reported decreased crusting and allergic mucin in patients treated with immunotherapy.

Although criteria for AFS include the absence of fungal invasion, several investigators [24–26] have examined the use of systemic and/or topical antifungal agents as adjuvants in the therapy of AFS. Again, treatment proposals for AFS have stemmed from evidence regarding the successful treatment of ABPA: Denning and colleagues [24] used itraconazole systemically and demonstrated improvement in a modest number of patients. Kuhn and Swain [13] tested amphotericin B and itraconazole in vitro against several typical allergic fungal agents and concluded good in vitro susceptibilities in five of six common isolates; however, in vivo testing was not performed. Rains and Mineck [27] published a review of 139 patients treated with surgery, high-dose itraconazole, short burst of corticosteroids, and nasal corticosteroids. Although there was no control group or comparison group, good control and low adverse side effects were reported with their treatment paradigm. Because of confounding variables, adverse side effects, expense, and because prospective studies evaluating the use of high-dose antifungal medication are lacking, inclusion of antifungal therapy in the treatment of AFS—systemic or topical—has met with lukewarm enthusiasm [26,28].

Invasive Fungal Sinusitis

Characteristics of Fungus

Invasive forms of fungal sinusitis principally stem from the saprophytic (obtaining nutrients from dead or decaying matter) Zygomycetes class of fungi, which is characterized by rapidly growing and reproducing species that are coenocytic (wide, ribbon-like) and largely aseptate. The predominant orders of fungi in the Zygomycetes class are Mucorales and Entomophthorales; however, Mucorales is by and large responsible for the invasive disease seen in human beings, which highlights the inaccuracy recognized by Greenberg et al. [29,30] of calling invasive fungal sinusitis mucormycosis rather than zygomycosis. To add another layer of confusion, invasive fungal sinusitis caused by *Aspergillus* species (members of the Ascomycota phylum and Eurotiales order) causes neither zygomycosis nor mucormycosis. Responsible genera within Mucorales include *Mucor*, *Rhizopus*, *Rhizomucor*, *Cunninghamella*, and *Absidia*, to name a few. The hallmark of this form of fungal sinusitis is tissue invasion, and more specifically, angioinvasion. According to the original deShazo [1,2] classification, these fungi become manifest in acutely invasive and chronically invasive forms.

Acute Invasive Fungal Sinusitis

As previously mentioned, the hallmark of invasive fungal sinusitis is tissue or blood vessel invasion. The acute form of invasive fungal sinusitis is rapidly progressive and lethal if not properly identified and promptly treated. The invasion of these molds cause tissue necrosis and blood vessel thrombosis. The saprophytic nature of these fungi contributes to the acceleration of disease within necrotic tissue, and, as detailed later, explains the poor tissue bioavailability of antifungal agents delivered in the absence of radical debridement.

Populations at risk for acute invasive fungal sinusitis include diabetic patients presenting in diabetic ketoacidosis, immunocompromised patients receiving immunosuppressive therapy for solid organ transplant, patients receiving high-dose corticosteroids, patients receiving the iron chelator deferoxamine, neutropenic patients, and patients undergoing bone marrow transplantation. Impairment of the host neutrophilic response and phagocytosis appears to be the central cause of disease progression. Immunocompetent patients exhibiting a robust neutrophilic response do not acquire invasive fungal sinusitis in the absence of large inoculation such as in a traumatic situation. Patients meeting criteria for these conditions who present with clinical or radiographic evidence of rhinosinusitis should be approached with a high level of suspicion for acute invasive fungal sinusitis until proven otherwise.

Recent concern has arisen in patients with human immunodeficiency virus (HIV) and acquired immunodeficiency syndrome (AIDS) and their risk for acute invasive fungal sinusitis. In the absence of neutropenia, concomitant diabetic ketoacidosis, or other forms of immunosuppression, acute invasive fungal sinusitis is uncommon in patients with AIDS, [31,32] because HIV chiefly affects T-lymphocytes and the host response to invasive fungal elements is primarily neutrophilic. Nevertheless, the patient with AIDS and symptoms or signs of acute rhinosinusitis should be approached with caution, and comorbid risk factors for acute invasive sinusitis should be identified.

Diagnosis

The rapid diagnosis of acute invasive fungal sinusitis is critical to the successful treatment of this disease. Several authors [1,29,33–35] have proposed algorithms for the diagnosis of acute invasive fungal sinusitis. The *sine qua non* feature of the diagnosis is the demonstration of fungal invasion. A positive fungal culture in a patient with suspected invasive fungal sinusitis is insufficient. Studies have shown that when invasive fungal sinusitis has been identified clinically, cultures were sensitive in 52% of cases at autopsy and in only 30% of surgical specimens [36]. Furthermore, *Mucor* species have been identified in cases of allergic fungal sinusitis and comprise part of the array of testing for allergic disease [26]. Cultures help to speciate organisms; however, the timeline associated with this is insufficient to help initiate the treatment of acute invasive fungal sinusitis. Nevertheless, a culture showing a *Zygomycetes* species in an otherwise sterile area or if obtained in the setting of tissue necrosis should be viewed with concern. Because of these considerations, a tissue biopsy is paramount. Necrotic tissue has been shown to be more yielding than viable tissue [29]. Gillespie and colleagues [35] have recommended the anterior-inferior portion of the middle turbinate as a suitable site for biopsy if the middle turbinate shows signs of invasive disease: discoloration, ulceration, etc. In their series, biopsy of the middle turbinate had 75% sensitivity and 100% specificity for acute invasive fungal sinusitis.

Clinical examination of the patient with the rigid endoscope reveals a spectrum of findings in the patient with acute disease: tissue necrosis ranging from the pale and ischemic mucosa to the frankly necrotic tissue, anesthesia of the affected regions, and absence of bleeding in the setting of biopsy or manipulation. The overlying skin or oral mucosa can demonstrate ischemia (Fig. 14.4), erythema, desquamation, or ecchymosis depending on the degree of extranasal infection. Concomitant orbital invasion may reveal proptosis, ecchymosis, blurry vision, ophthalmoplegia, or blindness. These clinical findings should raise suspicion for acute invasive fungal sinusitis with extranasal involvement in the right clinical setting.

Computed tomography and magnetic resonance (MR) imaging have been utilized to confirm the diagnosis of acute invasive fungal sinusitis. DelGaudio and coworkers [37] compared the CT findings in patients with acute invasive fungal sinusitis to

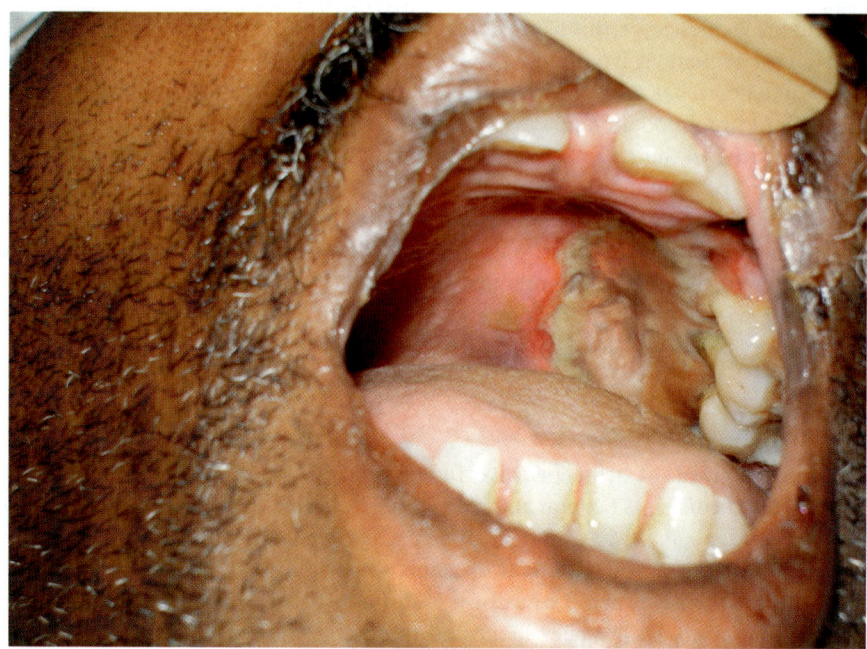

Fig. 14.4 A patient presenting with diabetic ketoacidosis, left nasal congestion, left midface pressure, and loose teeth. Inspection of his oral cavity revealed ischemic-appearing mucosa of the hard palate. Biopsy of the palate and middle turbinate revealed aseptate, 90° branching hyphae invading the soft tissue

immunocompromised patients with sinusitis but no evidence of invasive disease. Although they found unilateral thickening on CT images to be common in patients with invasive disease compared to their controls, findings were otherwise nonspecific. MR imaging (Fig. 14.5) can help identify orbital and intracranial involvement, [38] as these findings would significantly alter the course of therapy. On T_1-weighted images, infarcted tissue appears hypointense to muscle and fails to enhance when imaged with gadolinium. The combination of imaging augments the diagnosis and helps with surgical planning.

Treatment

The treatment of invasive fungal sinusitis involves three elements: (1) reversal of the underlying medical condition, (2) surgical eradication of the disease, and (3) prolonged intravenous antifungal therapy.

Most patients presenting with acute invasive fungal sinusitis either are diabetic or are immunosuppressed in some fashion. Consultation with an endocrinologist for the rapid reversal of hyperglycemia is essential to maintain a euglycemic state during therapy. A number of authors [39,40] have found that patients with diabetes presenting with sinonasal mucormycosis fare better than patients with

Fig. 14.5 A T$_1$-weighted
MRI showing invasive fungal
sinusitis after the
administration of contrast.
Areas of invasive fungal
sinusitis do not take up
contrast. Note the orbital
invasion detailed in the image

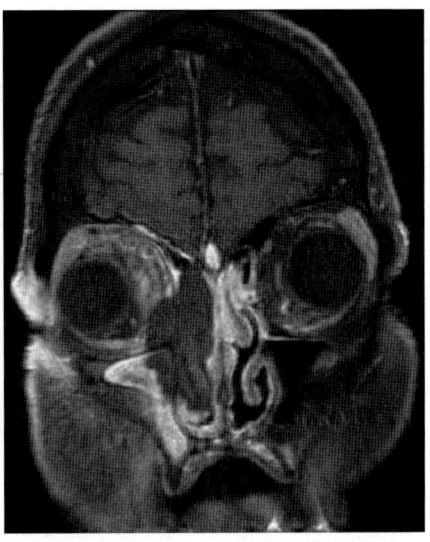

mucormycosis due to immunosuppression. If acceptable, immunosuppressive therapy should be stopped. Because acute invasive fungal sinusitis is highly fatal in the neutropenic patient, the risk of organ rejection or relapse of autoimmune disease, etc., should be secondary.

Because tissue infected with invasive fungal disease typically is ischemic, antibiotic delivery to the affected site is compromised. Therefore, radical debridement of the sinonasal cavity is indicated. Consideration should be given to the extent of the disease before operation because disseminated disease cannot be cured by surgery. Furthermore, rhinocerebral zygomycosis may not be amenable to surgical therapy if extensively involving the brain. Gillespie and colleagues have proposed an algorithm [34] that begins with endoscopy and frozen section diagnosis of suspected disease. When identified, prompt surgical debridement is indicated. If the disease is limited to the sinonasal cavity, extirpation may be performed endoscopically. Often open approaches involving maxillectomy with skin excision or orbital exenteration are required (Fig. 14.6). If the disease is limited to the sinonasal cavity, orbital exenteration is not required [41]. When clinical or radiographic evidence of orbital invasion is present, orbital exenteration should be considered. Hargrove and colleagues [42] reviewed the literature regarding the indications for orbital exenteration; however, their extensive research could not identify clear indications for orbital exenteration, despite such clinical findings as orbital cellulitis, proptosis, and ophthalmoplegia. Hargrove and coworkers did, however, identify that those patients who presented with fever benefited from orbital exenteration when compared to patients who did not present with fever. The reasons were unclear from their investigation; however, they proposed more advanced disease was present to illicit fever. Additionally, febrile patients were more likely to have a fatal outcome than patients

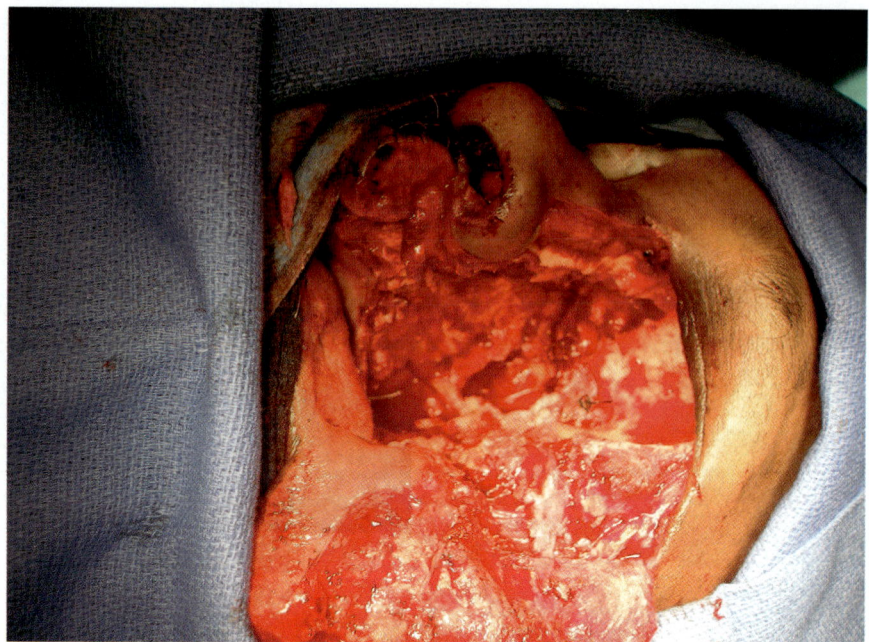

Fig. 14.6 The same patient as in Figure 14.4 after undergoing a total maxillectomy with orbital exenteration. Mucor was identified in all surgical specimens, including the globe

who were afebrile. Therefore, the decision to exenterate must be made on an individual basis and approached with sensitivity.

Systemic therapy with antifungal antibiotics should be administered promptly when acute invasive fungal sinusitis is identified. Amphotericin B is the drug of choice for the treatment of acute invasive fungal sinusitis [43]. Amphotericin B is administered beginning at 1.0 to 1.5 mg/kg/day; however, doses of 4 to 8 mg/kg/day are more typical for invasive disease. A broad range of *Mucorales* species demonstrate in vitro MIC_{50} susceptibilities to amphotericin B as low as 0.125 mg/L [29]. Despite maximal surgical therapy and concomitant administration of amphotericin B, as many as 20% to 30% of patients succumb to their disease. Amphotericin B is more commonly administered in a lipid complex or liposomal formulation; these formulations have been proven to lower the incidence of renal failure and need for hemodialysis. However, the cost of administration is significantly higher than that attributed to the deoxycholate form of amphotericin B. The failure rates of amphotericin B as well as the significant side effects (renal failure, anaphylaxis) have prompted investigators to evaluate other antifungal agents such as caspofungin, voriconazole, itraconazole, and posaconazole for the initial or prolonged treatment of acute invasive fungal sinusitis. In vitro testing has shown that *Mucorales* species do not show good susceptibilities to caspofungin and voriconazole. These drugs, however, do show strong activity against *Aspergillus* species; and when acute invasive fungal sinusitis is known to be caused by *Aspergillus*, caspofungin and voriconazole represent strong therapeutic drugs. Although *Mucorales* species show initial susceptibilities to itraconazole, the effect is not sustained, thus rendering itraconazole a poor choice for acute invasive fungal sinusitis. However, several studies [29,30,44–46] have shown that posaconazole, an extended traizole that inhibits ergosterol synthesis, demonstrates similar in vitro and in vivo susceptibilities to *Aspergillus* and *Mucorales* when compared to amphotericin B. This susceptibility is also maintained over the duration of treatment. Posaconazole is administered in oral formulation to a cumulative dose of 800 mg/day and metabolized by the CYP3A4 system. It is currently recommended as salvage therapy for amphotericin B failures or in patients who require long-term maintenance dosing.

Despite maximal treatment and reversal of underlying medical problems, patients with acute invasive fungal sinusitis have a 30% to 60% mortality rate, indicating the serious nature of the disease.

Chronic Invasive Fungal Sinusitis

Although members of the Zygomycetes class are by and large responsible for the acutely invasive form of this disease, the hyaline mold *Aspergillus*, specifically *A. fumigatus* and *A. flavus*, is more commonly isolated in chronically invasive forms. This rare subset of invasive fungal sinusitis can occur in immunocompetent patients [1,47,48] and span months before a proper diagnosis is made.

Diagnosis

The presentation of chronic invasive fungal sinusitis is usually similar to that of CRS: pressure, nasal discharge, headache, etc. However, slowly progressive features that share more in common with an invasive picture (proptosis, visual changes, cranial nerve palsy, and soft tissue cellulitis) can become manifest as well. As with acute invasive fungal sinusitis, CT and MR imaging are helpful in establishing the diagnosis. The usual features of CRS are seen on CT images in addition to bony erosion and differential densities within the affected sinuses. Similarly, MR imaging is complementary and can help identify orbital and intracranial involvement.

As with acute invasive fungal sinusitis, formal diagnosis involves the analysis of frozen or permanent biopsy specimens that demonstrate tissue invasion or necrosis in the presence of fungal hyphae. Additionally, a noncaseating granulomatous form of chronically invasive fungal sinusitis is characterized by tissue necrosis, vasculitis, eosinophilic infiltration, and giant cell proliferation. Granulomatous forms typically become manifest in immunocompetent patients and seem to be much more common in the northern African regions than elsewhere.

Treatment

Because chronic invasive fungal sinusitis can present in patients with intact immune systems, an underlying medical comorbidity may not be present to treat as with acute invasive fungal sinusitis. Patients presenting with diabetes or an immunocompromised state should have their medical illnesses addressed to the extent that is permissible. Fundamental to the treatment of chronic invasive fungal sinusitis is surgical debridement. Because of the uncommon nature of this disease, the optimal combination of surgery and adjuvant antifungal therapy is not known. However, eradication of macroscopic disease with postoperative surveillance and administration of amphotericin B is advocated [47,48]. No studies have been performed evaluating the efficacy of other antifungal therapies in the treatment of chronic invasive fungal sinusitis; however, since *Aspergillus* is the primary agent responsible for chronic invasive fungal sinusitis, other antifungals may be considered for salvage therapy. Caspofungin has demonstrated excellent in vitro and in vivo activity against *Aspergillus* in a murine model, and it can be used in combination with voriconazole for the treatment of invasive *Aspergillus* [49]. Voriconazole, posaconazole, and ravuconazole all demonstrate strong in vitro and in vivo activity against many *Aspergillus* species as well [49].

Patients with granulomatous forms of chronic fungal sinusitis have been treated with surgical debridement and long-term itraconazole with good results. Recurrence is not unusual, however. Long-term follow-up is necessary in patients with chronic invasive fungal sinusitis in order to identify relapse.

Conclusion

Fungal sinusitis can be subdivided into noninvasive and invasive forms. Although the two basic forms are vastly different, similar species may cause significantly different forms of disease. While noninvasive forms may go months to years without proper diagnosis and treatment and be complicated by drawn-out courses of medical and surgical therapy, invasive forms can be rapidly progressive and deadly if not identified promptly and treated aggressively.

References

1. deShazo RD, O'Brien M, Chapin K, et al. A new classification and diagnostic criteria for invasive fungal sinusitis. Arch Otolaryngol Head Neck Surg 1997;123:1181–1188.
2. deShazo RD, Chapin K, Swain RE. Fungal sinusitis. N Engl J Med 1997;337:254–259.
3. Ferreiro JA, Carlson BA, Cody DT III. Paranasal sinus fungus balls. Head Neck 1997;19:481–486.
4. Safirstein BH. Allergic bronchopulmonary aspergillosis with obstruction of the upper respiratory tract. Chest 1976;70:788–790.
5. Millar J, Johnston A, Lamb B. Allergic aspergillosis of the maxillary sinuses [abstract]. Thorax 1981;36:710.
6. Bent JP III, Kuhn FA. Diagnosis of allergic fungal sinusitis. Otolaryngol Head Neck Surg 1994;111:580–588.
7. Ferguson BJ. Eosinophilic mucin rhinosinusitis: a distinct clinicopathological entity. Laryngoscope 2000;110:799–813.

8. Carney AS, Tan LW, Adams D, et al. Th2 immunological inflammation in allergic fungal sinusitis, nonallergic eosinophilic fungal sinusitis, and chronic rhinosinusitis. Am J Rhinol 2006;20:145–149.
9. Pant H, Kette FE, Smith WB, et al. Eosinophilic mucus chronic rhinosinusitis: clinical subgroups or a homogeneous pathogenic entity? Laryngoscope 2006;116:1241–1247.
10. Eliashar R, Levi-Schaffer F. The role of the eosinophil in nasal diseases. Curr Opin Otolaryngol Head Neck Surg 2005;13:171–175.
11. Collins M, Nair S, Smith W, et al. Role of local immunoglobulin E production in the pathophysiology of noninvasive fungal sinusitis. Laryngoscope 2004;114:1242–1246.
12. Ponikau JU, Sherris DA, Kern EB, et al. The diagnosis and incidence of allergic fungal sinusitis. Mayo Clin Proc 1999;74:877–884.
13. Kuhn FA, Swain R Jr. Allergic fungal sinusitis: diagnosis and treatment. Curr Opin Otolaryngol Head Neck Surg 2003;11:1–5.
14. Marple BF, Mabry RL. Comprehensive management of allergic fungal sinusitis. Am J Rhinol 1998;12:263–268.
15. Waxman JE, Spector JG, Sale SR, et al. Allergic *Aspergillus* sinusitis: concepts in diagnosis and treatment of a new clinical entity. Laryngoscope 1987;97:261–266.
16. Schubert MS. Allergic fungal sinusitis: pathogenesis and management strategies. Drugs 2004;64:363–374.
17. Kupferberg SB, Bent JP III, Kuhn FA. Prognosis for allergic fungal sinusitis. Otolaryngol Head Neck Surg 1997;117:35–41.
18. Kinsella JB, Bradfield JJ, Gourley WK, et al. Allergic fungal sinusitis. Clin Otolaryngol Allied Sci 1996;21:389–392.
19. Schubert MS. Medical treatment of allergic fungal sinusitis. Ann Allergy Asthma Immunol 2000;85:90–97; quiz 97–101.
20. Mabry RL, Mabry CS. Allergic fungal sinusitis: the role of immunotherapy. Otolaryngol Clin N Am 2000;33:433–440.
21. Bassichis BA, Marple BF, Mabry RL, et al. Use of immunotherapy in previously treated patients with allergic fungal sinusitis. Otolaryngol Head Neck Surg 2001;125:487–490.
22. Folker RJ, Marple BF, Mabry RL, et al. Treatment of allergic fungal sinusitis: a comparison trial of postoperative immunotherapy with specific fungal antigens. Laryngoscope 1998;108:1623–1627.
23. Mabry RL, Manning SC, Mabry CS. Immunotherapy in the treatment of allergic fungal sinusitis. Otolaryngol Head Neck Surg 1997;116:31–35.
24. Denning DW, Van Wye JE, Lewiston NJ, et al. Adjunctive therapy of allergic bronchopulmonary aspergillosis with itraconazole. Chest 1991;100:813–819.
25. Bent JP III, Kuhn FA. Antifungal activity against allergic fungal sinusitis organisms. Laryngoscope 1996;106:1331–1334.
26. Marple BF. Allergic fungal rhinosinusitis: current theories and management strategies. Laryngoscope 2001;111:1006–1019.
27. Rains BM 3rd, Mineck CW. Treatment of allergic fungal sinusitis with high-dose itraconazole. Am J Rhinol 2003;17:1–8.
28. Ferguson BJ. What role do systemic corticosteroids, immunotherapy, and antifungal drugs play in the therapy of allergic fungal rhinosinusitis? Arch Otolaryngol Head Neck Surg 1998;124:1174–1178.
29. Greenberg RN, Scott LJ, Vaughn HH, et al. Zygomycosis (mucormycosis): emerging clinical importance and new treatments. Curr Opin Infect Dis 2004;17:517–525.
30. Greenberg RN, Mullane K, van Burik JA, et al. Posaconazole as salvage therapy for zygomycosis. Antimicrob Agents Chemother 2006;50:126–133.
31. Prabhu RM, Patel R. Mucormycosis and entomophthoramycosis: a review of the clinical manifestations, diagnosis and treatment. Clin Microbiol Infect 2004;10(suppl 1):31–47.
32. Hejny C, Kerrison JB, Newman NJ, et al. Rhino-orbital mucormycosis in a patient with acquired immunodeficiency syndrome (AIDS) and neutropenia. Am J Ophthalmol 2001;132:111–112.

33. Gillespie MB, O'Malley BW Jr, Francis HW. An approach to fulminant invasive fungal rhinosinusitis in the immunocompromised host. Arch Otolaryngol Head Neck Surg 1998;124:520–526.

34. Gillespie MB, O'Malley BW. An algorithmic approach to the diagnosis and management of invasive fungal rhinosinusitis in the immunocompromised patient. Otolaryngol Clin N Am 2000;33:323–334.

35. Gillespie MB, Huchton DM, O'Malley BW. Role of middle turbinate biopsy in the diagnosis of fulminant invasive fungal rhinosinusitis. Laryngoscope 2000;110:1832–1836.

36. Tarrand JJ, Lichterfeld M, Warraich I, et al. Diagnosis of invasive septate mold infections. A correlation of microbiological culture and histologic or cytologic examination. Am J Clin Pathol 2003;119:854–858.

37. DelGaudio JM, Swain RE Jr, Kingdom TT, et al. Computed tomographic findings in patients with invasive fungal sinusitis. Arch Otolaryngol Head Neck Surg 2003;129:236–240.

38. Press GA, Weindling SM, Hesselink JR, et al. Rhinocerebral mucormycosis: MR manifestations. J Comput Assist Tomogr 1988;12:744–749.

39. Blitzer A, Lawson W, Meyers BR, et al. Patient survival factors in paranasal sinus mucormycosis. Laryngoscope 1980;90:635–648.

40. Yohai RA, Bullock JD, Aziz AA, et al. Survival factors in rhino-orbital-cerebral mucormycosis. Surv Ophthalmol 1994;39:3–22.

41. Kohn R, Hepler R. Management of limited rhino-orbital mucormycosis without exenteration. Ophthalmology 1985;92:1440–1444.

42. Hargrove RN, Wesley RE, Klippenstein KA, et al. Indications for orbital exenteration in mucormycosis. Ophthalmol Plast Reconstr Surg 2006;22:286–291.

43. Herbrecht R, Letscher-Bru V, Bowden RA, et al. Treatment of 21 cases of invasive mucormycosis with amphotericin B colloidal dispersion. Eur J Clin Microbiol Infect Dis 2001;20:460–466.

44. Herbrecht R. Posaconazole: a potent, extended-spectrum triazole anti-fungal for the treatment of serious fungal infections. Int J Clin Pract 2004;58:612–624.

45. Rutar T, Cockerham KP. Periorbital zygomycosis (mucormycosis) treated with posaconazole. Am J Ophthalmol 2006;142:187–188.

46. Sun QN, Najvar LK, Bocanegra R, et al. In vivo activity of posaconazole against *Mucor* spp. in an immunosuppressed-mouse model. Antimicrob Agents Chemother 2002;46:2310–2312.

47. Busaba NY, Colden DG, Faquin WC, et al. Chronic invasive fungal sinusitis: a report of two atypical cases. Ear Nose Throat J 2002;81:462–466.

48. Washburn RG, Kennedy DW, Begley MG, et al. Chronic fungal sinusitis in apparently normal hosts. Medicine (Baltim) 1988;67:231–247.

49. Boucher HW, Groll AH, Chiou CC, et al. Newer systemic antifungal agents: pharmacokinetics, safety and efficacy. Drugs 2004;64:1997–2020.

Chapter 15
Complications of Rhinosinusitis

Benjamin S. Bleier and Erica R. Thaler

Rhinosinusitis is a common disease annually affecting one in eight individuals in the United States [1]. While the majority of rhinosinusitis cases are uncomplicated and can be managed successfully with outpatient medical therapy, in a small percentage of patients the infectious process may extend beyond the anatomic boundaries of the sinuses, thus mandating prompt initiation of more aggressive therapy.

Complications typically occur in the setting of acute or acute-on-chronic rhinosinusitis; and the incidences tend to be highest in the winter months, echoing seasonal increases in the rates of upper respiratory infections [2]. Children and adolescent males, in particular, represent a vulnerable population that have a differentially higher incidence of rhinosinusitis-related complications, largely because of anatomic factors. Although patient outcomes have improved dramatically in the postantibiotic era, morbidity and mortality rates associated with intracranial complications remain as high as 40% [3], and thus early recognition and treatment of this disease process is critical.

Complications of rhinosinusitis may be categorized as distant and local (Table 15.1). Distant complications include both pulmonary and systemic sequelae—such as asthma, bronchitis, and sepsis—and are beyond the scope of this chapter. Local complications can be broken down into intracranial, orbital, and bony processes. The pathophysiology of each of these subcategories may be understood in the context of anatomy of the paranasal sinuses and the site-specific barriers to infectious spread present in each sinus [1].

Anatomy

The human paranasal sinuses are composed of air spaces lined by ciliated respiratory epithelium, which are separated from the orbits and intracranial compartments by

E.R. Thaler
Department of Otorhinolaryngology – Head and Neck Surgery, University of Pennsylvania, Philadelphia, PA, USA
e-mail: erica.thaler@uphs.upenn.edu

E.R. Thaler, D.W. Kennedy (eds.), *Rhinosinusitis*, DOI: 10.1007/978-0-387-73062-2_15,   239
© Springer Science+Business Media, LLC 2008

Table 15.1 Local and distant complications of sinusitis

Distant
    Pulmonary
        Asthma
        Bronchitis
    Systemic
        Sepsis
        Toxic shock
Local
    Orbital (Chandler Classification)
        I. Preseptal cellulitis
        II. Orbital cellulitis
        III. Subperiosteal abscess
        IV. Orbital abscess
        V. Cavernous sinus thrombosis
    Intracranial
        Meningitis
        Epidural abscess
        Subdural abscess
        Intracerebral abscess
        Dural sinus thrombosis
            Superior sagittal sinus
            Cavernous sinus
    Bony
        Pott's puffy tumor

Source: Adapted from Younis et al. [1] and Giannoni et al. [15]

thin bony partitions. Extension of rhinosinusitis beyond these natural boundaries may result from either direct spread or vascular thrombophlebitis.

Direct spread of infection may progress through bony defects that result from natural causes or traumatic fractures [2]. Natural defects include congenital dehiscences and the presence of bony sutures or neurovascular foramina, all of which may allow for the direct transmission of infection. Additionally, the cribriform plate is pierced by numerous olfactory filae, which are associated with small veins and perineural spaces, both of which may also be vulnerable to bacterial spread [4].

The venous system supplying both the intracranial and intraorbital compartments represents another important potential route through which disease can spread. These veins comprise an extensive valveless network that allows for the propagation of retrograde thrombophlebitis from an infected sinus. For example, the superior ophthalmic vein communicates with the angular, supraorbital, and supratrochlear veins before crossing over the optic nerve to drain into the cavernous sinus via the superior orbital fissure. The ethmoid venous system also anastomoses with the superior ophthalmic vein and may pierce the cribriform plate in one of several areas to join with veins draining the frontal lobe. Similarly, the diploic veins of Breschet provide a route of unimpeded retrograde vascular spread of disease. The preponderance of the diploic venous system in male adolescents has been implicated as the explanation for the differentially high rate of rhinosinusitis complications within this patient population [1].

Orbital Complications

Complications related to rhinosinusitis most commonly involve the orbit and are generally associated with ethmoid disease [5]. In the preantibiotic era, 20% of patients' orbital sequelae would develop blindness in the ipsilateral eye, and a 17% mortality rate was noted, largely secondary to meningitis [6]. While these rates have decreased dramatically in recent years, orbital involvement continues to carry significant morbidity, with a 10% risk of blindness reported in the early 1990s [7].

The contents of the orbit are normally isolated from an adjacent sinus infection by a thin bony plate derived from the ethmoid bone known as the lamina papyracea (os planum) and the underlying periorbita (orbital periosteum). The periorbita continues anteriorly and becomes contiguous with the orbital septum at the orbital rim. The orbital septum fuses with the tarsal plates of the superior and inferior lids, thereby protecting the intraorbital structures from infections arising anterior to the eyelid. Extension of rhinosinusitis into the orbit therefore requires a breech in these normal anatomic boundaries, which may result from direct bacterial invasion through a traumatic or congenital dehiscence, or through retrograde thrombophlebitis most commonly through ethmoidal vessels.

If a potential orbital complication of rhinosinusitis is suspected, a contrast-enhanced computed tomography (CT) scan with fine axial and coronal cuts through the brain and maxillofacial complex is indicated [8]. These scans provide excellent bony detail of the relevant anatomy and allow for the delineation of a potential abscess, which will appear as a hypodense area with rim enhancement and local mass effect [9]. In addition, several studies have found a high coincidence between orbital and intracranial complications, and thus the intracranial compartment should be evaluated in all these patients. Intraconal inflammation will appear as a poorly defined infiltration of the orbital fat with relative obliteration of the extraocular musculature. Cavernous sinus thrombosis may be suggested on contrast-enhanced CT by poor venous enhancement; however, for this particular complication, magnetic resonance imaging (MRI) with gadolinium enhancement is the imaging study of choice.

The microbiology of orbital complications tends to reflect the organisms responsible for the precipitating rhinosinusitis (Table 15.2). The most valid cultures are those taken directly from the involved sinus at the time of surgical drainage. Although endoscopically guided cultures of the ipsilateral middle meatus may provide relevant data, random samples taken from nasal or nasopharyngeal secretions are of little value [10]. Commonly involved organisms include *Streptococcus* species, *Staphylococcus* species, and anaerobic microorganisms [2,11]. Immunocompromised populations are also affected by the same organisms, although they are additionally vulnerable to fungus and other atypical pathogens.

In 1937, Hubert [12] first proposed a classification schema for orbital complications, which was later modified by Chandler et al. [13] to the system most commonly

Table 15.2 Microbiology of complicated sinusitis

Acute sinusitis
Streptococcus pneumoniae
Haemophilus influenzae
Other *Streptococcus* species
Anaerobes
Staphylococcus aureus

Orbital complications
S. pneumoniae
Other *Streptococcus* species
S. aureus
Anaerobes
Gram-negative rods

Meningitis
S. pneumoniae
S. aureus
Other *Streptococcus* species
Anaerobes (i.e., *Fusobacterium* sp.)
Gram-negative rods

Intracranial abscess (commonly polymicrobial)
Anaerobes
S. aureus
S. pneumoniae
Staphylococcus epidermidis
Gram-negative bacilli

Pott's puffy tumor (commonly polymicrobial)
Streptococcus sp.
S. aureus
Anaerobes

Listed in order of prevalence.
Source: Adapted from Oxford and McClay [2], Giannoni et al. [15], and Osborn and Steinberg [19].

used currently. The Chandler classification divides orbital complications into five categories of escalating severity utilizing anatomic and pathophysiological criteria that provide a convenient manner with which to guide therapy.

Preseptal cellulitis is the most common orbital complication and represents inflammation isolated to the soft tissues anterior to the orbital septum. The swelling and edema are thought to result from impaired venous drainage related to obstruction of ethmoidal vessels by perivascular inflammation and direct pressure. Despite the often dramatic presentation with significant edema, vision and extraocular motion are typically spared [14].

Orbital cellulitis represents an extension of the infection into the postseptal, intraconal space (Fig. 15.1). This complication is associated with diffuse inflammation of the orbital contents and often presents with a preseptal component. Features that distinguish this entity from an isolated preseptal cellulitis include restriction of extraocular motion and occasional vision impairment.

Subperiosteal abscess represents a coalescence of infection or phlegmon into a true abscess that develops between the lamina papyracea and the periorbita

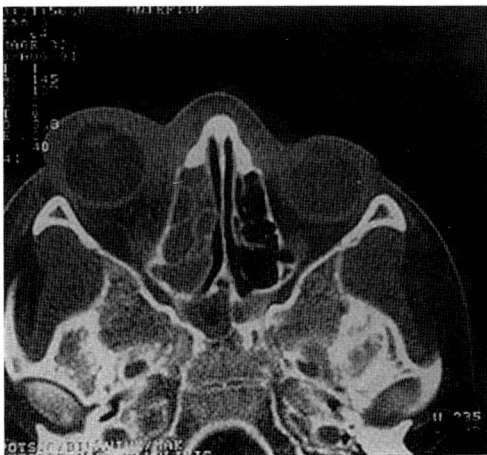

Fig. 15.1 Axial computed tomography (CT) scan (precontrast) demonstrating a right-sided orbital cellulitis with soft tissue edema and proptosis

(Fig. 15.2). The abscess most commonly derives from ethmoidal disease, but it may occur along the orbital roof as a result of frontal rhinosinusitis. Symptoms include inferior and lateral compression of the globe, proptosis, and impairment of extraocular motion. Additionally, the abscess may rupture anteriorly through the orbital septum, resulting in accumulation of purulent debris in the preseptal space.

If the abscess extends laterally into the orbital contents, an orbital abscess results, which presents dramatically with severe exopthalmos, chemosis, and ophthalmoplegia. Visual impairment is a hallmark of this process, and, if untreated, rapid development of irreversible blindness may ensue.

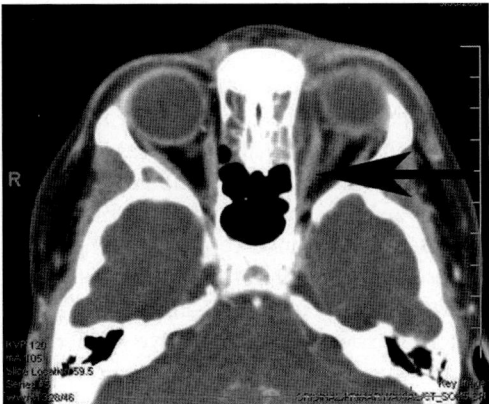

Fig. 15.2 Axial CT scan with contrast (soft tissue windows) demonstrating a left-sided subperiosteal abscess with rim enhancement, compression of the left medial rectus muscle, and adjacent bilateral ethmoid sinusitis

Cavernous sinus thrombosis represents a retrograde extension of orbital disease into the cavernous sinus through the valveless ophthalmic veins, and straddles the classification of orbital and intracranial complications. This entity presents with bilateral orbital pain, chemosis, proptosis, and ophthalmoplegia. The cardinal feature of cavernous sinus thrombosis is the rapid progression to the contralateral eye through extension of the phlebitis, which may then lead to meningismus, meningitis, and, ultimately, sepsis [15].

Treatment of orbital sequelae is largely dictated by the type of complication and presenting symptoms. All treatment algorithms involve medical therapy including antibiotics, nasal decongestants, and saline irrigations. The role of anticoagulation in cavernous sinus thrombosis remains controversial as data is lacking within the literature. The indications for surgical intervention include 20/60 or worse visual acuity on initial exam, progression of symptoms despite 48 h of aggressive medical therapy, and CT evidence of abscess. Of note, in the setting of a subperiosteal abscess without visual impairment, some authors advocate high-dose intravenous antibiotics alone and reserve surgery for patients who fail to improve within 24 hours [9].

The goal of surgery in these patients is to drain both the abscess as well as the precipitating sinus complex. A variety of options exist with respect to surgical approach in the management of these complications. While there is no consensus regarding the efficacy of traditional open versus endoscopic approaches [9], many authors advocate utilizing endoscopic techniques when possible, citing decreased postoperative pain and shorter hospital stays [16].

Intracranial Complications

Intracranial complications of rhinosinusitis have enjoyed a decrease in morbidity and mortality in recent decades. Bradley et al. [17] published a fourfold decrease in intracranial abscesses between 1940 and 1980, attributed largely to the widespread use of antibiotics. While the incidence of intracranial involvement in patients hospitalized for rhinosinusitis has been reported at 3.7% to 11% [1], mortality rates have dropped to 2% to 7% [2] from near 100% for subdural empyema in the preantibiotic era. The use of CT is also believed to have contributed significantly to the improvement in morbidity by allowing for much earlier diagnosis in what may often be otherwise asymptomatic intracranial involvement [18].

As with orbital disease, intracranial complications differentially affect children over adults. This finding is attributable to both the elaboration of the valveless venous system in children as well as the relative vulnerability of the pediatric cranial arachnoid to direct bacterial invasion [2]. Although ethmoid rhinosinusitis is causative in most orbital complications, intracranial involvement tends to derive from frontal and, less commonly, sphenoid disease. These sinuses do not begin to develop until later in childhood and early adolescence, thereby placing older children at higher risk for these types of complications.

Intracranial complications exhibit a seasonal variance that correlate with spikes in rates of upper respiratory infection and acute rhinosinusitis seen in the winter months. The microbiology of these complications also reflects those of the underlying rhinosinusitis, with *Streptococcus pneumoniae* being the most common pathogen cultured from patients with meningitis. Intracranial abscesses tend to be polymicrobial with cultures demonstrating *Streptococcus* and *Staphylococcus* species, anaerobic gram-positive cocci, and gram-negative bacilli. While no single species appears to be predominant, members of the *Streptococcus milleri* group tend to be overrepresented [19]. Of note, operative cultures fail to demonstrate growth in 7% to 53% of samples, owing largely to preoperative administration of empiric intravenous antibiotics; thus, coverage must often be directed toward the suspected causative pathogens in the absence of definitive culture results [20].

Definitive symptoms of intracranial extension may be cryptic, and late findings of seizure and focal neurological deficits portend a poor outcome. Other symptoms include sinonasal complaints, frontal or retro-orbital headache, photophobia, nuchal rigidity, and papilledema. Frontal lobe involvement is classically associated with a silent course, and the general practitioner must maintain a high level of clinical suspicion to refer these patients promptly for appropriate imaging studies.

Although most patients will initially be sent for CT imaging, gadolinium-enhanced MRI remains superior in the early diagnosis of intracranial extension of disease. This modality may also be combined with magnetic resonance angiography/venography to diagnose the presence of a dural sinus thrombosis during the same study. One series of 25 patients with intracranial disease attributed their favorable morbidity rates to the widespread use of MRI in their patient population [14].

As with orbital disease, several anatomic barriers exist to help prevent the spread of infection from the sinonasal complex to the sterile intracranial space. As the infection breaches each successive obstruction, morbidity and mortality increase despite optimal medical and surgical interventions.

Meningitis represents the most common manifestation of intracranial involvement. Although the adult arachnoid mater is relatively resistant, the pediatric leptomeninges is not as developed, placing children at a higher risk for spread of infection. In isolated meningitis, intravenous antibiotics with good cerebrospinal fluid penetration may be all that is required. However, surgery should be considered if there is no clinical improvement within 48 h. Despite treatment, neurological sequelae are not uncommon, and up to a 25% incidence of postmeningitic hearing loss has been reported [1].

Epidural abscess is the next most common intracranial complication and typically occurs in the setting of frontal rhinosinusitis. Infection is transmitted to the epidural space through the diploic system or via direct extension, and the abscess develops insidiously as the loosely adherent frontal dura is dissected off the skull by hydrostatic forces [1]. On CT, the abscess appears as a crescent-shaped mass overlying the inner table of the skull, while MRI will demonstrate an extraaxial low-attenuation lesion. Treatment involves high-dose intravenous antibiotics with concomitant surgical drainage of the involved sinus and abscess cavity as a combined procedure typically involving both an otolaryngologist and a neurosurgeon.

Once the infection breaches the dura, a subdural abscess may develop, which is associated with a 25% to 35% mortality rate and carries a 30% rate of permanent neurological sequelae [1]. Subdural abscesses derived from rhinosinusitis typically result from frontal disease, and collections are classically located over the frontal lobe convexity [21]. In contrast to an epidural collection, the only subdural anatomic barriers to spread of disease are the arachnoid granulations, and thus the abscess may rapidly extend over the cortex and interhemispheric area [19]. CT may sometime miss these lesions, and MRI will demonstrate a low T_1 and high T_2 signal with peripheral enhancement on postgadolinium studies [21]. Clinically, patients can deteriorate quickly, with early signs of headache, fever, and lethargy rapidly progressing to seizure and coma. Of note, lumbar puncture is contraindicated in these patients as herniation secondary to mass effect has been reported in the early literature. Treatment involves urgent surgical drainage, and high-dose intravenous antibiotics complemented by steroids and anticonvulsants [15].

Intracerebral abscess represents extension of the disease into the brain parenchyma itself. MRI demonstrates a cystic lesion with strong T_2 enhancement, which is typically found in the frontal or frontoparietal lobes. Of note, lesions localized to the frontal lobe may be associated with only minor alterations in mood and behavior. Treatment echoes that of a subdural abscess; however, intracerebral disease has a worse outcome with permanent neurological sequelae rates including hemiparesis, aphasia, and deafness approaching 60% [14,22].

Venous sinus thrombosis results from retrograde thrombophlebitis, which leads to venous stasis, thrombosis, infarction, and subsequent cerebral inflammation [19]. Sagittal sinus thrombosis typically derives from frontal disease, while cavernous sinus thrombosis is more often associated with sphenoid rhinosinusitis. Cavernous sinus thrombosis results in obstruction of the superior ophthalmic vein leading to chemosis and proptosis, which are exacerbated by the lack of lymphatic drainage from the orbit. The use of anticoagulation is controversial secondary to concerns over intracranial bleeding from cerebral venous infarction or intracavernous carotid rupture. However, in one series of 176 cases, anticoagulants were used in all cases of venous sinus thrombosis and no complications were recorded [4]. If anticoagulation is employed, it is typically used until complete radiographic elimination of the thrombus is recorded.

Bony Complications

In 1775, Sir Percivall Pott, a leading surgeon at St. Bartholomew's Hospital in 18th-century London [23], described a patient with localized forehead swelling, which became known as "Pott's puffy tumor." While initially ascribed to a complication of trauma, in 1879 Thomas and Nel clarified that the swelling in fact resulted from an underlying frontal rhinosinusitis [24]. Frontal sinus disease may extend both intracranially, as previously described, as well as anteriorly through

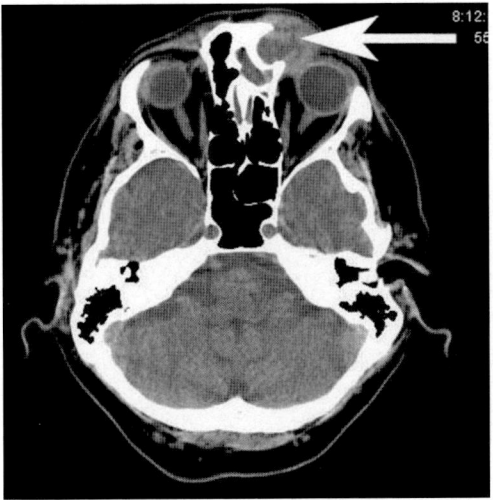

Fig. 15.3 Axial CT scan demonstrating erosion of the anterior table of the frontal sinus with extension of the abscess into the anterior soft tissues (*white arrow*)

direct or vascular extension (Fig. 15.3). The anterior table of the frontal sinus may become involved as an osteomyelitis, and, as the infection extends, a subpericranial abscess can develop, which manifests clinically as a doughy mass over the forehead (Figs. 15.4 and 15.5). While uncommon in the postantibiotic era, this disease is often associated with orbital or intracranial disease [1].

CT imaging is indicated in these patients; however, if intracranial extension is suspected, MRI should be added to the diagnostic workup. Treatment involves 3 to 6 weeks of antibiotics along with drainage of the abscess and involved sinus.

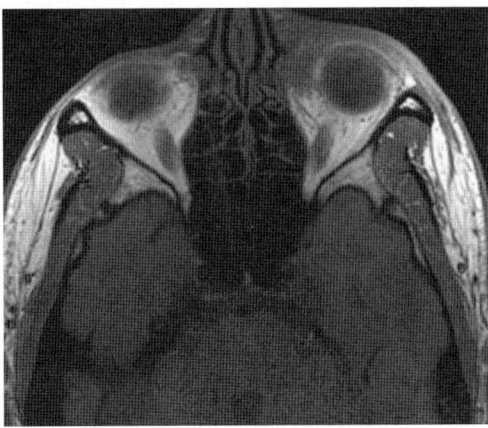

Fig. 15.4 Axial T_1-weighted, precontrast magnetic resonance (MR) image of a left subperiosteal abscess

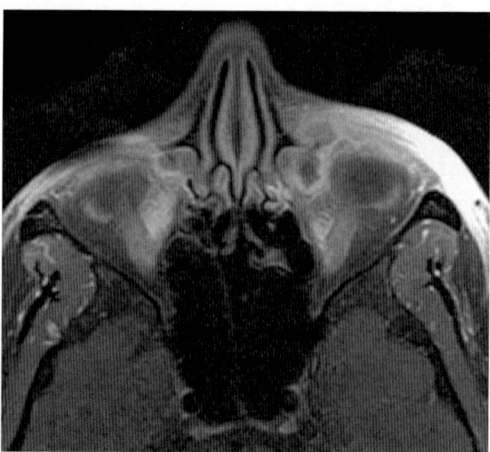

Fig. 15.5 Axial T$_1$-weighted, postcontrast MR image of a left subperiosteal abscess

Management of the offending frontal sinus is directed by degree of bony destruction by the underlying disease. An intact sinus cavity may be managed by open or endoscopic sinusotomy, and some surgeons advocate stenting to ensure frontal outflow patency. If significant anterior or posterior frontal table destruction is noted on CT, frontal obliteration or cranialization should be considered [15].

Conclusion

Complications of rhinosinusitis are uncommon in the postantibiotic era; however, they continue to carry significant morbidity, and favorable outcomes are critically dependent on early intervention. The presentation and severity of complications are dictated by anatomic considerations, and adolescent males comprise the most vulnerable population. The general practitioner must be able to recognize the symptoms heralding complicated rhinosinusitis to make a timely diagnosis and initiate appropriate treatment.

References

1. Younis RT, Lazar RH, Anand VK. Intracranial complications of sinusitis: a 15-year review of 39 cases. Ear Nose Throat J 2002;81(9):636–638, 640–642, 644.
2. Oxford LE, McClay J. Complications of acute sinusitis in children. Otolaryngol Head Neck Surg 2005;133(1):32–37.
3. Maniglia AJ, Goodwin WJ, Arnold JE, et al. Intracranial abscesses secondary to nasal, sinus, and orbital infections in adults and children. Arch Otolaryngol Head Neck Surg 1989;115(12):1424–1429.
4. Gallagher RM, Gross CW, Phillips CD. Suppurative intracranial complications of sinusitis. Laryngoscope 1998;108(11 pt 1):1635–1642.

5. Mortimore S, Wormald PJ. The Groote Schuur hospital classification of the orbital complications of sinusitis. J Laryngol Otol 1997;111(8):719–723.
6. Lazar RH, Periera KD, Younis RT. Sinusitis and complications of sinusitis In: de Souza C, Stankiewicz J, Pellitteri PK (eds) Textbook of Pediatric Otorhinolaryngology-Head and Neck Surgery. San Diego: Singular Publishing, 1999.
7. Patt BS, Manning SC. Blindness resulting from orbital complications of sinusitis. Otolaryngol Head Neck Surg 1991;104(6):789–795.
8. Singh B, Van Dellen J, Ramjettan S, et al. Sinogenic intracranial complications. J Laryngol Otol 1995;109(10):945–950.
9. Sobol SE, Marchand J, Tewfik TL, et al. Orbital complications of sinusitis in children. J Otolaryngol 2002;31(3):131–136.
10. Wald ER. Epidemiology, pathophysiology and etiology of sinusitis. Pediatr Infect Dis 1985;4(6 suppl):S51–S54.
11. Giannoni C, Sulek M, Friedman EM. Intracranial complications of sinusitis: a pediatric series. Am J Rhinol 1998;12(3):173–178.
12. Hubert L. Orbital infections due to nasal sinusitis. NY State J Med 1937;37:1559–1563.
13. Chandler JR, Langenbrunner DJ, Stevens ER. The pathogenesis of orbital complications in acute sinusitis. Laryngoscope 1970;80(9):1414–1428.
14. Germiller JA, Monin DL, Sparano AM, et al. Intracranial complications of sinusitis in children and adolescents and their outcomes. Arch Otolaryngol Head Neck Surg 2006;132(9):969–976.
15. Giannoni CM, Weinberger DG. Complications of rhinosinusitis. In: Bailey BJ, Johnson JT (eds) Head and Neck Surgery-Otolaryngology. Philadelphia: Lippincott Williams & Wilkins, 2006.
16. Arjmand EM, Lusk RP, Muntz HR. Pediatric sinusitis and subperiosteal orbital abscess formation: diagnosis and treatment. Otolaryngol Head Neck Surg 1993;109(5):886–894.
17. Bradley PJ, Manning KP, Shaw MD. Brain abscess secondary to paranasal sinusitis. J Laryngol Otol 1984;98(7):719–725.
18. Small M, Dale BA. Intracranial suppuration 1968–1982: a 15-year review. Clin Otolaryngol Allied Sci 1984;9(6):315–321.
19. Osborn MK, Steinberg JP. Subdural empyema and other suppurative complications of paranasal sinusitis. Lancet Infect Dis 2007;7(1):62–67.
20. Dill SR, Cobbs CG, McDonald CK. Subdural empyema: analysis of 32 cases and review. Clin Infect Dis 1995;20(2):372–386.
21. Kaufman DM, Litman N, Miller MH. Sinusitis: induced subdural empyema. Neurology 1983;33(2):123–132.
22. Spires JR, Smith RJ, Catlin FI. Brain abscesses in the young. Otolaryngol Head Neck Surg 1985;93(4):468–474.
23. Flamm ES. Percivall Pott: an 18th century neurosurgeon. J Neurosurg 1992;76(2):319–326.
24. Thomas JN, Nel JR. Acute spreading osteomyelitis of the skull complicating frontal sinusitis. J Laryngol Otol 1977;91:55–62.

Chapter 16
Adjunctive Surgical Therapies in the Treatment of Rhinosinusitis

Joel Guss and Erica R. Thaler

Rhinosinusitis refers to any inflammatory condition of the nose and paranasal sinuses. Although the terms rhinitis and sinusitis are often used independently, the term rhinosinusitis reflects an understanding that most pathological processes will affect the entire mucous membrane of the nose and sinuses. Rhinosinusitis represents a heterogeneous group of diseases and is the end result of a myriad of pathophysiological processes that include infection, allergy, autoimmunity, environmental exposure, structural abnormalities, hormonal effects, and genetic disease. The interaction of multiple processes in each individual patient further complicates the understanding and management of the disease.

Rhinosinusitis is very common. Approximately 32 million adults in the United States received a diagnosis of rhinosinusitis in 1998, reflecting 16% of the adult population [1]. Approximately 40 million Americans are estimated to be affected by allergic rhinitis each year, with half of these experiencing symptoms during 4 or more months of the year [2]. The direct health care costs associated with the management of sinusitis in the United States exceed $6 billion annually [1]. The indirect cost of rhinosinusitis, including missed days of work or school and decreased productivity while at work, may far exceed even this number. Further, these figures do not account for the costs of treating possible complications of rhinosinusitis such as asthma, otitis media, and sleep-disordered breathing.

Rhinosinusitis also has a profound impact on quality of life that has long been overlooked. For example, in 2006 a large-scale survey of patients with allergic rhinitis found that 40% thought the disease impacted their life a "moderate amount" or "a lot" [3]. While nasal congestion, postnasal drip, rhinorrhea, and headache were labeled "extremely bothersome" by the largest number of subjects, the psychosocial morbidity of the disease appeared to be great as well. Forty-four percent of patients claimed they were frequently tired during allergy season, while 29% and 13%, respectively, frequently felt miserable and depressed.

E.R. Thaler
Department of Otorhinolaryngology, Head and Neck Surgery, The University of Pennsylvania, Philadelphia, PA, USA
e-mail: erica.thaler@uphs.upenn.edu

E.R. Thaler, D.W. Kennedy (eds.), *Rhinosinusitis*, DOI: 10.1007/978-0-387-73062-2_16,   251
© Springer Science+Business Media, LLC 2008

The high prevalence of rhinosinusitis as well as the powerful socioeconomic and quality-of-life burden it exerts has fueled the development of many alternative surgical techniques aimed at its management.

Anatomy and Physiology

The anatomy and physiology of the nose are key in understanding the causes and treatments of rhinosinusitis. Nasal airflow begins at the nares and the vestibule. Although the rigidity of the lower lateral cartilages maintains the structure of this space, the soft tissues are susceptible to collapse, especially with high inspiratory flows. Distally, the internal nasal valve is the narrowest point in the nasal airway. It is a triangular space composed of the caudal edge of the upper lateral cartilage, the nasal septum, and the anterior edge of the inferior turbinate. Both bony and cartilaginous abnormalities of the external nose and septum as well as mucosal thickness overlying the inferior turbinates can affect airflow resistance at this site.

While intuition might lead one to presume that air follows the shortest path to the nasopharynx along the floor of the nose, in reality, the shape of the nasal vestibule, nasal valve, and lateral nasal wall actually guide the flow of air superiorly across the upper surface of the inferior and middle turbinates. The lateral nasal wall is composed of large folds of mucosa and bone; these are the inferior, middle, and superior turbinates. The olfactory mucosa is located in the superior nasal vault.

The nasal mucosa overlying the turbinates is heavily influenced by autonomic innervation supplied by the Vidian nerve. Dysregulation of autonomic input is being studied as a contributing factor in rhinosinusitis [4]. Afferent innervation is provided by the second division of the trigeminal nerve. Sensory input can result in poorly understood reflexes with profound effects on distant sites such as the cardiac and respiratory systems [4]. A nasal cycle exists in the majority of individuals whereby resistance to airflow alternates between the two sides of the nose.

The nasal septum is a midline structure composed anteriorly of a quadrangular cartilage and posteriorly of bone. Deviations from the midline, as well as spurs from the bony septum, can lead to airflow obstruction.

Finally, air flows through the choanae into the nasopharynx. The downward sloping roof of the nasopharynx contains lymphoid tissue commonly known as the adenoid or pharyngeal tonsil. Although adenoid tissue typically regresses during late childhood and adolescence, it may persist through adulthood and, occasionally, contribute to airway obstruction and inflammation.

Adjunctive Surgical Therapies

Preoperative Considerations

Accurate diagnosis of the specific cause of a patient's disease is the cornerstone of providing successful treatment. This is particularly challenging in patients with rhinosinusitis, because as previously stated, the end disease is usually the result of multiple pathophysiological processes. Nonetheless, surgically reducing the size of the inferior turbinate will not cure nasal obstruction in a patient with undiagnosed adenoid hypertrophy.

Diagnosis begins with a careful medical history and physical examination of the head, neck, and chest. History should elicit the age of onset, frequency, severity, and duration of symptoms, as well as seasonality and eliciting factors such as environmental exposure. The laterality of symptoms should be noted. The efficacy of previous treatments—such as antibiotics, nasal or systemic steroids, and antihistamines—is important. Exposure to tobacco smoke (both primary and secondary), chronic nasal cocaine use, and abuse of topical nasal decongestants should be elicited. Patients with allergic rhinitis will usually have a family history positive for atopy.

Physical examination may reveal so-called adenoid facies in patients with lifelong nasal obstruction. Signs of allergic rhinitis include darkening of the skin under the eyes (or "allergic shiners") and a transverse crease over the supratip of the nose. The external nose should be examined for asymmetry and collapse during quiet and deep inspiration. The modified Cottle maneuver is performed by using a cerumen loop to support the external and internal nasal valves and observe for improved airflow. Anterior rhinoscopy with a nasal speculum may detect septal deviation, turbinate hypertrophy, and clear or purulent rhinorrhea.

Nasal endoscopy is critical in evaluating the patient with symptoms and signs of rhinosinusitis. It may be performed with a flexible fiberoptic or a rigid endoscope. The nasal cavities should be examined both before and after decongestion of the mucosa. The floor of the nose, middle meatus, sphenoethmoidal recess, and nasopharynx are sequentially examined for the presence of anatomic abnormalities, inflamed mucosa or polyps, and purulent secretions. The size of the adenoid is assessed as well.

Based on the history and examination, laboratory and radiographic studies are carefully selected. Allergy testing, either by skin or radioallergosorbent testing (RAST), should be ordered in patients with suspected allergic rhinoconjunctivitis to aid in allergen avoidance and for possible immunotherapy. Computed tomography (CT) scans are the most commonly employed imaging modality and can detect both soft tissue and bony changes of the sinonasal cavities. CT scanning also allows for study of the patient's anatomy before surgical intervention. Magnetic resonance imaging (MRI) provides greater soft tissue but poorer bony detail. Imaging is rarely obtained in the acute setting unless a complication of sinusitis is suspected.

Before offering surgical treatment of the patient's disease, efforts at less risky medical management should be maximized. These approaches are detailed in Chapter 6. Of note, most forms of chronic rhinosinusitis are lifelong diseases, and medical treatments such as oral corticosteroids or repeated courses of antibiotics carry risks as well. The discussion regarding the risks and benefits of surgery must be individualized for each patient.

Surgical Procedures

Surgery of the External Nose and Nasal Septum

Although collapse of the nasal valves and deviations of the nasal septum are not forms of rhinosinusitis, they are common causes of nasal obstruction and are often misdiagnosed. For example, it is not uncommon for patients with collapse of the internal nasal valve and no evidence of rhinitis to be treated with long courses of intranasal steroids and decongestants with no improvement.

Collapse of the nasal valves is a dynamic process that occurs on moderate or deep inspiration secondary to Bernoulli forces. External valve (nostril margin) collapse is typically seen in patients with narrow slit-like nostrils and thin alar sidewalls, but may also be a complication of facial paralysis [5]. Internal valve collapse usually results from overly aggressive resection of cartilage during rhinoplasty, especially in patients with short nasal bones and long weak upper lateral cartilages [6]. Such patients often benefit from external taping devices such as Breathe Right nasal strips [7].

Surgically, external valve collapse can be corrected by bolstering the flaccid alar soft tissues with cartilaginous alar batten grafts as described by Toriumi et al. [5] Cartilage is usually harvested from the auricle or the nasal septum, shaped into a curved rectangle, and placed into a pocket on the inner aspect of the ala with the convex surface facing outward. In Toriumi's original series, 98% of patients noted improvement in nasal breathing, with the average patient rating nasal breathing as severely obstructed preoperatively and mildly obstructed postoperatively [5].

Surgical correction of internal valve collapse involves widening the angle between the caudal edge of the lower lateral cartilage and the nasal septum to increase the area of the airway; this is typically done by placing two strips of cartilage between the dorsal septum and the upper lateral cartilage, called spreader grafts, as described by Sheen [8]. In one study, 22 of 25 (88%) of patients with internal valve collapse reported significant improvement with spreader grafts, and 13 of 14 (93%) patients with both internal and external valve collapse improved with a combination of alar batten and spreader grafts [9].

Deviation of the nasal septum is another common cause of nasal obstruction (Fig. 16.1). The anterior cartilaginous septum is most common deviated, although the posterior bony septum may be affected as well. The abnormality may be congenital or a result of trauma, although the patient may not recall a specific traumatic event. Septoplasty involves the resection of the deviated portion of the septum, which may or may not then be straightened and regrafted into the nose. An incision is made through the mucosa and perichondrium of the anterior septum, and mucoperichondrial and mucoperiosteal flaps are elevated on either side of the cartilaginous and bony septum. The deviated cartilage and bone is resected and the flaps are replaced. Surgeons differ in their use of stents and nasal packing during healing. The endoscope can be helpful in minimizing the amount of normal septum resected.

One prospective study administered a disease-specific quality-of-life questionnaire before and after septoplasty to 59 patients who failed medical treatment, and

Fig. 16.1 Image shows
extreme septal deviation to
the right

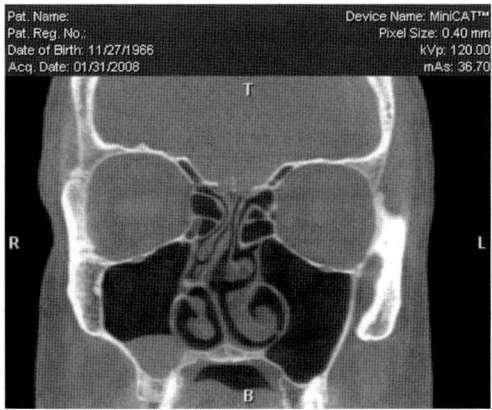

found significant improvement at both 3 and 6 months postoperatively [10]. Inter-estingly, this study found no correlation between the physician's assessment of the degree of obstruction and the patient's baseline and postoperative quality-of-life scores. Another similar study of 93 patients found a clinically significant improve-ment in quality-of-life scores in 71% of patients, and also documented a smaller but significant decrease in medication usage postoperatively [11]. The most common long-term complications of septoplasty include septal perforation and external nasal deformity if the dorsal and caudal septal struts are overresected.

Surgery of the Inferior Turbinate

Inferior turbinate hypertrophy is another common cause of nasal obstruction. The anterior face of the inferior turbinate makes up the "floor" of the internal nasal valve, the narrowest portion of the nasal airway. This position allows the inferior turbinate to obstruct nasal airflow significantly when enlarged. While acute inflam-mation results primarily in mucosal edema, chronic rhinitis can lead to fibrosis and dilation of venous sinuses [12] that may not respond to medical treatment. The most common causes of inferior turbinate hypertrophy are allergic and nonallergic rhinitis.

The turbinates serve to warm and humidify air and to guide its laminar flow through the nose. The importance of the inferior turbinate in nasal physiology is underscored by the observation that on a side opposite a septal deviation, there is compensatory enlargement of the middle turbinate to fill the nasal cavity [13]. Conversely, complete resection of the inferior turbinates is thought to be associated with a chronic disease known as atrophic rhinitis that is characterized by chronic mucosal dryness, crusting, and foul drainage [14], but a clear cause-and-effect rela-tionship has not been proven [15]. Additional complications of turbinate surgery include bleeding and crusting in the immediate postoperative period, and scarring or synechiae formation within the nose.

Given the morbidity associated with total resection of the turbinates, a variety of more conservative surgical approaches have emerged. The philosophy underlying all these procedures is that reducing the size of the turbinate while maintaining its overall structure and function will result in an improved nasal airway with fewer adverse effects. The procedures include partial resection, lateral outfracturing, laser cautery, electrocautery, cryotherapy, submucosal resection, radiofrequency ablation, and coblation. While much has been published about turbinate surgery, long-term data regarding efficacy and safety—as well as prospective randomized studies comparing different techniques—are lacking.

Simple outfracture or lateralization of the inferior turbinate is thought to improve the dimensions of the nasal airway without disturbing the mass of the inferior turbinate. Although this technique may be a helpful adjunct to other forms of turbinate reduction surgery, it does not appear to be effective alone [16].

Partial resection or "trimming" of the inferior turbinate involves cutting the free edge of the turbinate with either scissors or with the aid of powered instrumentation. No guidelines exist regarding how much tissue must be resected to provide an adequate nasal airway and, conversely, how much should be preserved to preserve normal nasal physiology. While several studies have demonstrated good results with this technique [17,18], one small long-term study found significant recurrence of symptoms in patients 7 or more years after surgery [19].

Although partial resection does preserve some normal turbinate, it still results in a large edge of raw tissue that is susceptible to bleeding, crusting, and scar formation. Thus, some surgeons advocate submucosal resection of turbinate bone and connective tissue while preserving the mucosal cover. One long-term prospective study found this technique to be very effective, even at 6 years of follow-up, and to be associated with far less bleeding, crusting, scarring, and atrophy than total turbinectomy [20]. Use of the microdebrider (an instrument with a rotating knife and suction at its tip) for submucous resection has been described [21].

Less invasive surgery on the inferior turbinate involves techniques whereby, instead of resecting tissue, destructive energy is administered to the turbinate to cause scarring and shrinkage. In one set of procedures, radiofrequency energy is applied to the submucosal tissues of the turbinate via an electrode. The heat generated causes obliteration of venous sinuses and fibrosis that anchors the mucosa to the underlying bone [22]. There may also be damage to overlying glandular elements, thus improving rhinorrhea as well [22]. Energy can be provided in the form of an electrical current (conventional diathermy), high-frequency radio waves (radiofrequency tissue reduction), or coblation. These procedures are all quite safe and easy to perform, even in an office setting, but results regarding efficacy are quite mixed. Review of the literature is plagued by inconsistent surgical techniques and patient selection.

Submucosal diathermy relieved symptoms of nasal obstruction 1 year postoperatively in 70% of patients in one study, but about 18% of patients required another surgical procedure within that year [23]. Another study showed no difference between airway resistance preoperatively and 15 months postoperatively [24].

Radiofrequency turbinoplasty (RFT) was shown to be better than placebo in improving subjective nasal obstruction at 8 weeks in a randomized blinded study, although both the placebo and treatment arms improved significantly compared to preoperative data [25]. The same group found sustained benefit at 2 years of follow-up [26]. Another randomized study found RFT to be equivalent to submucosal turbinate resection in precipitating marked improvement in nasal obstruction 3 months postoperatively [27].

Coblation uses a plasma field created by radiofrequency current between bipolar electrodes to ablate tissue [28]. One study found submucosal coblation of the inferior turbinate to be less effective than partial resection with a microdebrider at 1 year follow-up [18]. Another study found significant improvement in nasal symptoms at 6 months follow-up [28].

In summary, techniques involving application of submucosal radiofrequency energy appear effective in the short term, but long-term data are lacking. These operations are likely to be less effective than those that resect a portion of the turbinate. On the other hand, they are simple to perform in an office setting with inexpensive equipment and carry little risk.

Lasers have also been widely used in turbinate reduction. The effect of a laser applied to a tissue depends primarily on the wavelength of the laser and the optical properties of the tissue. For example, the CO_2 laser has a wavelength of 10,600 nm and is highly absorbed by water. Since epithelial surfaces have high water content, the energy of this laser is all deposited superficially. It is, therefore, used for cutting and superficial vaporization. The argon and potassium-titanyl-phosphate (KTP) lasers have wavelengths in the visible light spectrum and are primarily absorbed by endogenous chromophores. Energy from these lasers penetrates deeper into tissues and preferentially coagulates vascular structures such as the venous sinuses of turbinates while preserving surrounding tissue. The infrared light of the diode and neodymium-yttrium aluminum garnet (Nd:YAG) lasers is poorly absorbed by water and tissues, resulting in even deeper penetration [29].

All these lasers have been shown in some studies to be reasonably effective in improving nasal obstruction in patients with allergic and vasomotor rhinitis [30–34], while other studies have shown less impressive results [35]. Laser treatment of the turbinate, again, appears to be less effective than turbinate resection, as demonstrated by the only large prospective randomized study comparing several modalities for treating large inferior turbinates [20]. On the other hand, it can be safely performed with topical or local anesthesia in the office setting.

Ultraviolet Phototheraphy

Another interesting application of electromagnetic radiation in the nose has been the use of ultraviolet (UV) light phototheraphy. The goal is not to structurally alter the nose as with the laser, but instead to immunomodulate the inflammatory response in the mucosa. UV light has long been known to have powerful immunomodulatory capabilities and is widely used in dermatology. Its effects include induction of apoptosis of T lymphocytes, depletion of antigen-presenting cells in tissues, and inhibition of inflammatory mediators [36]. UV irradiation of a skin site before allergen skin prick testing will reduce the size of the resulting wheal [36].

Despite its success in treating diseases of the skin and oral cavity, UV therapy has to date not been extensively studied in the nose. One study examined psoralen plus UV light (PUVA), which entailed treatments four times a week for 3 weeks for 13 patients with medication-refractory allergic rhinitis, and found improvement in all subjective nasal symptoms during the course of the study [37]. There were no controls, and the duration of improvement was not specified. Another randomized blinded study also found significant subjective improvement, as well as a decrease in nasal lavage eosinophil counts, in patients treated with a combination of UV-A, UV-B, and visible light over control; although, once again, patients were only followed during the 3-week treatment period [38]. Treatment with an ultraviolet xenon chloride laser was also demonstrated as effective [39]. There were no complications other than nasal dryness in any of these studies.

UV phototherapy for rhinitis is clearly in its infancy (all the studies cited were conducted by a single group). Its safety profile regarding possible induction of mucosal malignancy must be established as well. Nonetheless, it is exciting technology as it holds the ability to affect the underlying inflammatory process in many patients with rhinosinusitis without resorting to systemic medications such as steroids.

Balloon Sinuplasty

Functional endoscopic surgery of the paranasal sinuses (FESS) is described in detail in Chapter 7. The major goals of such surgery are to enlarge the natural ostia of the sinuses to improve drainage and ventilation, as well as to remove diseased mucosa and bone. Introduction of the endoscope to paranasal sinus surgery was an enormous advancement. It obviates the need for external facial incisions and allows excellent visualization of the nasal microanatomy to allow precise removal of diseased tissue while preserving normal mucosa and anatomic landmarks.

In an attempt to make endoscopic sinus surgery even less invasive, there has been recent interest in the use of balloon catheters to dilate the natural ostia of the sinuses to improve drainage and ventilation (Fig. 16.2). Bolger and Vaughan [40] first demonstrated the feasibility of this approach in cadavers using the Balloon Sinuplasty system (Acclarent, Menlo Park, CA, USA). In this system, a guidewire is passed through an ostium under fluoroscopic guidance. A balloon catheter is then fed over the guidewire and inflated to dilate the ostium. In the cadaver study, all attempted ostial dilations were successful; and follow-up CT scan and gross dissection demonstrated no violation of the orbit or skull base and minimal mucosal injury.

More recently, the system was examined prospectively in a noncontrolled multicenter study of 115 patients [41]. Included patients were adults without extensive polyposis or previous sinus surgery. In 6 patients, no diseased sinus could be

Fig. 16.2 Fluoroscopic view of balloon dilating the right frontal recess

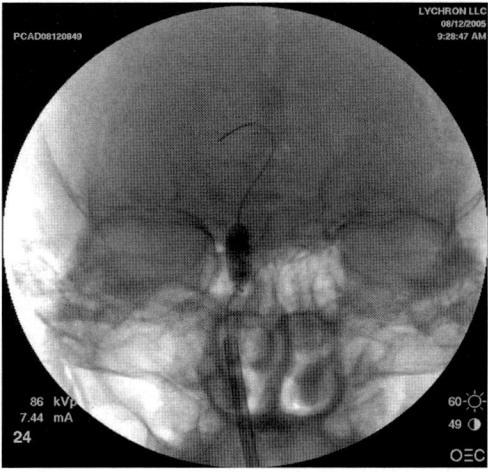

cannulated with the system. Of the remaining patients, half had only balloon dilations performed, while half had a combination of traditional FESS and balloon dilations. On average, 3.1 sinuses were dilated in each patient. In the 95 patients (323 sinuses) that completed the 24 weeks of follow-up, 80.5% of sinuses were patent on endoscopy, 1.6% were nonpatent, and 17.9% could not be visualized during the in-office examination. During the course of the study, 3 patients underwent revision surgery. Disease-specific quality-of-life questionnaire scores improved during the postoperative period. There were no major complications. Average radiation exposure approximated that of a chest CT scan.

Balloon dilation is promising in that it may allow dilation of an isolated obstructed ostium without extensive dissection. Such disease, however, is found in a small minority of rhinosinusitis patients [42]. The technique also does not address the ethmoid sinuses and does not remove irreversibly inflamed mucosa and bone [41]. This limitation not only leaves behind diseased ethmoid cells, but also makes care, monitoring, and culturing of treated sinuses difficult postoperatively [42]. For example, in the aforementioned study, nearly one in five dilated ostia could not be visualized postoperatively, despite the fact that half the patients had traditional FESS in addition to balloon dilation. In addition, the authors admit that balloon dilation is not appropriate in the presence of extensive polypoid disease [41]. Further investigation to define the efficacy of, and indications for, this procedure are necessary.

Office Treatment of Sinonasal Polyps

As endoscopic technology has improved and surgeons have become more facile with nasal endoscopic surgery, many have begun performing increasingly complex procedures in the office setting without sedation. Removal of sinonasal polyps in the office is particularly attractive as it would allow immediate relief of nasal obstruction without the need for general anesthesia. Many patients with nasal polyps suffer from recurrent disease and require multiple surgical procedures throughout their lifetimes. These individuals could clearly benefit from having their disease managed in such a manner.

The major limitations of office-based sinonasal surgery are patient discomfort and a limited ability to manage complications such as bleeding. The potential for cardiovascular complications such as vasovagal syncope from intranasal manipulation or, conversely, tachyarrhythmias from injection of vasoconstrictors to the highly vascular nasal mucosa must be considered as well.

Imaging of the paranasal sinuses with fine-cut CT scanning should be performed before resection of polyps, particularly in patients who have not had previous surgery or those with unilateral findings. A meningoencephalocele (herniation of dura or brain tissue into the nose through a skull base defect) can present as an obstructing nasal mass. In addition, large inflammatory polyps can erode the orbit or skull base. Only polyps far from these high-risk areas should be addressed in the office [43].

The nasal cavity is topically anesthetized using an aerosolized spray or cotton pledgets soaked in a mixture of a local anesthetic (such as lidocaine or Pontocaine) and a decongestant (such as oxymetazoline or phenylephrine). Additional anesthesia can be obtained by injection of 1% lidocaine with epinephrine 1:100,000 near the anterior and posterior insertions of the middle turbinate to target the anterior ethmoid and sphenopalatine neurovascular bundles, respectively. Alternatively, a sphenopalatine block can be performed by injection through the greater palatine foramen intraorally.

Traditionally, sinonasal polyps were resected using a wire snare [43]. Today, endoscopic forceps and even powered instrumentation are more commonly employed [43,44]. To date, no large studies examining either the efficacy or the safety of office-based polypectomy have been conducted.

Sinonasal polyps have also been treated with office injection of corticosteroids in an attempt to avoid surgical resection in patients who fail medical treatment with topical corticosteroids. Both oral and topical corticosteroids have been shown to be very effective in improving symptoms and in reducing polyp size in patients with sinonasal polyposis [45–47]. Despite their efficacy, the use of systemic steroids is limited by their adverse effects. Injection of polyps with steroids has, to date, not been studied in any detail. One retrospective descriptive study identified 68 patients who failed medical treatment with topical steroids and did not undergo surgery after receiving intranasal steroid injections [48]. No further outcome data are presented for this patient population. The study also found steroid injection of polyps to be safe, with only one complication (transient diplopia) occurring in almost 1500 injections.

Adenoidectomy

The hypertrophic adenoid pad found in children is thought to contribute to the pathophysiology of rhinosinusitis by acting as a bacterial reservoir, as well as obstructing the clearance of nasal secretions to the pharynx [49]. Surgeons generally prefer to avoid sinus surgery in children because there is evidence that it may interfere with facial skeletal growth [50]. This concern has led some surgeons to consider adenoidectomy as a potential initial surgical treatment in children who fail medical management.

One study prospectively followed a cohort of 37 children and found a significant decrease in the number of office visits for new episodes of rhinosinusitis after adenoidectomy [51]. Another prospective nonrandomized study compared adenoidectomy to FESS in children and found the latter to be superior based on a symptom questionnaire completed by the children's caregivers and the need for further surgery [52]. Don et al. examined a protocol in which children with chronic sinusitis who failed at least 3 to 4 weeks of oral antibiotics were taken to the operating room for antral puncture and placement of an intravenous catheter with or without adenoidectomy. Adenoidectomy was performed at the surgeon's discretion [49]. The outcomes were equivalent in patients who did and did not undergo adenoidectomy, although in the group that did not undergo adenoidectomy, over half the children had undergone the procedure in the past.

Adenoidectomy is generally a safe procedure in children. It is performed transorally under general endotracheal anesthesia. Cold instrumentation, cautery, and powered debridement have all been used. The major short-term complications are pain, nausea, dehydration, and bleeding [53]. Long-term complications are uncommon and include velopharyngeal insufficiency that is usually transient, velopharyngeal stenosis, and eustachian tube dysfunction [53].

The precise role of adenoidectomy in managing medically refractive chronic sinusitis in children needs to be determined. Its favorable safety profile over FESS, as well as its ability to treat coexisting otitis media and sleep disordered breathing, make adenoidectomy an attractive surgical option. Nonetheless, no evidence currently exists that demonstrates that adenoidectomy is superior to watchful waiting in managing chronic sinusitis.

Vidian Neurectomy

The Vidian nerve carries autonomic innervation to the sinonasal mucosa. Imbalanced sympathetic and parasympathetic activity is generally thought to be the underlying cause of vasomotor or nonallergic rhinitis [54]. Surgical ligation of the Vidian nerve or Vidian neurectomy for the treatment of chronic vasomotor rhinitis was first described by Golding-Wood in the 1960s [55]. While there was initially significant interest in the procedure, it was generally abandoned for reasons of technical difficulty and complications, including dry eye in up to a third of patients [56]. Dry eye results from disruption of the parasympathetic innervation of the lacrimal gland.

Nonetheless, the procedure appears to be effective. One review of 276 patients found excellent results in 88% of patients, although the study was retrospective and results were rated by the physician [57]. Use of the surgical endoscope allows the procedure to be performed more precisely with visualization and section of the nerve via a transnasal approach [56]. In a recent series of 9 patients (14 procedures) with a mean follow-up period of 2 years, patients experienced significant improvement in nasal obstruction and rhinorrhea [56]. Postnasal drip and sneezing did not improve, however, and only half the patients rated their surgery as "successful." Only 1 patient required long-term use of lubricating eye drops for dry eyes.

Conclusion

A large variety of surgical procedures are available to treat patients with chronic rhinosinusitis who fail medical management. As technology and our understanding of the pathophysiology of sinonasal disease advance, more such procedures will be developed. The goal of all of these surgeries is to provide patients with improved quality of life while minimizing invasiveness and reducing complications. The key to successful treatment lies in accurately diagnosing the precise cause of each patient's symptoms so that the appropriate intervention can be applied.

References

1. Anand VK. Epidemiology and economic impact of rhinosinusitis. Ann Otol Rhinol Laryngol Suppl 2004;193:3–5.
2. Nathan RA. The burden of allergic rhinitis. Allergy Asthma Proc 2007;28(1): 3–9.
3. HealthStar Communications, Inc. in partnership with Schulman, Ronca and Bucuvalas, Inc. Allergies in America: a landmark survey of nasal allergy sufferers. Executive Summary. 2006.
4. Kim D, Baraniuk JN. Neural aspects of allergic rhinitis. Curr Opin Otolaryngol Head Neck Surg 2007;15(4):268–273.
5. Toriumi DM, Josen J, Weinberger M, et al. Use of alar batten grafts for correction of nasal valve collapse. Arch Otolaryngol Head Neck Surg 1997;123(8):802–808.
6. Boccieri A, Marco C, Pascali M. The use of spreader grafts in primary rhinoplasty. Ann Plastic Surg 2005;55(2):127–131.
7. Gosepath J, Mann WJ, Amedee RG. Effects of the Breathe Right nasal strips on nasal ventilation. Am J Rhinol 1997;11(5):399–402.
8. Sheen JH. Spreader graft: a method of reconstructing the roof of the middle nasal vault following rhinoplasty. Plastic Reconstr Surg 1984;73(2):230–239.
9. Khosh MM, Jen A, Honrado C, et al. Nasal valve reconstruction: experience in 53 consecutive patients. Arch Facial Plast Surg 2004;6(3):167–171.
10. Stewart MG, Smith TL, Weaver EM, et al. Outcomes after nasal septoplasty: results from the Nasal Obstruction Septoplasty Effectiveness (NOSE) study. Otolaryngol Head Neck Surg 2004;130(3):283–290.
11. Siegel NS, Gliklich RE, Taghizadeh F, et al. Outcomes of septoplasty. Otolaryngol Head Neck Surg 2000;122(2):228–232.
12. Berger G, Gass S, Ophir D. The histopathology of the hypertrophic inferior turbinate. Arch Otolaryngol Head Neck Surg 2006;132(6):588–594.
13. Akoglu E, Karazincir S, Balci A, et al. Evaluation of the turbinate hypertrophy by computed tomography in patients with deviated nasal septum. Otolaryngol Head Neck Surg 2007;136(3):380–384.
14. Moore GF, Freeman TJ, Ogren FP, et al. Extended follow-up of total inferior turbinate resection for relief of chronic nasal obstruction. Laryngoscope 1985;9(pt 1):1095–1099.

15. Jackson LE, Koch RJ. Controversies in the management of inferior turbinate hypertrophy: a comprehensive review. Plast Reconstr Surg 1999;103(1):300–312.
16. Thomas PL, John DG, Carlin WV. The effect of inferior turbinate outfracture on nasal resistance to airflow in vasomotor rhinitis assessed by rhinomanometry. J Laryngol Otol 1988;102(2):144–145.
17. Wexler D, Braverman I. Partial inferior turbinectomy using the microdebrider. J Otolaryngol 2005;34(3):189–193.
18. Lee JY, Lee JD. Comparative study on the long-term effectiveness between coblation- and microdebrider-assisted partial turbinoplasty. Laryngoscope 2006;116(5):729–734.
19. Carrie S, Wright RG, Jones AS, et al. Long-term results of trimming of the inferior turbinates. Clin Otolaryngol Allied Sci 1996;21(2):139–141.
20. Passali D, Bernstein JM, Passali FM, et al. Treatment of inferior turbinate hypertrophy: a randomized clinical trial. Ann Otol Rhinol Laryngol 2003;112(8):683–688.
21. Friedman M, Tanyeri H, Lim J, et al. A safe, alternative technique for inferior turbinate reduction. Laryngoscope 1999;109(11):1834–1837.
22. Farmer SEJ, Eccles R. Understanding submucosal electrosurgery for the treatment of nasal turbinate enlargement. J Laryngol Otol 2007;121(7):615–622.
23. Fradis M, Malatskey S, Magamsa I, et al. Effect of submucosal diathermy in chronic nasal obstruction due to turbinate enlargement. Am J Otolaryngol 2002;23(6):332–336.
24. Jones AS, Lancer JM. Does submucosal diathermy to the inferior turbinates reduce nasal resistance to airflow in the long term? J Laryngol Otol 1987;101(5):448–451.
25. Nease CJ, Krempl GA. Radiofrequency treatment of turbinate hypertrophy: a randomized, blinded, placebo-controlled clinical trial. Otolaryngol Head Neck Surg 2004;130(3):291–299.
26. Porter MW, Hales NW, Nease CJ, et al. Long-term results of inferior turbinate hypertrophy with radiofrequency treatment: a new standard of care? Laryngoscope 2006;116(4): 554–557.
27. Cavaliere M, Mottola G, Iemma M. Comparison of the effectiveness and safety of radiofrequency turbinoplasty and traditional surgical technique in treatment of inferior turbinate hypertrophy. Otolaryngol Head Neck Surg 2005;133(6):972–978.
28. Bhattacharyya N, Kepnes LJ. Clinical effectiveness of coblation inferior turbinate reduction. Otolaryngol Head Neck Surg 2003;129(4):365–371.
29. Janda P, Sroka R, Baumgartner R, et al. Laser treatment of hyperplastic inferior nasal turbinates: a review. Lasers Surg Med 2001;28(5):404–413.
30. Wang HK, Tsai YH, Wu YY, et al. Endoscopic potassium-titanyl-phosphate laser treatment for the reduction of hypertrophic inferior nasal turbinate. Photomed Laser Surg 2004;22(3): 173–176.
31. Elwany S, Thabet H. Endoscopic carbon dioxide laser turbinoplasty. J Laryngol Otol 2001;115(3):190–193.
32. Janda P, Sroka R, Tauber S, et al. Diode laser treatment of hyperplastic inferior nasal turbinates. Lasers Surg Med 2000;27(2):129–139.
33. Ferrie E, Armato E, Cavaleri S, et al. Argon plasma surgery for treatment of inferior turbinate hypertrophy: a long-term follow-up in 157 patients. ORL J Otorhinolaryngol Relat Spec 2003;65(4):206–210.
34. Lippert BM, Werner JA. Comparison of carbon dioxide and neodymium: yttrium-aluminum-garnet lasers in surgery of the inferior turbinate. Ann Otol Rhinol Laryngol 1997;106(12):1036–1042.
35. DeRowe A, Landsberg R, Leonov Y, et al. Subjective comparison of Nd:YAG, diode, and CO_2 lasers for endoscopically guided inferior turbinate reduction surgery. Am J Rhinol 1998;12(3):209–212.
36. Kemeny L, Loreck A. Ultraviolet light phototherapy for allergic rhinitis. J Photochem Photobiol B. 2007;87(1):58–65.
37. Csoma Z, Koreck A, Ignacz F, et al. PUVA treatment of the nasal cavity improves the clinical symptoms of allergic rhinitis and inhibits the immediate-type hypersensitivity reaction in the skin. J Photochem Photobiol B 2006;83(1):21–26.

38. Koreck AI, Csoma Z, Bodai L, et al. Rhinophototherapy: a new therapeutic tool for the management of allergic rhinitis. J Allergy Clin Immunol 2005;115(3):541–547.
39. Csoma Z, Ignacz F, Bor Z, et al. Intranasal irradiation with the xenon chloride ultraviolet B laser improves allergic rhinitis. J Photochem Photobiol B 2004;75(3):137–144.
40. Bolger WE, Vaughan WC. Catheter-based dilation of the sinus ostia: initial safety and feasibility analysis in a cadaver model. Am J Rhinol 2006;20(3):290–294.
41. Bolger WE, Brown CL, Church CA, et al. Safety and outcomes of balloon catheter sinusotomy: a multicenter 24-week analysis in 115 patients. Otolaryngol Head Neck Surg 2007;137(1):10–20.
42. Lanza DC, Kennedy DW. Balloon Sinuplasty: not ready for prime time. Ann Otol Rhinol Laryngol 2006;115(10):789–790; discussion 791–792.
43. Armstrong M. Office-based procedures in rhinosinusitis. Otolaryngol Clin N Am 2005;38(6):1327–1338.
44. Krouse JH, Christmas DA. Powered nasal polypectomy in the office setting. Ear Nose Throat J 1996;75(9):608–610.
45. Alobid I, Benitez P, Pujols L, et al. Severe nasal polyposis and its impact on quality of life. The effect of a short course of oral steroids followed by long-term intranasal steroid treatment. Rhinology 2006;44(1):8–13.
46. Stjarne P, Blomgren K, Caye-Thomasen P, et al. The efficacy and safety of once-daily mometasone furoate nasal spray in nasal polyposis: a randomized, double-blind, placebo-controlled study. Acta Otolaryngol. 2006;126(6):606–612.
47. Small CB, Hernandez J, Reyes A, et al. Efficacy and safety of mometasone furoate nasal spray in nasal polyposis. J Allergy Clin Immunol 2005;116(6):1275–1281.
48. Becker SS, Rasamny JK, Han JK, et al. Steroid injection for sinonasal polyps: the University of Virginia experience. Am J Rhinol 2007;21(1):64–69.
49. Don DM, Yellon RF, Casselbrant ML, et al. Efficacy of a stepwise protocol that includes intravenous antibiotic therapy for the management of chronic sinusitis in children and adolescents. Arch Otolaryngol Head Neck Surg 2001;127(9):1093–1098.
50. Mair EA, Bolger WE, Breisch EA. Sinus and facial growth after pediatric endoscopic sinus surgery. Arch Otolaryngol Head Neck Surg 1995;121(5):547–552.
51. Ungkanont K, Damrongsak S. Effect of adenoidectomy in children with complex problems of rhinosinusitis and associated diseases. Int J Pediatr Otorhinolaryngol 2004;68(4):447–451.
52. Ramadan HH. Adenoidectomy vs. endoscopic sinus surgery for the treatment of pediatric sinusitis. Arch Otolaryngol Head Neck Surg 1999;125(11):1208–1211.
53. Johnson LB, Elluru RG, Myer CM. Complications of adenotonsillectomy. Laryngoscope 2002;112(8 pt 2 suppl 100):35–36.
54. Jaradeh SS, Smith TL, Torrico L, et al. Autonomic nervous system evaluation of patients with vasomotor rhinitis. Laryngoscope 2000;110(11):1828–1831.
55. Golding-Wood PH. Observations on petrosal and Vidian neurectomy in chronic vasomotor rhinitis. J Laryngol Otol 1961;75:232–247.
56. Robinson SR, Wormald PJ. Endoscopic Vidian neurectomy. Am J Rhinol 2006;20(2):197–202.
57. Fernandes CM. Endoscopic transseptal Vidian neurectomy. J Laryngol Otol 1994;108(7):569–573.

Index

A

Abscess
  epidural, 245–246
  intracerebral, 37, 152–153, 246
  intracranial, 219–220, 244–246
  orbital, 153, 218–219
  subdural, 219, 246
  subperiosteal, 217, 218, 242–243, 244,
    247, 248
Acinar cell carcinoma, 162
Acquired immunodeficiency syndrome
  (AIDS), 9, 23, 231
Acupuncture, 133–134, 137, 138
Acute bacterial rhinosinusitis
  allergic rhinitis as risk factor for, 32
  complications of, 152–153
  definition of, 18, 65
  diagnosis of, 18, 69
    inflammation markers in, 33
  differentiated from viral rhinosinusitis,
    32, 70
  microbiology of, 18–20, 30
  pathophysiology of, 30–31
  prevalence of, 4
  spontaneous resolution of, 70
  symptoms of, 209–210
  treatment of
    medical management, 19–20, 65–74
    sinonasal culture-directed, 33
  viral infections as risk factor for, 17, 18,
    66, 69
Acute rhinosinusitis, 29–38
  average annual episodes of, 96
  complicated, 37
  definition of, 29–30
  diagnosis of
    in children, 209–211
    diagnostic criteria for, 29–30, 31–38
    imaging-based, 34–37, 150

  microbiology of, 4–5
  recurrent, 21, 22
    in children, 216
    eosinophil content in, 115
    relationship to chronic rhinosinusitis,
      69–70
  signs and symptoms of, 30, 31–33
  treatment of, 120–128, 129, 136
  See also Acute bacterial rhinosinusitis;
    Viral rhinosinusitis
Adenocarcinoma, 162, 177
Adenoid cystic carcinoma, 162, 178
Adenoidectomy, 216, 260–261
Adenoid facies, 253
Adenoid hypertrophy, 253
  differentiated from rhinosinusitis, 208
  as nasal obstruction and inflammation
    cause, 48, 252
  treatment of, 215, 260–261
Adenovirus, 30, 66
Adolescents
  allergic rhinitis in, 108
  frontal sinus development in, 145
  rhinosinusitis in
    complications of, 37, 205, 219
    differential diagnosis of, 208
Agger nasi cells, 146
Airflow, nasal, 252
Air pollution, as rhinosinusitis risk factor,
  4, 8, 96
Airways hyperresponsiveness, 188–189
Albuterol, 196
Allergic fungal rhinosinusitis, *see* Fungal
    rhinosinusitis/sinusitis, allergic
Allergic response, as type I hypersensitivity
    reaction, 110
Allergic rhinitis, 6–7, 107–108
  as acute bacterial rhinosinusitis risk
    factor, 32

Printed in the United States of America